CASE REVIEW
Musculoskeletal Imaging

Series Editor

David M. Yousem, MD, MBA
Professor of Radiology
Director of Neuroradiology
Russell H. Morgan Department of Radiology and Radiological Science
The Johns Hopkins Medical Institutions
Baltimore, Maryland

Other Volumes in the CASE REVIEW Series

Brain Imaging
Breast Imaging
Cardiac Imaging
Gastrointestinal Imaging, Second Edition
General and Vascular Ultrasound, Second Edition
Genitourinary Imaging, Second Edition
Head and Neck Imaging, Second Edition
Nuclear Medicine
Obstetric and Gynecologic Ultrasound, Second Edition
Pediatric Imaging
Spine Imaging, Second Edition
Thoracic Imaging
Vascular and Interventional Imaging

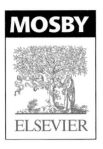

Joseph S. Yu, MD
Professor of Radiology
Vice Chair for Education
Section Chief for Musculoskeletal Radiology
Ohio State University Medical School
Columbus, Ohio

CASE REVIEW

Musculoskeletal Imaging

SECOND EDITION

CASE REVIEW SERIES

WE
18.2
Y94m
2008

1600 John F. Kennedy Blvd.
Suite 1800
Philadelphia, PA 19103-2899

MUSCULOSKELETAL IMAGING: CASE REVIEW, Second Edition   ISBN: 978-0-323-05242-9
Copyright © 2008, 2001 by Mosby, Inc., an affiliate of Elsevier Inc.

Library of Congress Cataloging-in-Publication Data

Yu, Joseph.
Musculoskeletal imaging : case review / Joseph S. Yu. — 2nd ed.
      p. ; cm.
   Includes bibliographical references and index.
   ISBN 978-0-323-05242-9
1. Musculoskeletal system—Imaging—Case studies. I. Title.
   [DNLM: 1. Musculoskeletal Diseases—diagnosis—Case Reports. 2. Musculoskeletal Diseases—diagnosis—Examination Questions. 3. Musculoskeletal System—radiography—Case Reports.
4. Musculoskeletal System—radiography—Examination Questions. 5. Diagnosis,
Differential—Case Reports. 6. Diagnosis, Differential—Examination Questions. 7. Diagnostic Imaging—Case Reports. 8. Diagnostic Imaging—Examination Questions. WE 141 Y94m 2008]
RC925.7.Y8 2008
616.7'07572—dc22   2007030153

Acquisitions Editor: Maria Lorusso
Developmental Editor: Colleen McGonigal
Project Manager: Bryan Hayward
Design Direction: Steven Stave

Printed in the United States of America.

Last digit is the print number: 9 8 7 6 5 4 3 2

To my daughter Sarah for her enthusiasm and her determination to succeed; to Cindy for her love and companionship; to Jim and John for their support; and to Mom and Dad, who taught me to aim high.

I have been very gratified by the popularity and positive feedback that the authors of the Case Review Series have received on publication of the first edition volumes. Reviews in journals and word-of-mouth comments have been uniformly favorable. The authors have done an outstanding job in filling the niche of an affordable, easy-to-read, case-based learning tool that supplements the material in *THE REQUISITES* series.

While some students learn best in a noninteractive study-book mode, others need the anxiety or excitement of being quizzed, being put on the hot seat. Recognizing this need, the publisher and I selected the format for the Case Review Series to simulate the Boards experience by showing a limited number of images needed to construct a differential diagnosis and asking a few clinical and imaging questions (the only difference being that the Case Review books give you the correct answer and immediate feedback!). Cases are scaled from relatively easy to very hard to test the limit of the reader's knowledge. In addition, a brief authors' commentary, a cross-reference to the companion *REQUISITES* volume, and an up-to-date literature reference are also provided for each case.

Because of the popularity of the series, we have been rolling out the second editions of the volumes. The expectation is that the second editions will bring the material to the state-of-the-art, introduce new modalities and new techniques, and provide new and even more graphic examples of pathology.

This volume of the Case Review Series, *Musculoskeletal Imaging* by Dr. Joseph Yu, is the latest of the second editions. Dr. Yu has updated his edition with new and improved cases, discussions, and techniques. Musculoskeletal imaging has seen an enormous growth in volume of cases as well as in fellowship trained specialists in the field. At the same time, this is an area where turf wars have been raging, with nonradiology physicians purchasing imaging modalities and entering the field. It behooves our specialty to have knowledgeable, well-trained experts in this area to provide quality interpretations and added value in demonstrating the pathology. We need to be ahead of the curve in bringing MR spectroscopy, diffusion imaging, elastography, molecular imaging, and other advanced techniques to the subspecialty to maintain our edge. Learn this material well grasshopper! I am also sure that residents preparing for the oral Boards will find that this volume is a treasure trove of quality material that will serve them well in Louisville or wherever Boards will be held in the future . . . and beyond.

I am pleased to present for your viewing pleasure the latest volume of the second editions of the Case Review Series, joining the previous second editions of *Gastrointestinal Imaging* by Robert D. Halpert; *General and Vascular Ultrasound* by William D. Middleton; *Genitourinary Imaging* by Ronald J. Zagoria, William W. Mayo-Smith, and Julia R. Fielding; *Head and Neck Imaging* by David M. Yousem and Carol da Motta; *Obstetric and Gynecologic Ultrasound* by Karen L. Reuter and T. Kemi Babagbemi; and *Spine Imaging* by Brian Bowen, Alfonso Rivera, and Efrat Saraf-Lavi.

David M. Yousem, MD

When I was asked to contribute a second edition of *Musculoskeletal Imaging: Case Review*, the only dilemma that I encountered was whether to write an entirely new book with all new topics or keep the topics that I had presented in the first edition but emphasize different aspects of each subject. I decided to find a balance between these two extremes, since many of the subjects broached in the first edition are considered to be essential core material in orthopedic radiology and therefore appropriate for the second edition. However, in this edition, you will find 110 entirely new topics, a different point of emphasis in the majority of the remaining 90 topics, nearly 600 new board-type questions, and over 200 new references; in other words, 80% of the text material is brand new! Furthermore, all of the images have been replaced with new ones so that each chapter has a fresh, new look.

There are two notable differences in this edition. First, I have incorporated musculoskeletal ultrasound cases, which were lacking in the first edition. I am very grateful and indebted to Jon A. Jacobson, M.D., Director of the Musculoskeletal Division at the University of Michigan, who provided me with all of the ultrasound cases in this current edition. As a recognized authority in musculoskeletal ultrasound, and author of *Fundamentals of Musculoskeletal Ultrasound* (Saunders), his contribution greatly enhanced this project. Second, at the direction of David M. Yousem, M.D., Case Review Series Editor, I have brought this edition in line with others in the series to allow referral to the third edition of *THE REQUISITES: Musculoskeletal Imaging* by Manester, May, and Disler.

I would like to thank the staff at Elsevier and in particular Maria Lorusso for her excellent editorial management. I would like to thank my partner Dr. Marcella Dardani for providing me with many of the cases. As always, I am especially grateful to all residents and fellows, past and present, for being receptive to my teachings.

I am grateful for the constant support that my wife, Cindy, has given me throughout my career and the many sacrifices she has made to allow me to thrive in academia. And to Sarah, who approaches everything new with utter enthusiasm, I thank her for teaching the meaning of *"No Fear!"*

Joseph S. Yu, MD

One of the most difficult challenges in life is discovering the things that motivate you and help keep you going. We are faced with this dilemma in nearly every facet of our daily lives, whether it is professionally or at home.

Education is one of my passions. Early in my medical training, I discovered that teaching fulfilled me, and it was at that time that I decided to set a career path in academia. Nearly a decade has now passed and I find myself undaunted by the constant renewal of residents going through our program and the task of taking them from a neophyte clinician to a competent radiologist. I find myself refreshed and rejuvenated by the enthusiasm and inquisitive nature of those whom I am surrounded by, and it is this curiosity that keeps me motivated to maintain a constant vigilance for updated information to pass on.

I am thankful to have had the opportunity to contribute to the Case Review Series. I like the format provided in this series because it engages the reader to commit to a diagnosis or formulate a list of differential possibilities before divulging the answer. Not meant to be a comprehensive text, it still allows emphasis of important concepts regarding the entity covered in each chapter. The questions are meant to simulate those that one may encounter in an examination. In keeping with the theme of Dr. Yousem, author of the first book in the Case Review Series, *Head and Neck Imaging*, I have not cited articles that are necessarily "classics" in musculoskeletal imaging but have emphasized the recent literature. I have chosen representative cases from different areas of osteoradiology and have made an attempt to include as many imaging modalities as possible, with one notable exception—ultrasound. I admit that we rarely perform sonography for musculoskeletal conditions in my institution, so I have little experience with and even less accessibility to such cases.

I want to thank Dr. Donald Resnick, a teacher and colleague who continues to inspire me to reach for new heights. Under the tutelage of Dr. Resnick and his partners, Dr. Mini Pathria and the late Dr. David Sartoris, I gained valuable experience in both teaching and learning. I want to thank Dr. Javier Beltran for instilling in me the desire to become just like him, an accomplished osteoradiologist, when I was a second-year resident. I want to thank my partners, Drs. Carol Ashman and Marcella Dardani, for helping me compile an excellent teaching file from which to draw my cases for this book. I especially want to thank all residents and fellows, past and present, for nurturing my need to teach and responding favorably to my style of teaching.

I also would like to thank my chairman, Dr. Dimitrios Spigos, and all my colleagues for their support. I want to thank Liz Corra and Stephanie Donley of W. B. Saunders for their excellent editorial management. I want to thank Nydic Open MRI of Cleveland, Boardman, and Kettering for providing me with many of the cases shown in this book and for continuing to keep my teaching file well stocked. And to Theron Ellinger and John Croyle for their excellent photographic support, and Sandy Baker for her secretarial assistance, my gratitude.

Most of all, I want to thank Cindy, my wife, for enduring my idiosyncrasies during this year and for helping and encouraging me to finish despite many distractions. And lastly, to the jewel of my life, my daughter Sarah, thanks for your understanding during the times that I could not play with you.

Joseph S. Yu, MD

Opening Round

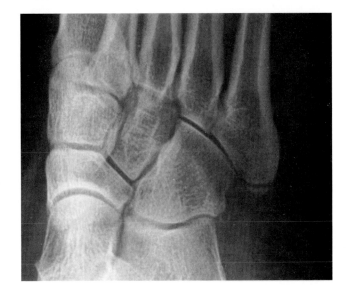
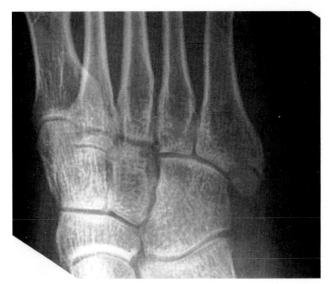
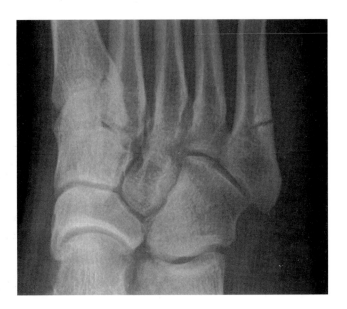
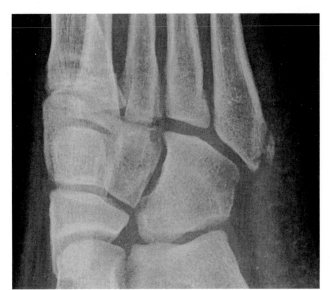

You are shown four radiographs of fifth metatarsal fractures.

1. What is the injury?
2. What is the injury?
3. What is the injury?
4. What is the injury?

Fractures of the Fifth Metatarsal Base

1. Avulsion fracture at the insertion of the lateral cord of the plantar fascia.

2. Avulsion fracture at the insertion of the peroneus brevis tendon.

3. Jones fracture, an impaction fracture of the fifth metatarsal, often beginning as a stress fracture.

4. There is no injury. This is the normal developing apophysis of the base of the fifth metatarsal bone.

References

Vu D, McDiarmid T, Brown M, Aukerman DF: Clinical inquiries. What is the most effective management of acute fractures of the base of the fifth metatarsal? *J Fam Pract* 55:713–717, 2006.

Yu JS: Pathologic and post-operative conditions of the plantar fascia: Review of MR imaging appearances. *Skeletal Radiol* 29:491–501, 2000.

Cross-Reference

Musculoskeletal Imaging: THE REQUISITES, 3rd ed, pp 256, 258, and 277–279.

Comment

Fractures of the fifth metatarsal base are common but they are not all the same. The fractures often have implications to ambulation and the potential for morbidity if improperly treated. Therefore, it is important to identify the structure that has contributed to the fracture, if any, or the mechanism of injury that may help to identify other injuries in the ankle or foot. There are several structures that converge at the base of the fifth metatarsal bone and these all have different contributions to the injuries that are shown. The lateral cord of the plantar fascia and the peroneus brevis tendon both attach to different portions of the tubercle of the metatarsal base. Both are avulsion fractures that are the result of ankle supination injuries, but the position of the forefoot, whether plantar or dorsiflexed, influences which structure is likely to avulse the bone. In general, peroneal brevis avulsion fractures are larger and intra-articular. Jones fracture occurs about 1.5 cm to 2 cm distal to the tuberosity and often develops as a stress fracture, requiring surgical treatment in a majority of cases. Remember, the developing apophysis has a sagittally oriented growth plate so that the ossification center has a longitudinal orientation.

Notes

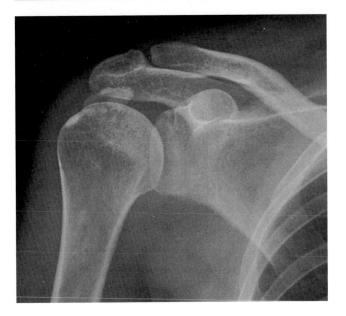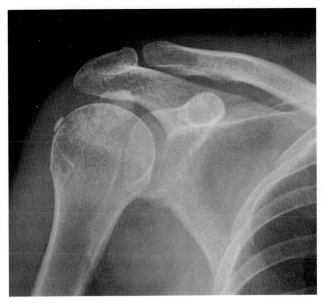

1. Where are these calcifications located?

2. Are patients more likely to be symptomatic when the calcifications are ill defined or sharply defined?

3. Once a calcification is identified, does it ever change in appearance?

4. What pathologic cascade causes the structural damage in the joint?

Calcific Tenditinis and Bursitis

1. The larger calcific deposit is likely in the subacromial/ subdeltoid bursa while the smaller calcification is likely within the infraspinatus tendon.

2. Ill-defined calcifications indicate calcium resorption, the active phase of the disease.

3. Yes, frequently these calcifications may be resorbed, become denser, increase in size, or change in position.

4. Hydroxyapatite crystals are released into the synovial fluid, which become engulfed by fixed macrophage-like synovial cells that release the enzymes collagenase and protease. These enzymes attack the periarticular tissues, including the rotator cuff, destabilizing the joint and causing progressive joint destruction. This releases more crystals into the fluid.

Reference

Ishii H, Brunet JA, Welsh RP, Uhthoff HK: "Bursal reactions" in rotator cuff tearing, the impingement syndrome, and calcifying tendinitis. *J Shoulder Elbow Surg* 6:131–136, 1997.

Cross-Reference

Musculoskeletal Imaging: THE REQUISITES, 3rd ed, pp 342–343.

Comment

Calcific tendinitis and subacromial/subdeltoid bursitis are two manifestations of a spectrum of conditions caused by the deposition of calcium hydroxyapatite crystal in the soft tissues. The shoulder joint is the articulation most commonly involved although virtually any joint may be affected. Periarticular deposits of these crystals often are asymptomatic but when it is associated with acute inflammation, patients complain of severe pain, swelling, occasional erythema, and fever, as with a septic joint.

Deposits consisting of granular inclusions of calcium hydroxyapatite are associated with necrosis and inflammation. Radiographically, these deposits appear ill defined and cloudlike initially, but become denser and more sharply defined. Ill-defined deposits show histologic evidence of calcium resorption, and correlate with symptomatic episodes. The insertion of the supraspinatus tendon is the most frequent site involved. Structural damage can produce degenerative changes in the joint and rotator cuff defects. Radiographic findings include loss of joint space, destruction of bone, subchondral sclerosis, intra-articular debris, and joint disorganization. Rotator cuff tears cause superior migration of the humeral head, which often contacts the inferior surface of the acromion process. Because these deposits may become extruded from the tendon into the surrounding bursa, both tendinitis and bursitis can coexist in the joint.

Notes

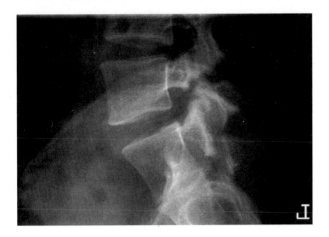

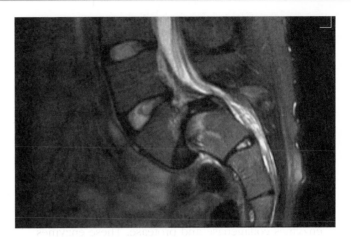

1. The radiograph was taken about 7 years prior to the magnetic resonance image. What has happened?

2. List several proposed etiologies for the underlying condition.

3. Is herniation of the thecal sac a common associated finding? What is the tissue seen anteriorly?

4. Why do degenerative changes occur in the disk?

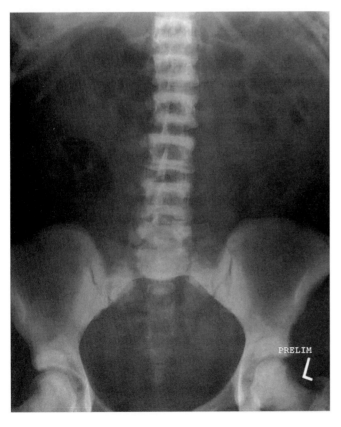

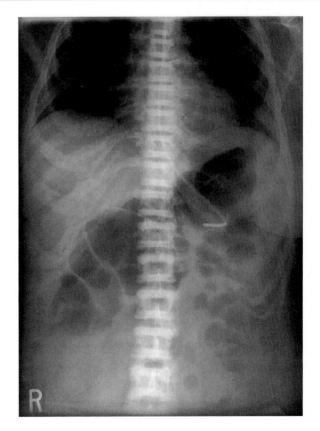

1. What is the disease? List some cranial abnormalities.

2. What common complication occurs in the mandible?

3. Why is this not renal osteodystrophy?

4. What is the differential for dense metaphyseal bands?

CASE 3

Spondylolisthesis

1. The patient developed grade 3 spondylolisthesis of L5 on S1 owing to spondylolysis of L5.

2. Both congenital (hypoplasia or aplasia) and acquired (pseudoarthrosis secondary to fracture from repeated trauma or underlying bone disease) theories have been proposed but the cause is unknown.

3. No, the dura of the thecal sac is firm and does not adhere to the posterior margin of the vertebral body; thus it remains posteriorly positioned. The enlarged epidural space fills with fat.

4. Facet instability results in weakening of the disk and, ultimately, loss of height and degeneration.

Reference

Jinkins JR, Matthes JC, Sener RN, et al: Spondylolysis, spondylolisthesis, and associated nerve root entrapment in the lumbosacral spine: MR evaluation. *AJR Am J Roentgenol* 159:799–803, 1992.

Cross-Reference

Musculoskeletal Imaging: THE REQUISITES, 3rd ed, pp 590–591.

Comment

Spondylolysis refers to a defect through the pars inter-articularis of a vertebra. The cause of this defect is not known. The pars interarticularis bridges the superior and inferior articular processes, depicted by uninterrupted cortices and continuous bone marrow. In patients with spondylolysis, an obliquely oriented cleft bisects the pars as seen on the lateral radiograph. The incidence of spondylolysis increases with age and has been estimated to be about 5% in the general population. The L5 vertebra is the most common location for a spondylolysis, followed in incidence by the L4 vertebra. Together, these two levels account for over 90% of cases.

When the defect is bilateral, it can be associated with spondylolisthesis. This condition is graded according to the degree of slippage: Grade 1, less than 25% slippage; Grade 2, 25% to 50% slippage; Grade 3, 50% to 75% slippage; and Grade 4, greater than 75% slippage. In severe spondylolisthesis, several characteristic changes occur including erosion of the inferior endplate of the subluxed vertebra and rounding of the superior endplate of inferior vertebra, degeneration of the disk, anterior and posterior prominence of the disk, and hypertrophy of the anterior epidural fat.

Notes

CASE 4

Osteopetrosis

1. Osteopetrosis. Hydrocephalus, optic nerve atrophy, facial paralysis, deafness, subarachnoid hemorrhage, and obliteration of the sinuses.

2. Osteomyelitis.

3. The sacroiliac joints appear normal and there are areas in the endplates that are not involved.

4. Heavy metal poisoning, hypothyroidism, scurvy, congenital syphylis, healed rickets, and systemic illness.

Reference

Greenspan A: Sclerosing bone dysplasias—a target-site approach. *Skeletal Radiol* 20:561–583, 1991.

Cross-Reference

Musculoskeletal Imaging: THE REQUISITES, 3rd ed, pp 386–388 and 627–629.

Comment

Osteopetrosis, or Albers-Schonberg disease, is a rare hereditary bone disease caused by lack of absorption of the primary spongiosa in the process of enchondral bone formation. It is suspected that an underlying enzyme deficiency is responsible for this lack of absorption because the vascular mesenchyme that erodes the spongiosa fails to form. Clinically, the disease varies in its severity and age of presentation. Two forms of osteopetrosis are recognized. The congenital form is inherited as an autosomal recessive and is lethal. Hepatosplenomegaly and anemia are characteristic of this form and the infant, if not stillborn at birth, fails to thrive. The tarda form is inherited as an autosomal dominant and is clinically benign, although pathologic fractures are a prominent feature of the disease. Organomegaly and anemia do not occur. Poor dentition may lead to osteomyelitis of the maxilla and mandible. The key to this case is that the bones are too dense. Radiographically, osteopetrosis is characterized by a symmetric, generalized increase in bone density with loss of distinction between the cortical and medullary bone, particularly in tubular bones. Failure of tubulation results in an Erlenmeyer flask deformity. A "bone-in-bone" appearance may be evident in the long bones and spine. A characteristic finding in the spine is increased density only at the endplates (sandwich vertebrae sign). However, typically, there are areas of normal bone that remain, particularly in the anterior aspect of the endplates. The increased density in the skull affects both the base and calvarium, obliterating the diploic space.

Notes

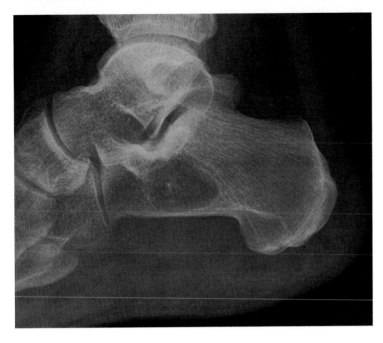

1. What is your differential diagnosis?

2. How can you differentiate the lesions you are considering on magnetic resonance imaging?

3. Which lesion becomes more distinctive with generalized osteopenia?

4. Is an angiolipoma malignant?

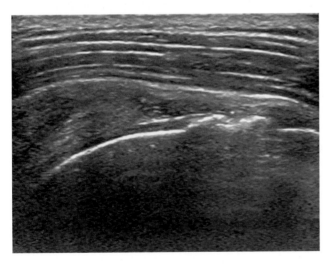 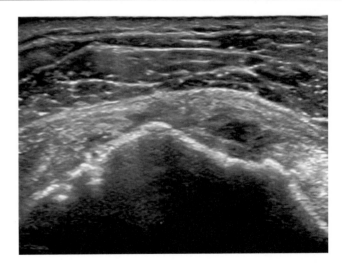

1. You are shown longitudinal (right side is lateral) and transverse (right side is anterior) sonograms of the antero-lateral shoulder. What are the findings?

2. What does this mean?

3. What is the cartilage interface sign? Does this patient have it?

4. Why must the transducer be perpendicular to the tendon?

CASE 5

Intraosseous Lipoma

1. Intraosseous lipoma, simple bone cyst, and normal trabecular variation (pseudocyst).

2. A lipoma appears bright on T1W images. A cyst is bright on T2W images. A pseudocyst has normal marrow signal intensity.

3. A calcaneal pseudocyst is generally less prominent and less well defined than the other two lesions. It also tends to become more conspicuous with osteopenia.

4. No, but it can be infiltrative and invade locally, and recur after excision.

Reference

Yu JS, Vitellas K: The calcaneus: Applications of MR imaging. *Foot Ankle Int* 17:771–780, 1996.

Cross-Reference

Musculoskeletal Imaging: THE REQUISITES, 3rd ed, pp 475–478.

Comment

An intraosseous lipoma may be detected in patients of all ages. Histologically, this neoplasm is identical to an extraosseous lipoma, comprised of mature adipose cells that are separated into lobules by fibrovascular septations. Two thirds of patients present with localized pain, which varies in duration. The most common location for this tumor is in the long bones of the lower extremity, with nearly 50% of cases involving the femur, tibia, and fibula. The calcaneus is the most common tarsal bone involved, accounting for 15% of all cases of intraosseous lipomas. A typical lesion appears well marginated, radiolucent, and surrounded by a thin rim of sclerosis. Lobulations are common at the margins of the lesion. In the calcaneus, it depicts a triangular configuration, typically residing in between the major trabeculations of the bone and sharing a similar location with simple cysts. A central nidus of dystrophic calcification (this patient has a small one) is common, which is nearly pathognomonic for this neoplasm. Unequivocal diagnosis is readily provided by T1W magnetic resonance images. The high signal intensity of the lipoma is demarcated from the fat in the bone marrow by a low signal intensity rim. Fat saturation is a good technique for confirmation of the tumor histology.

Notes

CASE 6

Rotator Cuff Tear (Supraspinatus)

1. Hypoechoic region in the rotator cuff that extends from the bursa to the articular surface.

2. Complete tear of the supraspinatus tendon with retraction.

3. The hyperechoic interface between the joint fluid and the hyaline cartilage beneath the rotator cuff tear is from increased through-transmission of the ultrasound beam. Yes.

4. Even slight angulation can create artifactual hypoechoic to anechoic defects, simulating tears.

References

Jacobson JA, Lancaster S, Prasad A, et al: Full-thickness and partial-thickness supraspinatus tendon tears: Value of US signs in diagnosis. *Radiology* 230:234–242, 2004.

Moosikasuwan JB, Miller TT, Burke BJ: Rotator cuff tears: Clinical, radiographic and US findings. *Radiographics* 25:1591–1607, 2005.

Cross-Reference

Musculoskeletal Imaging: THE REQUISITES, 3rd ed, pp 92–98.

Comment

This patient has a full-thickness tear of the supraspinatus tendon, which allows communication between the glenohumeral joint and the subacromial bursa. Sonography of the shoulder is an excellent and rapid method for evaluating abnormalities of the rotator cuff. The supraspinatus tendon appears hyperechoic and fibrillar, positioned directly on the humerus. A thin anechoic rim of cartilage covers the hyperechoic bone cortex. The deltoid muscle, which is hypoechoic, is just deep to the subcutaneous fat. Beneath it is a thin anechoic bursa with surrounding hyperechoic peribursal fat. Medially, the supraspinatus muscle is interposed between the trapezius muscle and the scapula. Full-thickness rotator cuff tears appear as hypoechoic or anechoic defects in which fluid has replaced the torn tendon. This fluid accentuates the through-transmission of the ultrasound beam, accentuating the cartilage that appears hyperechoic. This creates the appearance of a double cortex, with two hyperechoic parallel lines, or the cartilage interface sign. Compression may produce herniation of the peribursal fat into the tendon gap, called the sagging peribursal fat sign. Nonvisualization of the tendon indicates a very large, retracted tendon. Atrophy of the muscle may increase the overall echogenicity of the muscle.

Notes

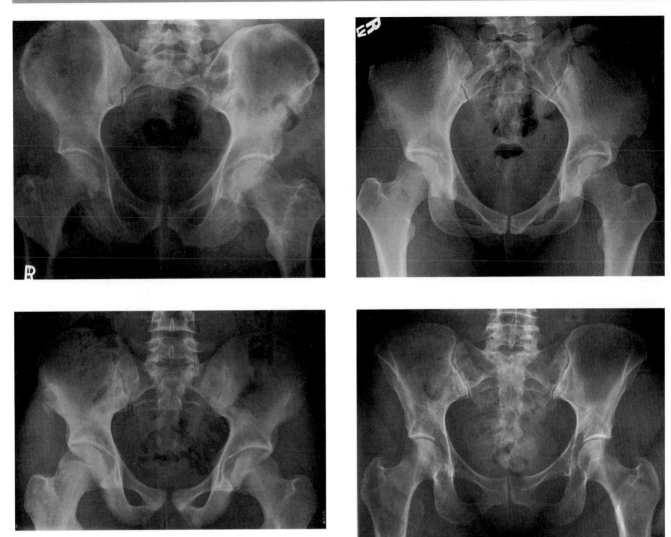

These four patients presented with hip or pelvic pain and/or swelling.

1. Identify the abnormality and what structure is injured. Would you biopsy?

2. Identify the abnormality and what structure is injured. Would you biopsy?

3. Identify the abnormality and what structure is injured. Would you biopsy?

4. Identify the abnormality and what structure is injured. Would you biopsy?

Pelvis Avulsion Fractures

1. Avulsion of the right ischial tuberosity; hamstring tendon. No.

2. Avulsion of the left anterior inferior iliac spine; rectus femoris origin. No.

3. Avulsion of the right anterior superior iliac spine; sartorius muscle. No.

4. Avulsion of the lesser trochanter of right femur; iliopsoas tendon. Yes, if patient has no other lesion.

Reference

Fernbach SK, Wilkinson RH: Avulsion injuries of the pelvis and proximal femur. *AJR Am J Roentgenol* 137:581–584, 1984.

Cross-Reference

Musculoskeletal Imaging: THE REQUISITES, 3rd ed, pp 187–189 and 200.

Comment

Avulsion injuries about the pelvis are not uncommon injuries in the adolescent or young adult athlete. The activities that are associated with such injuries include those that require repetitive to-and-fro adduction and abduction, or flexion and extension. Hurdlers, sprinters, and cheerleaders are especially susceptible to this type of injury, largely due to the stresses that are experienced at the origin and insertion sites of different muscle groups during their activity. An avulsion of the ischial tuberosity ossification center—the attachment of the hamstring muscle group—is one such injury. It is common in hurdlers. An avulsion of the rectus femoris muscle origin is another injury, often heralded by the presence of small flecks of bone adjacent to the superior acetabular rim (reflected head) or in the region of the inferior anterior iliac spine (straight head). Other common potential sites of avulsion in the pelvis and hips include the anterior superior iliac spine (origin of the sartorius muscle or tensor fasciae femoris), the apophysis of the lesser trochanter (insertion of the iliopsoas muscle), the greater trochanter (insertion of the gluteal musculature), the apophysis of the iliac crest (insertion of the abdominal musculature), and the parasymphyseal region of the pubis (origin of the adductor muscles). The radiographic hallmark of avulsion injuries is irregularity of the cortex at the site of avulsion and displaced pieces of bone of variable size. Follow-up radiographs may reveal hypertrophic new bone formation, which can be associated with marked skeletal overgrowth or deformity mimicking a neoplasm. Generally, only avulsions of the lesser trochanter yield a "knee jerk" response of neoplasm, which may require a biopsy.

Notes

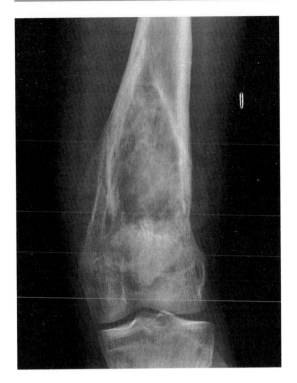 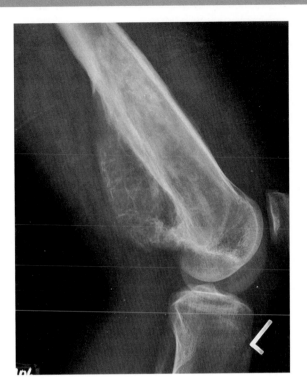

1. What is the likely diagnosis? What would you do next?

2. Can this lesion occur in the soft tissues?

3. Can this lesion appear cystic?

4. What are the surface subtypes and their typical locations?

Osteogenic Sarcoma

1. Conventional osteogenic sarcoma. Computed tomography (CT) or magnetic resonance imaging (MRI) of the femur to determine the extent of the lesion, biopsy, and then stage the patient.

2. Yes, but they are rare.

3. Yes, telangiectatic osteosarcoma is an osteolytic subtype that may appear benign, mimicking an aneurismal bone cyst (ABC) or giant cell tumor (GCT).

4. Periosteal osteosarcoma, diaphyseal; parosteal osteosarcoma, metaphyseal.

Reference

Murphey MD, Robbin MR, McRae GA, et al: The many faces of osteosarcoma. *Radiographics* 17:1205–1231, 1997.

Cross-Reference

Musculoskeletal Imaging: THE REQUISITES, 3rd ed, pp 429–433.

Comment

This patient presented with a painful mass; from a radiographic perspective, this case is straightforward. There is a large lytic mass in the distal femoral metaphysis associated with a prominent Codman's triangle at the margin of the tumor, manifested as a prominent triangular area of periosteal new bone. The key observation is the presence of an osseous matrix in the intramedullary region of the tumor, producing variable density in the involved portion of the distal femur. Osteosarcoma is the most common primary malignant neoplasm of bone in adolescents and young adults. The most common clinical presentation is pain at the tumor site. It usually begins as an insidious pain but progresses to become severe and constant. As the tumor grows, a palpable soft tissue mass develops and eventually breaks through the cortex, leading to a pathologic fracture. Although an osseous matrix characterizes this tumor, the radiographic appearance can range from densely blastic to nearly completely lytic. Osteoid can also be formed from cartilaginous tissue, which often is present in abundance in this tumor. Only 50% of tumors produce sufficient osteoid to be termed osteoblastic, whereas 25% produce predominantly cartilage (chondroblastic), and 25% produce predominantly spindle cells (fibroblastic).

Notes

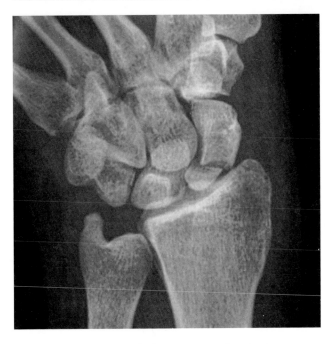 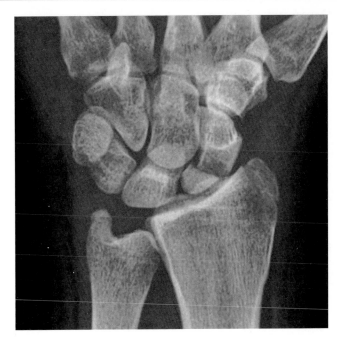

1. What is the most likely injury mechanism?

2. What would you anticipate seeing on a magnetic resonance imaging study?

3. Is this a surgical case? Explain.

4. What percentage of cases results in nonunion? What factors lead to this?

Scaphoid Fracture

1. Fall on outstretched hand.

2. Marrow edema in the radial styloid, scaphoid, capitate, and likely in the triquetrum and ulnar styloid, as well as fractures of the scaphoid waist and radial styloid (greater arc pattern).

3. Yes. It is displaced and it moves with ulnar and radial deviation.

4. Less than 10%. Delay in diagnosis and improper treatment.

Reference

Goldfarb CA, Yin Y, Gilula LA, et al: Wrist fractures: What the clinician wants to know. *Radiology* 219: 11–28, 2001.

Cross-Reference

Musculoskeletal Imaging: THE REQUISITES, 3rd ed, pp 143–145.

Comment

The most common carpal fracture is a scaphoid fracture, constituting about 60% to 70% of all fractures involving the carpus. Nearly 70% of scaphoid fractures occur at the waist and are nondisplaced. The most common mechanism of injury is a dorsiflexion injury. Over 90% of fractures of the scaphoid unite, but owing to the vascular distribution of this bone (the nutrient artery enters the distal scaphoid and traverses the waist before reaching the proximal pole), the risk of developing avascular necrosis (AVN) of the proximal pole is significant. The risk of AVN increases in frequency the more proximal the fracture is located and with more longitudinal orientation, occurring in 16% of patients with scaphoid nonunion. Nondisplaced fractures may be difficult to detect, and magnetic resonance imaging is advocated in patients with persistent pain.

Treatment is dependent on location, displacement, and associated soft tissue injuries. Nondisplaced fractures are generally treated by cast immobilization. Displaced fractures require reduction. If the reduction is unstable, surgical fixation is advocated to avoid the potential complication of nonunion and development of AVN. Instability is defined by persistent displacement greater than 1 mm, associated dorsal intercalated instability, persistent intrascaphoid angulation of 35 degrees on frontal view or 25 degrees on lateral view, and motion with ulnar and radial deviation.

Notes

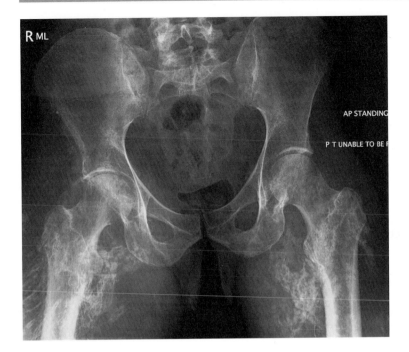

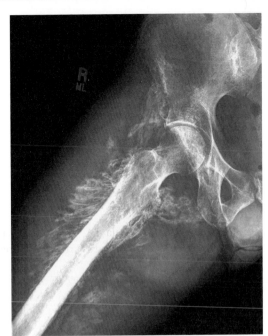

1. What is the most likely diagnosis?

2. What are some causes for this abnormality?

3. When do you think the initial insult occurred?

4. Why does calcific myonecrosis occur? Does it look like this?

Myositis Ossificans Traumatica

1. Myositis ossificans traumatica secondary to myonecrosis.

2. Any condition that leads to rhabdomyolysis, such as a crush injury, severe muscle strain, and electrocution.

3. A long time ago.

4. Compartment syndrome. No, it is generally a sheet of calcification in one of the compartments in the calf.

Reference

Yu JS: MR imaging of soft tissue trauma. *Emergency Radiol* 3:181–194, 1996.

Cross-Reference

Musculoskeletal Imaging: THE REQUISITES, 3rd ed, pp 523–526.

Comment

Myositis ossificans traumatica is a benign process characterized by the formation of an ossifying soft tissue mass or masses in skeletal muscle. The pathogenesis of myositis ossificans is unknown. About 80% of cases involve the large muscles of the extremities, but locations about the scapula, posterior part of the neck, thorax, abdominal wall, and hip have been described. Pain, swelling, and diminished range of motion are common clinical symptoms. The distribution in this patient is extensive, caused by a crush injury to both upper thighs from an industrial accident many years ago.

The radiographic findings parallel the histologic pattern of maturation. The initial radiographic finding is soft tissue swelling. After 3 weeks, floccular calcifications develop. At 6 to 8 weeks, lamellar bone with a well-defined cortex surrounds central radiolucent areas. In mature lesions, dense peripheral ossification is characteristic, often associated with a radiolucent zone separating the masses from the underlying cortex. The magnetic imaging features also depend on the stage of the lesion. Acute lesions are isointense to muscle on T1W images. On T2W images, the signal intensity is higher than that of fat, and the margins may appear heterogeneous owing to peripheral edema. Subacute lesions demonstrate a border of low signal intensity surrounding the lesion, corresponding to ossification. Centrally, the lesion may be isointense or slightly higher in signal intensity compared to muscle on T1W images, reflecting areas of fatty infiltration.

Notes

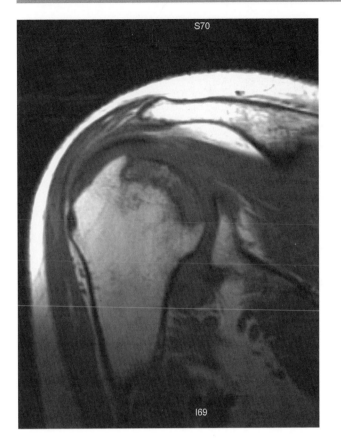 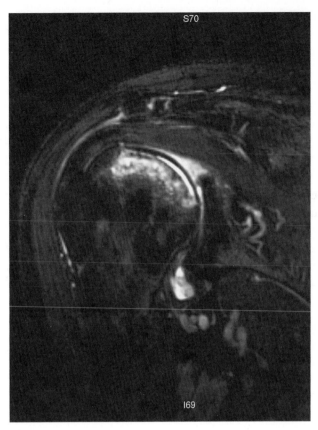

1. What is the diagnosis? What is the most likely cause?

2. What histopathologic factors contribute to the development of this disorder?

3. What does the high signal intensity beneath the cortex represent on the T2W image?

4. What is a finding that would indicate an acute event or exacerbation?

Avascular Necrosis of Humeral Head

1. Avascular necrosis of the humeral head. Corticosteroid use.

2. Thrombosis, embolism, or disruption of vascular supply, and weakening of the bone marrow from repetitive exposure to cytotoxic factors.

3. Subchondral collapse.

4. Surrounding bone marrow edema.

Reference

Lee JA, Farooki S, Ashman CJ, Yu JS: MR patterns of involvement of humeral head osteonecrosis. *J Comput Assist Tomogr* 26:839–842, 2002.

Cross-Reference

Musculoskeletal Imaging: THE REQUISITES, 3rd ed, pp 346–351.

Comment

Avascular necrosis indicates bone death, most commonly due to ischemia. Etiologic factors that contribute to its development in the humeral head include trauma, hematologic conditions (systemic lupus erythematosus, Gaucher's disease), Cushing's syndrome or exogenous corticosteroid administration, alcoholism, pancreatitis, pregnancy, and Caisson disease. In the shoulder, alcoholism and corticosteroid use are the most common causes. Magnetic resonance imaging is efficacious in assessing patients with shoulder pain and risk factors for developing avascular necrosis. In the acute phase of the disease, bone marrow edema involving the humeral head may be the only notable finding. In the absence of any risk factors, osteonecrosis is only one of a number of other potential diagnoses. As the ischemic process worsens, a "double line" sign becomes evident, a characteristic finding that is distinctive of this process. This sign, an irregular rim of low signal intensity on T1W images and paired rims of high and low signal intensities on T2W images, identifies the interface between viable and dying bone marrow. The high signal intensity rim is indicative of granulation tissue, and the adjacent low signal intensity rim reflects cellular debris, fibrous tissue, and reactive trabecular bone. The most common location is the superior aspect of the humeral head, and generally involves about 75% of the articular surface.

Notes

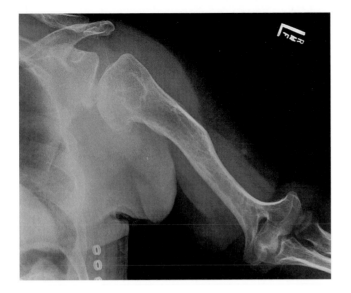

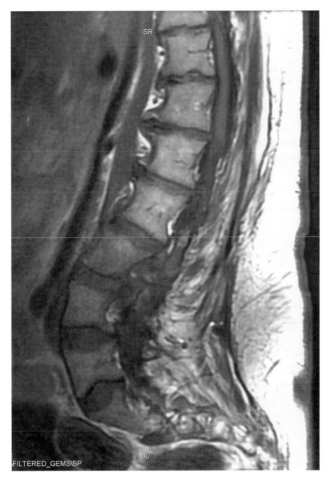

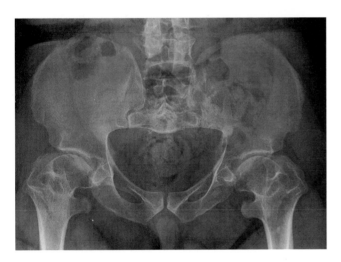

1. What is the diagnosis, and would you consider anything else?

2. Genetically, what is the risk for developing the homozygous form of the disease?

3. What are some characteristic findings in the skull? What can be a complication of this morphology?

4. What is a "trident hand" and when is this deformity typically seen?

C A S E 1 2

Achondroplasia

1. Achondroplasia. Usually the findings are distinctive, although milder forms of this dwarfism such as hypochondroplasia and chondrohypoplasia (spares the skull), and chondrodystrophia calcificans congenita (affects only one side) occasionally may be considered.

2. The same likelihood of having a normal offspring, 25%.

3. Large skull, frontal bossing, short skull base, anteriorly displaced foramen magnum. Hydrocephalus.

4. Divergence of the middle and ring fingers occurring in infants with achondroplasia.

Reference
Lemyre E, Azouz EM, Teebi AS, et al: Bone dysplasia series. Achondroplasia, hypochondroplasia and thanatophoric dysplasia: Review and update. *Can Assoc Radiol J* 50:185–197, 1999.

Cross-Reference
Musculoskeletal Imaging: THE REQUISITES, 3rd ed, pp 632–633.

Comment
Achondroplasia is a bone dysplasia characterized by rhizomelic, short-limbed dwarfism. Eighty to ninety percent of cases occur as a sporadic mutation and the remaining cases are inherited as autosomal dominant. The essential abnormality is a defect in enchondral bone formation affecting all bones formed in cartilage. It is the most common form of dwarfism with bone deformities that are evident at birth. Intelligence and life span are normal. In the tubular bones, ossification of the periosteum exceeds cartilaginous ossification causing the new bone to extend beyond the margins of the growth plate. The bone appears short and square with cupped ends. In the spine, the spinal canal is narrowed in both transverse and anteroposterior dimensions. Progressive narrowing of the interpediculate distance and shortening of the pedicles contribute to significant spinal stenosis. The vertebral bodies are also shortened in the anteroposterior dimension and show prominent posterior scalloping as shown in the T1W sagittal image. The lumbosacral lordosis is exaggerated resulting in a horizontal sacrum. In some patients, a progressive gibbus deformity at the thoracolumbar spine may compress the spinal cord. Classic findings are evident in the pelvis, where there is shortening of the iliac bones and narrowing of the sacrum. The morphologic changes in the innominate bones result in small and deep greater sciatic notches, squaring of the iliac wings, and flattening of the acetabular angles (champagne glass appearance).

Notes

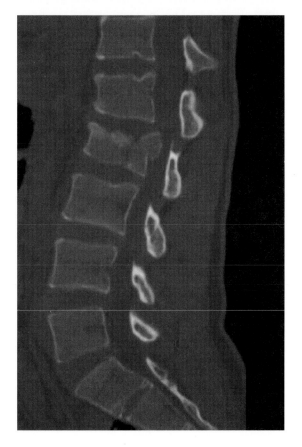 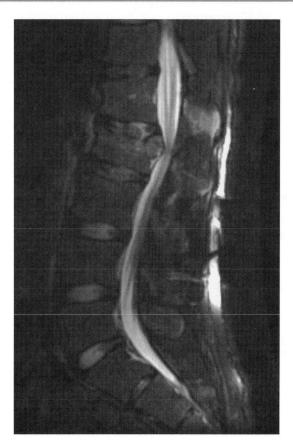

1. What is the mechanism of injury?
2. When is it considered a stable injury and when is it unstable?
3. What finding in this patient indicates its stability?
4. How frequent are neurologic deficits with this fracture?

Burst Fracture (L2 Vertebra)

1. Axial loading and flexion.

2. It is stable when it involves the anterior column only, and unstable with involvement of the middle and posterior columns.

3. Retropulsion of the middle column indicates that this is an unstable fracture.

4. About 50% of patients with an acute burst fracture suffer from a neurologic deficit. However, there is no direct relationship between the extent of spinal canal narrowing and the severity of the deficit.

Reference

Denis F: The three column spine and its significance in the classification of acute thoracolumbar spinal injuries. *Spine* 8:817–831, 1983.

Cross-Reference

Musculoskeletal Imaging: THE REQUISITES, 3rd ed, pp 175–177.

Comment

Compressive axial loading of the vertebral body, which produces end-plate failure and vertebral body collapse, is the principal cause of burst fractures of the spine. The force of the axial load dictates the morphology of the fracture. When the axial force is small, a simple compression fracture is produced. As the force increases, vertical fractures develop throughout the body. Assessment of spinal stability can be achieved by applying Denis's three-column model of the spine. In this model, the spine is divided into three columns: the anterior column comprises the anterior one half of the vertebral body and disc, anterior annulus fibrosus, and anterior longitudinal ligament; the middle column comprises the posterior vertebral body and disc, posterior annulus fibrosus, and posterior longitudinal ligament; and the posterior column comprises the posterior osseous and ligamentous structures. Unstable fractures are defined as injuries in which two of the three columns are involved. When the middle column is involved, the injury is usually unstable when caused by axial loading. As the axial load increases, there is displacement of the bone fragments and retropulsion into the spinal canal, resulting in cord compression. Ultimately, when the axial force overwhelms the pedicle junction, the interpedicular distance may widen, causing significant disruption of the posterior elements. Other associated findings include fracture and/or dislocation of the facet joints. Remember that the presence of a burst fracture indicates that there is a 40% chance that there is another fracture in the spine.

Notes

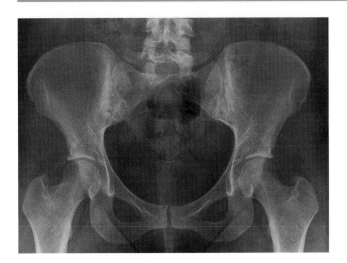 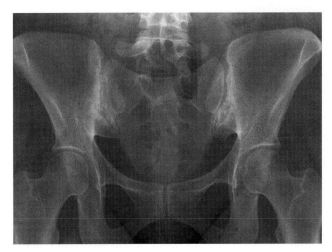

1. In this sacroiliac joint disorder, why is the iliac side more severely involved?

2. What inflammatory bowel diseases may be associated with this disorder?

3. Regarding sacroiliac joint ankylosis, which patient is more likely to develop it—one with enteropathic disease, psoriasis, or Reiter syndrome?

4. What is the second film projection called? How is it performed?

Sacroiliitis

1. The ilium has thinner cartilage than the sacrum, and also contains degenerative clefts and perpedicular splits in the cartilage.

2. Ulcerative colitis and Crohn's disease are the classic diseases but Whipple's disease, infectious colitis with *Salmonella*, *Shigella*, and *Yersinia*, and intestinal bypass surgery may also be associated with sacroiliitis.

3. One with enteropathic sacroiliitis.

4. A Ferguson view. AP radiograph of the pelvis with the tube angulated 25 to 30 degrees in a cephalad direction.

References

Battistone MJ, Manaster BJ, Reda DJ, Clegg DO: Radiographic diagnosis of sacroiliitis—are sacroiliac views really better? *J Rheumatol* 25:2395–2401, 1998.

Oostveen J, Prevo R, den Boer J, van de Laar M: Early detection of sacroiliitis on magnetic resonance imaging and subsequent development of sacroiliitis on plain radiography: A prospective, longitudinal study. *J Rheumatol* 26:1953–1958, 1999.

Cross-Reference

Musculoskeletal Imaging: THE REQUISITES, 3rd ed, pp 318–322.

Comment

The principal observation when evaluating sacroiliitis is the distribution of the disease. Typically, the synovial portion of the sacroiliac joint, found in the inferior one half to two thirds of the joint on frontal radiographs, is more severely involved than the ligamentous portion. Erosions involving the synovial articulation affect the iliac side more than the sacral articulation. In ankylosing spondylitis, the disease is generally bilateral and symmetric in distribution. Sacroiliitis associated with inflammatory bowel disease is usually bilateral and symmetric in distribution and cannot be differentiated from ankylosing spondylitis. Psoriatic arthropathy and Reiter syndrome result in osseous erosions and bony sclerosis that are similar to those seen in ankylosing spondylitis, although ankylosis is less common. The distribution may be bilateral and symmetric, bilateral and asymmetric, or unilateral. Osteoarthritis may involve one or both joints, and is manifested by joint space narrowing, osteophyte formation, and eburnation. When only one sacroiliac joint appears abnormal, one must always consider the possibility of infection, particularly if there is a history of intravenous drug abuse. In this situation, it is best to aspirate the joint, although magnetic resonance imaging and computed tomography may be noninvasive alternatives. Both cross-sectional imaging techniques allow for direct inspection of the joint surface and are better able to detect cartilaginous and osseous destruction than conventional radiography.

Notes

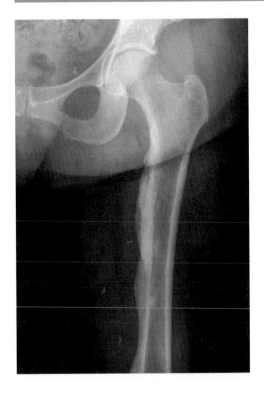 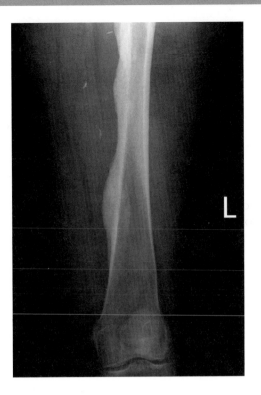

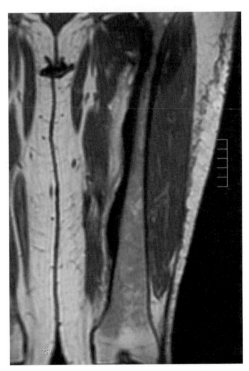

1. Is this disorder progressive?

2. List two lesions that are associated with this condition when it affects the axial skeleton.

3. Can this condition involve the soft tissues?

4. What is Voorhoeve's disease?

Melorheostosis

1. Yes. The hallmark of the disease is progressive hyperostosis of bone along sclerotomes (skeletal zones supplied by individual spinal sensory nerves).

2. Fibrolipomatous lesions and arteriovenous malformations.

3. Yes, but that is seen in more severe cases.

4. Osteopathia striata that appears as dense linear striations in the metaphyses of bones.

Reference

Yu JS, Resnick D, Vaughan L, et al: Melorheostosis with an ossified soft tissue mass: MR features. *Skeletal Radiol* 24:367–370, 1995.

Cross-Reference

Musculoskeletal Imaging: THE REQUISITES, 3rd ed, pp 629–631.

Comment

Melorheostosis, a rare noninheritable mesodermal disorder of unknown etiology, usually involves one bone or several bones distributed along the axis of a limb or along the distribution of a nerve. The hallmark of this process is progressive hyperostosis of bone. Melorheostosis usually is recognized in infancy and progresses during childhood and adult life. Chronic progressive pain in an affected limb is typical, and joint stiffness and decreased range of motion contribute to atrophy and weakness of the surrounding musculature. Para-articular soft tissue ossification is uncommon but may be seen in more severely affected persons. Associated soft tissue abnormalities include joint contractures, fibrosis and edema of the subcutaneous tissue, and varices. Pathologically, the sclerotic bone is composed of a mixture of immature and mature bone. Interlacing osteoid and thickened trabeculae eventually obliterate the Haversian system. Fibrous tissue can be seen within the marrow spaces surrounding areas of new bone proliferation. Dense linear hyperostosis resembling "flowing candle wax" is the radiographic hallmark of this disease. The hyperostosis may advance to the joint margin or even protrude into the joint. Thickening of the cortex and adjacent underlying trabeculae is best demonstrated on computed tomography, while soft tissue involvement is best depicted on magnetic resonance imaging. In this case, the findings are so characteristic that there really is no differential diagnosis.

Notes

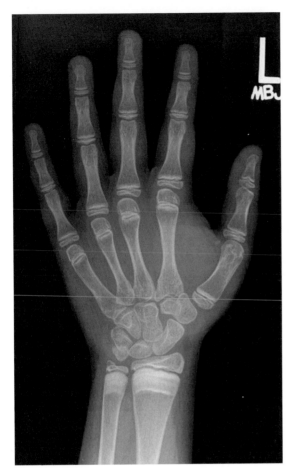 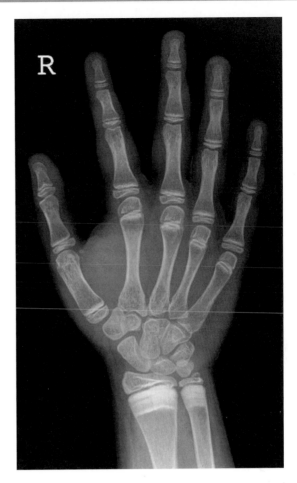

1. What is the differential diagnosis? The patient does not have a chronic systemic disease, so what is the most likely cause of the bands?

2. How is it diagnosed?

3. At what point do the bands occur?

4. What neurologic emergency may develop? How often does this occur?

Dense Metaphyseal Bands

1. Lead poisoning, radiation, rickets, osteopetrosis, chemotherapy, chronic disease, and treated leukemia. Lead poisoning.

2. Check the urine for porphyrin.

3. After the concentration of lead in the blood reaches 50 to 70 μg/dL.

4. Increased intracranial pressure that may require decompression craniotomy. In 10% of cases of chronic lead poisoning.

References

Raber SA: The dense metaphyseal band sign. *Radiology* 211:773–774, 1999.

Tuzun M, Tuzun D, Salan A, Hekimoglu B: Lead encephalopathy: CT and MR findings. *J Comput Assist Tomogr* 26:479–481, 2002.

Cross-Reference

Musculoskeletal Imaging: THE REQUISITES, 3rd ed, pp 387–388.

Comment

The finding of dense metaphyseal bands elicits a differential diagnosis that includes toxic poisoning as well as insult to the growth of the bone. Lead poisoning is the most common disease of toxic environmental origin in the United States today. It results from prolonged ingestion of lead-containing materials, such as paint, ceramics, and drinking water; inhalation of fumes from burning storage batteries, and occasionally from absorption of material from bullets or buckshot. It can be passed to the fetus if the mother is exposed. Clinically, lead is toxic to other organs as well, leading to fatigue, colic, constipation, anemia, peripheral neuropathy, and encephalopathy. The bands form after the blood concentration reaches 70 μg/dL but has been reported with lower concentrations (as low as 10 μg/dL). Some have hypothesized that the lead is laid down within the cartilaginous matrix, a process termed leadification, resulting in the formation of the bands, but they are more likely the result of calcium deposition. The condition is termed chondrosclerosis, depicted as the presence of trabeculae composed of calcified thick cartilaginous cores covered by thin sleeves of endosteal bone almost devoid of osteoblasts.

Notes

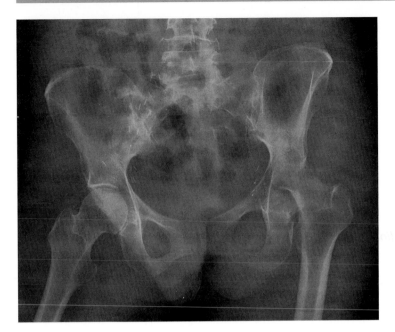 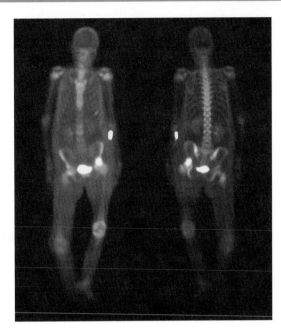

1. By what mechanisms could this joint have become this way?

2. Identify the potential sequelae of this process.

3. Early in the disease process, what else might you consider in the differential diagnosis?

4. What peculiar manifestations do intravenous drug abusers demonstrate?

Septic Arthritis

1. Hematogenous spread, direct extension, or direct implantation of bacteria into the joint.

2. Osteonecrosis, degenerative joint disease, and, occasionally, bony ankylosis. Systemic sepsis is also a very real concern.

3. Anything that causes synovial inflammation such as crystal deposition diseases (hydroxyapatite disease, gout, pseudogout), hemophilia, juvenile chronic arthritis, and neuroarthropathy.

4. Unusual locations (spine, SI joints) and unusual organisms (*Pseudomonas, Klebsiella, Serratia*).

References

Ma LD, Frassica FJ, Bluemke DA, Fishman EK: CT and MRI evaluation of musculoskeletal infection. *Crit Rev Diagn Imaging* 38:535–568, 1997.

Perry CR: Septic arthritis. *Am J Orthop* 28:168–178, 1999.

Cross-Reference

Musculoskeletal Imaging: THE REQUISITES, 3rd ed, pp 560–562.

Comment

Infection of a joint is a serious problem. It is a condition that should be diagnosed rapidly, particularly in immunocompromised patients. This patient demonstrates classic signs of advanced disease. *Staphylococcus* and *Gonococcus* are the infectious agents that are responsible for a majority of cases of septic arthropathy. Clinically, patients complain of pain, erythema, soft tissue swelling, and an effusion. Patients may present with leukocytosis and fever. You should always consider this diagnosis when inflammation is observed involving only one joint, especially if a recent invasive procedure has been performed in the vicinity of the joint. This patient, for instance, had previously undergone a coronary angiogram with a left femoral artery access site. The initial findings are related to synovial inflammation (focal periarticular osteopenia) but osseous destruction can be rapid once a pannus has formed. The joint, becomes irregularly narrowed as the pannus penetrates through the cartilage or into the recesses of the joint, producing central and marginal erosions. As cartilage destruction progresses, the joint narrowing becomes widespread. In the appendicular skeleton, periostitis in the periarticular region of the infected bone is a common finding although often subtle. The most important test that should be performed in patients suspected of having an infected joint is an aspiration. Although this procedure may not always identify the bacterial agent, it will demonstrate the presence of leukocytes, an elevated protein count, and low sugar level that is diagnostic of a septic arthropathy. Magnetic resonance imaging is useful for confirming the marrow edema and in further delineating the extent of soft tissue infection.

Notes

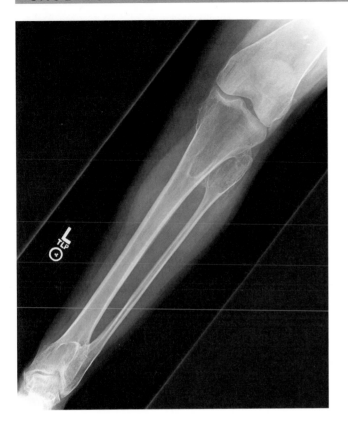 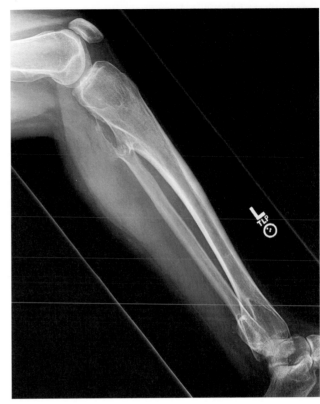

1. What is your diagnosis?

2. What are some potential complications seen in patients with this disorder?

3. A painful growth spurt of a lesion in a skeletally mature patient may be indicative of what condition?

4. Define Trevor's disease. Would you consider it in your differential diagnosis?

Hereditary Multiple Exostosis

1. Hereditary multiple exostosis.

2. Impairment of joint function, reactive bursal formation, and mechanical pressure on adjacent neurovascular structures or spinal cord.

3. Malignant transformation.

4. Exostoses involving the epiphyses (epiphyseal hemimelica dysplasia). No, the lesions extend beyond the epiphyses and have epicenters in the metaphyses.

References

Pierz KA, Stieber JR, Kusumi K, Dormans JP: Hereditary multiple exostoses: One center's experience and review of etiology. *Clin Orthop Relat Res* 401:49–59, 2002.

Stieber JR, Dormans JP: Manifestations of hereditary multiple exostoses. *J Am Acad Orthop Surg* 13:110–120, 2005.

Cross-Reference

Musculoskeletal Imaging: THE REQUISITES, 3rd ed, pp 447–449.

Comment

This patient demonstrates classic findings of hereditary multiple exostosis, also known as diaphyseal aclasis, an uncommon autosomal-dominant metaphyseal hyperplastic disorder characterized by the development of multiple osteochondromas. Most patients present with a discovery of a single or multiple painless masses near the joints, usually in the first decade of life. The lesions typically form and enlarge during growth until the skeleton is fully matured. Although some osteochondromas may be pedunculated, most are broad-based and sessile like those seen in this patient. Because these osteochondromas frequently involve a large circumference of the metaphyseal region, they can mimic a bone dysplasia. Undertubulation of the ends of the long bones often results in a broadened shaft, hence the term diaphyseal aclasis. When the lower extremities are asymmetrically affected, it can produce a compensatory scoliosis. Patients tend to be of short stature. A family history is identified in 70% of cases. Each patient may have few to several hundred lesions. The risk for sarcomatous transformation is about 2% to 5%, although the risk for proximal lesions has been reported to be as high as 10%. The risk for any one particular lesion is the same as for an isolated osteochondroma.

Notes

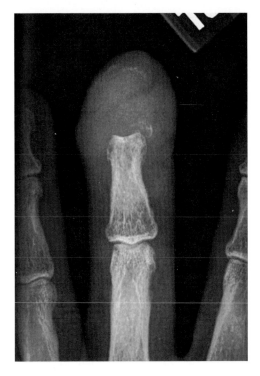 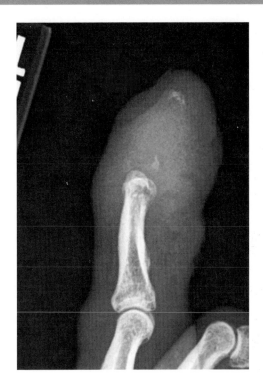

1. What conditions would you consider?

2. What radiographic study would you recommend next if this patient is new to your institution?

3. Describe the pathologic findings of an epidermoid cyst.

4. Why can a glomus tumor occur in the terminal phalanx?

CASE 20

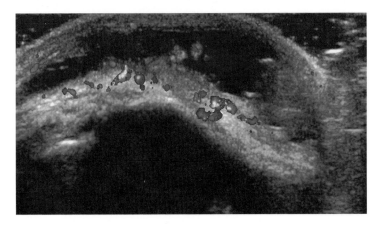 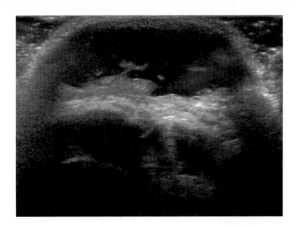

You are shown a longitudinal with Doppler (right side is distal) sonogram and transverse sonogram over the olecranon process of the elbow.

1. What are the findings?

2. What is the diagnosis? What is the differential diagnosis?

3. What are common treatment regimens for the specific types?

4. How often is olecranon bursitis seen in toddlers?

Lesions of the Distal Phalanx

1. Metastasis and osteomyelitis. Occasionally, multiple myeloma, aneurysmal bone cyst, giant cell tumor, and rarely, leprosy.

2. Chest radiograph to search for lung cancer since it is the most common source of metastasis to the phalanx.

3. Cavity filled with white, keratinous debris that is lined by stratified squamous epithelium and a thick layer of fibrous tissue.

4. Neuromyoarterial masses (glomus) are located in the fingertips, functioning as a temperature regulator.

Reference

Palmieri TJ: Common tumors of the hand. *Orthop Rev* 16:367–378, 1987.

Cross-Reference

Musculoskeletal Imaging: THE REQUISITES, 3rd ed, pp 331–333.

Comment

There is an aggressive lesion with an infiltrative soft tissue mass growing out of the bone. It has destroyed much of the medullary bone of the distal phalanx and disrupted the cortex in a circumferential fashion. The most likely consideration is a metastasis, although osteomyelitis is also a consideration if there are constitutional signs of infection or prior penetrating injury or ulcer. Although this patient had melanoma, the most common cause of metastasis to the distal phalanx is lung cancer. It can occasionally be the only location of metastasis. Leprosy is caused by *Mycobacterium leprae* and affects the skeleton in 3% to 5% of those infected. In the hand, osseous involvement represents contamination of the bone from infection of the soft tissues, tendon, tendon sheath, or skin.

Epidermoid cysts are uncommon bone lesions, hypothesized to occur as a result of intraosseous implantation of ectodermal tissue from either penetrating or blunt trauma. The terminal phalanx is the preferred site of involvement in the hand, and the cysts rarely exceed 2 cm in size. They can cause mild expansion of the bone and cortical thinning, which can lead to a fracture. A thin rim of sclerosis reflects the chronicity of this lesion. Glomus tumor arises from neuromyoarterial masses in the fingertips and generally is eccentrically located or entirely extraosseous.

Notes

Olecranon Bursitis

1. Anechoic distension of the olecranon bursa.

2. Olecranon bursitis. Trauma versus infection versus inflammatory processes (this patient had trauma).

3. Trauma-conservative treatment, infection-antibiotics and occasionally surgery, and inflammatory-intrabursal corticosteroid treatment.

4. Almost never since the olecranon bursa does not develop in children under the age of 7 years.

Reference

Finlay K, Ferri M, Friedman L: Ultrasound of the elbow. *Skeletal Radiol* 33:63–79, 2004.

Cross-Reference

Musculoskeletal Imaging: THE REQUISITES, 3rd ed, pp 114–116.

Comment

The superficial olecranon bursa resides directly posterior to the olecranon process of the proximal ulna. The bursa may become distended as a result of trauma or infection, or from a synovial inflammatory process such as gout. Clinical diagnosis is not difficult, and fluid in the bursa can be detected radiographically, although small volumes of fluid are generally confirmed either with magnetic resonance imaging or sonography. Both modalities are sensitive to effusions, synovial proliferation, calcifications, loose bodies, gouty tophi, and septic processes. Sonography has the advantage of dynamic imaging, while MR imaging allows direct inspection of the bone. Septic and nonseptic olecranon bursitis have a considerable imaging overlap and differentiation often requires either the use of intravenous contrast or direct aspiration.

On ultrasound, the bursa appears as hypoechoic clefts in the soft tissue, often bounded by a hyperechoic periphery. This patient shows characteristic findings of an uncomplicated, post-traumatic olecranon bursitis. There is distension of the bursa with anechoic fluid with posterior acoustic enhancement. The cortex of the olecranon process is hyperechoic and associated with acoustic shadowing. Long-standing effusions may result in debris or fibrous adhesions. Echogenic material within the bursa may indicate an inflammatory, hemorrhagic, or infectious etiology. Power Doppler often shows increased flow within the bursal synovial lining in inflammatory conditions.

Notes

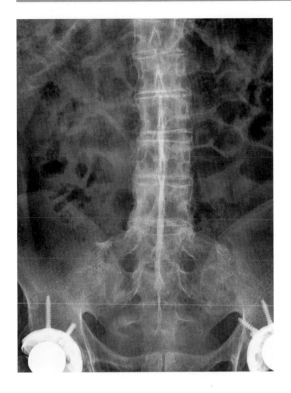
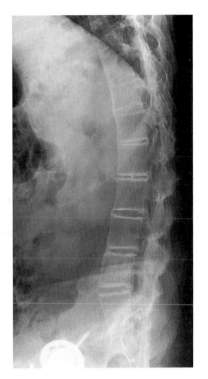
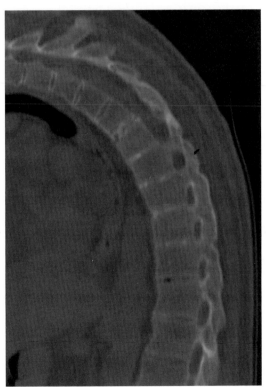

1. What are the radiographic findings that you observe?

2. List some extra-articular manifestations of this disease.

3. List some complications that can occur in this patient's spine.

4. Who is likely to have this disease?

Ankylosing Spondylitis

1. Syndesmophytes (bamboo spine), interspinous ligament ossification, and ankylosis of the sacroiliac joints.

2. Iritis, aortic insufficiency, and interstitial lung disease.

3. Pseudoarthrosis, fractures, atlantoaxial instability, spondylodiscitis, cord compression, and spinal stenosis.

4. Males between 15 and 35 years of age who are HLA-B27 positive.

Reference

Van der Linden S, van der Heijde D: Ankylosing spondylitis: Clinical features. *Rheum Dis Clin North Am* 24:663–676, 1998.

Cross-Reference

Musculoskeletal Imaging: THE REQUISITES, 3rd ed, pp 318–321.

Comment

This case is an "Aunt Minnie." The unmistakable features of ankylosing spondylitis (AS) are evident in both radiographs and the sagittal CT reformation. AS is the most common seronegative spondyloarthropathy and it has an overwhelming male predilection. The onset of the disease occurs between 15 and 35 years of age and over 90% are HLA-B27 positive. Clinically, these patients present with low back pain and stiffness. As the disease progresses, prominent thoracic kyphosis and limited lumbar lordosis become evident. The sacroiliac joint is classically the first site involved and sacroiliitis is a hallmark of the disease. Initial periarticular osteoporosis and superficial cortical erosions on the iliac side of the joint is followed by more dramatic erosive changes resulting in joint space widening. Eburnation develops as a dense ill-defined band of sclerosis. As proliferative changes become more prominent, irregular bony bridges eventually lead to complete joint ankylosis. All of these findings occur in both the ligamentous and synovial portion of the joint.

The term "bamboo spine" characterizes the presence of extensive formation of syndesmophytes (ossification of the annulus fibrosis). The "trolley-track" sign is seen in frontal radiographs and denotes three vertically oriented dense lines corresponding to ossification of the supraspinous and interspinous ligaments and apophyseal joint capsules. The trolley-track sign may be preceded by the "dagger" sign, which is a single radiodense line on frontal radiographs indicating ossification of the supraspinous and interspinous ligaments.

Notes

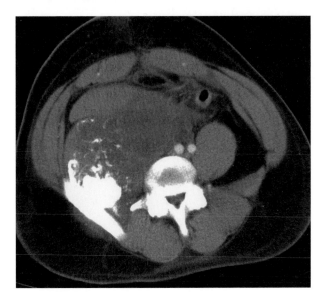 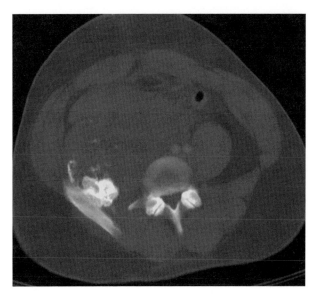

1. What is the most likely diagnosis?
2. What key observation enabled you to narrow your differential?
3. Is cortical thickening and expansion common?
4. What does the low attenuation area in the lesion represent? Is this common?

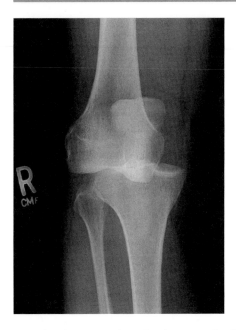 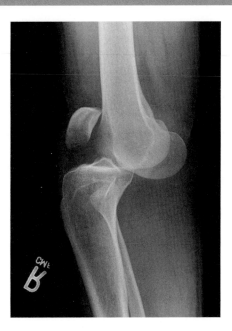

1. What happened to this knee and what is the most critical step in the evaluation of this extremity?
2. How are these injuries classified?
3. Which type(s) is/are considered the most severe?
4. What does a foot drop indicate? Is this injury permanent?

C A S E   2 2

Chondrosarcoma

1. Chondrosarcoma.

2. Chondroid calcifications in the form of rings and arcs within a soft tissue mass.

3. Yes, expansion and thickening of the cortex indicate tumor invasion.

4. Liquifaction and necrosis. Yes.

Reference

Murphey MD, Walker EA, Wilson AJ, et al: From the archives of the AFIP: Imaging of primary chondrosarcoma: Radiologic-pathologic correlation. *Radiographics* 23:1245–1278, 2003.

Cross-Reference

Musculoskeletal Imaging: THE REQUISITES, 3rd ed, pp 456–459.

Comment

Chondrosarcoma is a malignant tumor of cartilaginous origin. It may be a primary lesion or develop from a preexisting cartilage containing a lesion such as an osteochondroma or enchondroma. These tumors may be categorized according to their location (central, peripheral, juxtacortical), the degree of cellular differentiation (low grade, medium grade, high grade), or unusual histologic features (mesenchymal, clear cell). Central chondrosarcomas are more common than the peripheral type, and primary tumors are more common than secondary lesions. Chondrosarcomas may occur at any age but 50% of tumors affect people who are older than 40 years of age. Males and females are nearly equally affected. A dull ache or pain is the most common presenting complaint and it may be present for one to two years before the tumor is discovered. The majority of chondrosarcomas arise centrally with the pelvis and femur accounting for 40% of lesions, the spine and ribs accounting for 25%, and the shoulder and proximal humerus accounting for another 15%. The tumors are nearly always lobulated, and necrosis and liquefaction are common as is cortical thickening from tumor invasion. Eventually, the tumor will break through the cortex extending into the adjacent soft tissues. Chondroid matrix formation in 70% of cases is best detected by computed tomography. Magnetic resonance imaging depicts the high water content of these lesions as high signal intensity on T2W images and is an excellent modality for exact delineation of tumor extent.

Notes

C A S E   2 3

Complete Knee Dislocation

1. Complete knee dislocation; assess the vascular supply for injuries, particularly intimal tears of the popliteal artery.

2. By the position of the tibia relative to the femur.

3. Posterior or posterolateral dislocations tend to cause more soft tissue injuries including tears of both cruciate and collateral ligaments, meniscal tears, and frequent rupture of the popliteus complex.

4. An injury to the common peroneal nerve. Usually.

Reference

Yu JS, Goodwin D, Salonen D, et al: Complete dislocation of the knee: Spectrum of associated soft-tissue injuries depicted by MR imaging. *Am J Roentgenol* 164:135–139, 1995.

Cross-Reference

Musculoskeletal Imaging: THE REQUISITES, 3rd ed, p 223.

Comment

A dislocation of the knee is a severe injury that is caused by high-energy trauma. The incidence of complete knee dislocations reportedly is low, although any estimate is speculative because many dislocations reduce spontaneously at the scene of the injury. Therefore, a patient who had a knee dislocation may present with extensive ligamentous disruption without an obvious dislocation. There are five types of knee dislocations: anterior, posterior, lateral, medial, and posterolateral. Anterior and posterior dislocations account for the majority of dislocations. Both cruciate ligaments are likely to be torn although, in certain situations, the posterior cruciate ligament may be spared. Injuries involving both collateral ligaments and menisci are common. Injury to the popliteal tendon denotes a more severe mechanism of injury and is likely to be the result of posterior or posterolateral dislocation. A knee dislocation constitutes a true orthopedic emergency owing to the possibility of associated injuries to the popliteal artery or the common peroneal nerve. Vascular injuries occur in 33% to 40% of patients, and up to 50% of patients require an amputation when vascular lesions are not treated promptly. An emergent lower extremity angiogram is recommended to assess the vascular supply, even if a pulse is palpable in the foot since latent thrombosis may occur from an unsuspected intimal injury. Peroneal nerve injuries occur in 14% to 35% of patients and usually cause permanent defects.

Notes

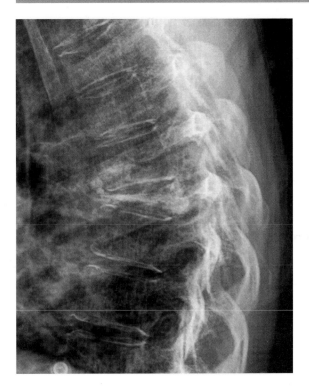 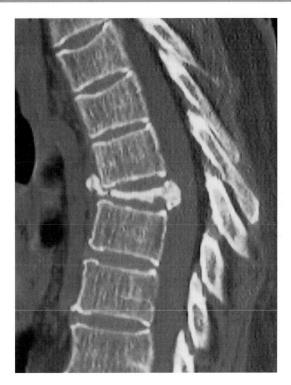

1. What is your differential diagnosis? Is age important?

2. Where is the most common location for an eosinophilic granuloma lesion?

3. How is this condition different from platyspondyly?

4. What sarcomatous lesion can present with this abnormality?

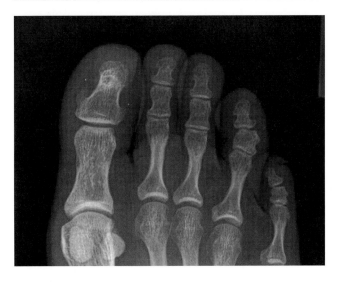 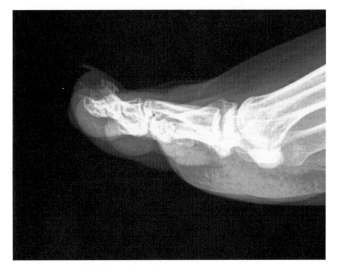

1. What is the diagnosis?

2. Is this lesion a true osteochondroma?

3. Why does it occur in the dorsum of the phalanx and not on the volar side?

4. What is the treatment? Can it recur?

CASE 24

Vertebra Plana

1. Metastasis, multiple myeloma, traumatic fracture, infection, and eosinophilic granuloma. Less likely, lymphoma, hemangioma, and underlying lesions such as an aneurysmal bone cyst. Yes, age is very important.

2. Skull, in the parietal bone.

3. In vertebra plana, the morphology of the vertebral body was at one time normal.

4. Ewing's sarcoma can rarely present with vertebra plana.

Reference

Baghaie M, Gillet P, Dondelinger RF, Flandroy P: Vertebra plana: Benign or malignant lesion? *Pediatr Radiol* 6:431–433, 1996.

Cross-Reference

Musculoskeletal Imaging: THE REQUISITES, 3rd ed, pp 521–522.

Comment

A flattened vertebral body is referred to as a vertebra plana, and the deformity is classically caused by eosinophilic granuloma (EG), although a number of other conditions can produce a flat vertebral morphology. The abnormality is not difficult to identify and the diagnosis can be relatively straightforward if certain conditions are applied. In young patients, consider EG, neuroblastoma metastasis, possibly infection, possibly trauma, and rarely Ewing's sarcoma; in elderly, consider metastasis, multiple myeloma, trauma, possibly infection, and possibly lymphoma. With normal disc space, consider EG, metastasis, multiple myeloma, possibly Paget's disease, and possibly compression fracture. With irregular or destroyed end plate(s), consider infection, tumor, possibly trauma, and possibly Scheuermann's disease. If there is decreased bone density, consider trauma, osteoporosis compression fracture, multiple myeloma, metastasis, osteogenesis imperfecta, and possibly osteomalacia. With increased bone density, consider tumor, trauma, possibly Paget's disease, and possibly hemangioma. If there are multiple vertebral bodies, consider metastasis, multiple myeloma, osteoporosis, and possibly EG. Remember, if you see intravertebral vacuum phenomenon in a collapsed vertebral body, the diagnosis is osteonecrosis (Kummel's disease).

Notes

CASE 25

Subungual Exostosis

1. Subungual exostosis. It mimics an osteochondroma.

2. No, it is a reactive cartilage metaplasia.

3. The periosteum is loose dorsally but very tightly adhered volarly.

4. Treatment consists of complete surgical excision of the lesion. Yes (10% to 50% recur).

References

Miller-Breslow A, Dorfman HD: Dupuytren's (subungual) exostosis. *Am J Surg Pathol* 12:368–378, 1988.

Murphey MD, Choi JJ, Kransdorf MJ, et al: Imaging of osteochondroma: Variants and complications with radiologic-pathologic correlation. *Radiographics* 20:1407–1434, 2000.

Cross-Reference

Musculoskeletal Imaging: THE REQUISITES, 3rd ed, pp 445–446.

Comment

Subungual exostosis, also known as Dupuytren exostosis, is a common, solitary lesion characterized by proliferating fibroblasts and cartilage metaplasia, which progresses to mature ossification. The cause is unknown, although trauma and infection have been proposed. Subungual exostosis arises from the dorsal aspect of the distal phalanx, likely related to the loose periosteum in this area, with a variable relationship to the nail bed. The typical clinical appearance is that of a mass under or adjacent to the nail bed present for weeks to months. The lesion may be painful and show secondary overlying skin ulceration. A preceding history of trauma, such as repetitive injury in athletes, is elicited in about one fourth of cases. Patients are affected in the 2nd and 3rd decades of life. Almost 90% involve the toes, with a curious predilection for the great toe accounting for nearly 80% of lesions. The distal phalanges of the fingers (thumb and index) are affected in 10% of cases, usually in the dominant hand. Radiographs show an ossific mass protruding from the bone without cortical and medullary continuity to the underlying bone. The base of the lesion may be broad or narrow. Unlike most osteochondromas in this region, subungual exostoses arise distal to the physeal scar, manifest in older patients, and are not associated with growth deformities.

Notes

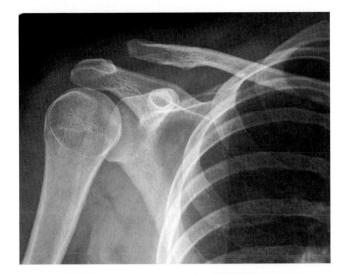

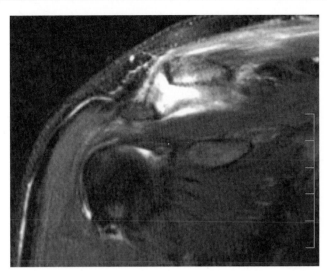

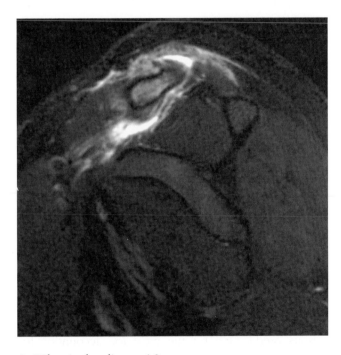

1. What is the diagnosis?

2. List some complications of this injury.

3. What is a "floating clavicle"?

4. What associated osseous injury may occur in pediatric patients?

Acromioclavicular Joint Separation/ Dislocation

1. Type 3 acromioclavicular (AC) joint dislocation.

2. Heterotopic calcification/ossification, post-traumatic osteolysis of the distal clavicle, and secondary osteoarthritis.

3. Simultaneous dislocation of the AC and sternoclavicular joints.

4. Avulsion of the coracoid process.

Reference

Rockwood CA, Jr: Subluxations and dislocations about the shoulder: Injuries to the acromioclavicular joint. In Rockwood CA, Green DP (eds): *Fracture in Adults*, 2nd ed. Philadelphia, JB Lippincott, 1984, pp 860–910.

Cross-Reference

Musculoskeletal Imaging: THE REQUISITES, 3rd ed, pp 76–77.

Comment

AC joint separations/dislocations occur from direct impaction to the point of the shoulder. The most widely used classification is the Allman classification, which identifies three different types. The radiographs appear normal in a type 1 separation. On magnetic resonance imaging, soft tissue swelling about the joint and an effusion may be evident and indicate a mild strain of the AC and coracoclavicular ligaments. In a type 2 injury, there is disruption of the AC ligament and partial disruption of the coracoclavicular ligaments, such that the clavicle migrates superiorly less than 5 mm or 50% of the width of the clavicle on weight-bearing views. In type 3 injuries, the AC and coracoclavicular ligaments are completely disrupted and there is clavicular migration exceeding 5 mm or 50% of the bone width as seen in this patient. The sagittal T2W MR image shows the disruption of the coracoclavicular ligaments with intervening hemorrhage. Interstitial edema in the surrounding connective tissues and muscles correspond to a more severe injury mechanism. Rockwood described three additional injury patterns. In type 4 injuries, the clavicle is displaced posteriorly into or through the trapezius muscle. In type 5 injuries, the clavicle migrates superiorly more than in a type 3 separation. In type 6 injuries, the clavicle dislocates inferiorly below the coracoid or acromion process.

Notes

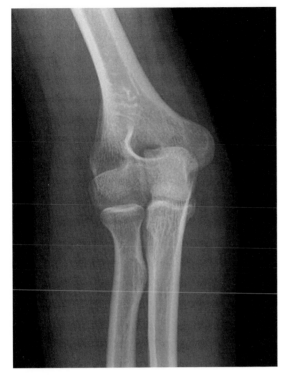

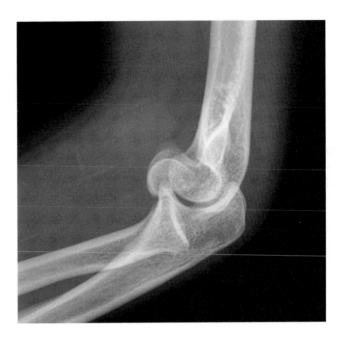

1. What is the diagnosis? What type?

2. What is the mechanism of injury?

3. What is a common associated injury?

4. Review the pattern of ossification in the elbow.

Capitellar Fractures

1. Capitellar fracture, type 1.

2. Fall on outstretched hand or a direct blow to the capitellum.

3. One-eighth of cases are associated with an ulnar collateral ligament rupture.

4. CRITOE approximates the age the ossification center becomes radiographically evident. C, capitulum (year 1); R, radial head (3 to 6 years); I, internal or medial epicondyle (5 to 7 years); T, trochlea (9 to 10 years); O, olecranon (6 to 10 years); and E, external or lateral epicondyle (9 to 13 years).

Reference

Sonin A: Fractures of the elbow and forearm. *Semin Musculoskeletal Radiol* 4:171–191, 2000.

Cross-Reference

Musculoskeletal Imaging: THE REQUISITES, 3rd ed, pp 131–132.

Comment

Capitellar fractures account for 1% of all elbow fractures but it remains a difficult diagnosis to make radiographically. The most common mechanism of injury is either a direct blow or a fall on the outstretched hand. Fractures of the capitellum are classified into three different types: Type 1, a fracture that involves most or all of capitellum; Type 2, a shearing injury producing an osteochondral defect; and Type 3, a comminuted fracture of the capitellum often associated with a radial head fracture. The difficulty with diagnosing these fractures is that the frontal projection often is not helpful. Type 1 fractures are readily apparent on lateral views because they are usually displaced. Type 3 fractures are best diagnosed by either computed tomography or magnetic resonance imaging. Type 2 fractures are most optimally depicted by magnetic resonance imaging, although it may require intra-articular contrast if the defect is purely cartilagenous. Treatment is aimed at restoring normal biomechanics of the elbow. If the fragment is sufficiently large, reduction and fixation with small screws, Herbert screws, or Kirschner wires have had good success. Excision is recommended when fragments are too small for fixation.

Notes

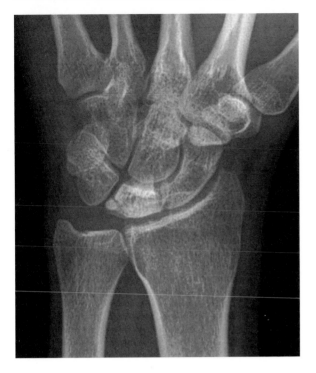 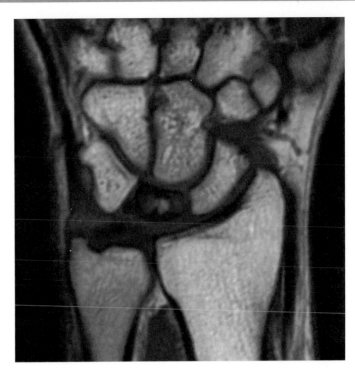

1. What is the diagnosis?

2. Can the process be interrupted with treatment?

3. What is the proposed cause of this condition?

4. Is this abnormality considered a "greater arc" injury?

Kienböck's Disease

1. Kienböck's disease.

2. Yes, with early diagnosis, collapse can be avoided.

3. Primary fracture, ligament disruption, or repetitive trauma interrupts blood supply to lunate.

4. No.

References

Gelberman RH, Bauman TD, Menon J, Akeson WH: The vascularity of the lunate bone and Kienböck's disease. *J Hand Surg* 5:272–278, 1980.

Lichtman DM, Alexander AH, Mack GR, Gunther SF: Kienböck's disease—update on silicone replacement arthroplasty. *J Hand Surg* 7[Am]:343–347, 1983.

Cross-Reference

Musculoskeletal Imaging: THE REQUISITES, 3rd ed, pp 145 and 351.

Comment

Isolated lunate fractures are uncommon; however, this carpal bone is susceptible to Kienböck's disease—avascular necrosis of the lunate. The loss of the blood supply to the lunate has been attributed to primary fracture, repetitive trauma causing microfractures, and traumatic injury to the ligaments that carry blood supply to the lunate. There is a statistical association among patients with an ulnar minus variant. The diagnosis is based on radiographic observations. Initially, the lunate may appear normal but with time the bone becomes increasingly sclerotic. This is followed by eventual loss of height, fragmentation, and subsequent collapse. Magnetic resonance imaging is useful in diagnosing the disease process earlier in patients with central wrist pain since marrow edema can be identified before sclerosis occurs.

Lichtman and colleagues devised a staging classification that identifies four different stages. In stage I, the radiographs are normal but magnetic resonance imaging may show areas of altered signal intensity or a subchondral fracture. In stage II, the density of the bone increases. In stage III, the subchondral bone collapses. Two subtypes exist in Stage III. In stage IIIA, there is lunate collapse but normal scaphoid rotation. In stage IIIB, the scaphoid rotation is fixed and there may be advanced capitate collapse. In stage IV, arthritic changes develop throughout the carpus.

Notes

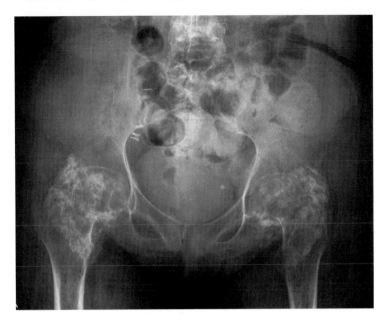

1. Name the process that you see and list the different types.
2. What type do you think this patient has and why?
3. Where do you usually see this process?
4. Can this process cause symptoms?

Heterotopic Ossification

1. Heterotopic ossification. There are three forms: traumatic, neurogenic, and myositis ossificans progressiva.

2. Neurogenic; she is extremely osteopenic because of paralysis from a spinal cord injury.

3. In addition to the hip, the shoulder, elbow, and knee are common locations.

4. Yes, pain and diminished range of motion. Swelling, fever, erythema, and a palpable mass may mimic an infection or deep venous thrombosis.

References

Balboni TA, Gobezie R, Mamon HJ: Heterotopic ossification: Pathophysiology, clinical features, and the role of radiotherapy for prophylaxis. *Int J Radiat Oncol Biol Phys* 65:1289–1299, 2006.

Shehab D, Elgazzar AH, Collier BD: Heterotopic ossification. *J Nucl Med* 43:346–353, 2002.

Cross-Reference

Musculoskeletal Imaging: THE REQUISITES, 3rd ed, pp 36–38.

Comment

Heterotopic ossification is a well-recognized condition characterized by the formation of mature, lamellar bone in the soft tissues. Three factors are required: an osteogenic precursor cell, an inducing agent(s), and an environment that permits the formation of new bone. There are three forms: traumatic (occurs after fractures and dislocations, or after procedures such as total hip replacements and internal fixation of fractures), neurogenic (occurs after traumatic brain injuries, spinal cord trauma, strokes, or infections and tumors that affect the central nervous system), and congenital. Myositis ossificans progressiva is a rare hereditary disease (autosomal dominant) characterized by the progressive deposition of heterotopic bone throughout the skeleton.

This patient had a traumatic spinal cord injury. Soft tissue ossification appears about 2 to 6 months following the initial insult. Common areas affected are the hips, shoulders, knees, and elbows and more than one site may be involved. Initially, the heterotopic ossification appears as an ill-defined radiodense area, lacking in trabeculation. As it enlarges, the cortex and trabeculation becomes apparent. Ultimately, complete ankylosis of a joint may occur. Treatment is aimed at two different goals. The first is prophylaxis and may include the administration of nonsteroidal anti-inflammatory drugs or radiation therapy. The second is aimed at restoring motion of the involved joint when the process is mature (based on the absence of activity on bone scintigraphy).

Notes

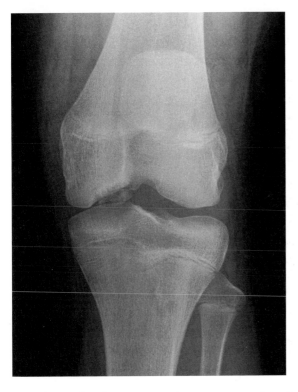
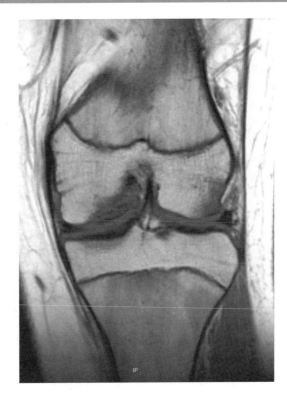

1. What is the diagnosis? Is this a common location?

2. What percentage of patients present with bilateral involvement?

3. Although the etiology of this lesion is unknown, how many patients reveal a history of trauma?

4. What is the most specific finding indicating fragment instability on magnetic resonance arthrography?

Osteochondritis Dissecans

1. Osteochondritis dissecans. Yes, 80% of lesions occur in the medial femoral condyle, but the lateral femoral condyle, patella, and trochlea of the femur are also potential sites.

2. Twenty-five percent are bilateral.

3. Nearly one half of patients.

4. Imbibition of contrast between the fragment and rest of femur. This finding correlates with a complete cleft surrounding the fragment.

Reference

Helgason JW, Chandnani VP, Yu JS: MR arthrography: A review of current technique and applications. *AJR Am J Roentgenol* 168:1473–1480, 1997.

Cross-Reference

Musculoskeletal Imaging: THE REQUISITES, 3rd ed, pp 53–58.

Comment

Osteochondritis dissecans refers to a condition that is characterized by the development of a devascularized fragment of bone, usually in the nonweightbearing surface of the medial femoral condyle. Radiographically, the lesion has a well-demarcated rim of sclerosis, which surrounds the abnormal marrow and extends to the articular cortex. Osteochondritis dissecans affects males two to three times more frequently than females, and most patients present in adolescence (mean age of 15 years). The size of the osteochondral lesion and the thickness of the surrounding sclerotic rim are helpful when trying to stage a lesion. In stage 1, a lesion measures approximately 1 to 3 cm in diameter and the articular cartilage overlying the defect is intact. In stage 2, the articular cartilage demonstrates a cleft or fissuring that extends to the cortex but there is no indication of loosening of the fragment. In stage 3, there is partial detachment of the osteochondral defect with a large cleft extending into the subchondral bone. In stage 4, the fragment is loose within the crater. Some investigators identify a fifth type in which there is a loose body and an empty crater. Magnetic resonance arthrography is the most accurate technique for establishing the stability of a lesion. Conventional T2W images may depict high signal intensity surrounding the osteochondral fragment but it may be difficult to differentiate granulation tissue from free fluid. Focal cystic lesions deep to the lesion are associated with instability of the fragment as is fluid imbibition between the fragment and the rest of the condyle.

Notes

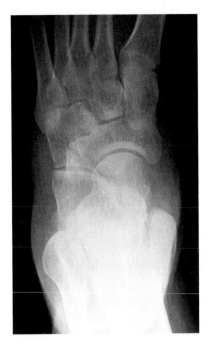 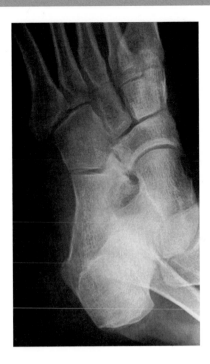

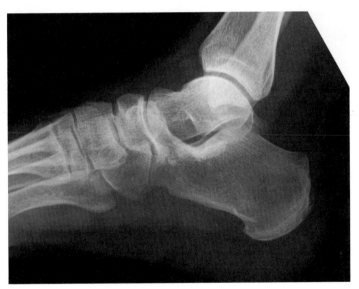

1. What is the diagnosis? What type is it?

2. What is the most common presenting symptom?

3. What is the preferred imaging technique for diagnosis and preoperative planning?

4. What is the "C" sign?

Calcaneonavicular Tarsal Coalition

1. Calcaneonavicular tarsal coalition. Fibrous.

2. Pain.

3. Magnetic resonance imaging allows for more flexibility in the imaging planes and is superior for establishing other causes of ankle pain.

4. A radiographic sign for subtalar coalition, seen on the lateral radiograph of the foot, which is formed by the continuous bone across the posterior margin of the middle facet.

Reference

Emery KH, Bisset GS, III, Johnson ND, Nunan PJ: Tarsal coalition: A blinded comparison of MRI and CT. *Pediatr Radiol* 28:612–616, 1998.

Cross-Reference

Musculoskeletal Imaging: THE REQUISITES, 3rd ed, pp 616–621.

Comment

A tarsal coalition is common, occurring in 1% of the population. It can be osseous, fibrous, or cartilaginous. Most are due to failure of segmentation of the bones of the foot in utero but they also occur as part of various syndromes. Clinically, coalitions may cause pain and decreased range of motion, usually noted in the second decade of life as the child becomes more active and progression of ossification of the growth centers continues in the foot. Coalitions often occur in both feet, and, occasionally, more than one type of coalition may be seen in one foot. Both computed tomography and magnetic resonance imaging are very good for detecting tarsal coalitions and are advocated for preoperative evaluation. A calcaneonavicular coalition is best seen on an oblique radiograph of the foot. In an osseous coalition, there is complete osseous bridging between the calcaneus and navicular bones. In fibrous and cartilaginous coalitions, there is close approximation of the two tarsal bones with deformation, an irregular cortical margin and sclerosis. The elongated anterior process of the calcaneus resembles the snout of an anteater on a lateral radiograph. A talar beak may be present. Magnetic resonance imaging may show intervening high signal intensity tissue on T2W images and bone edema.

Notes

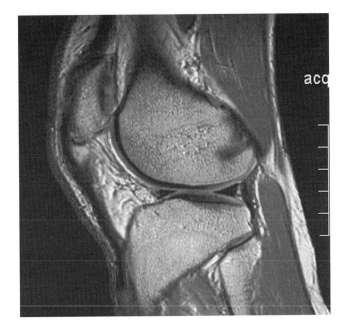
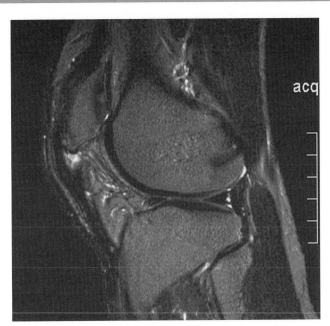
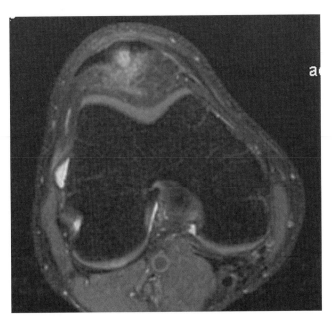
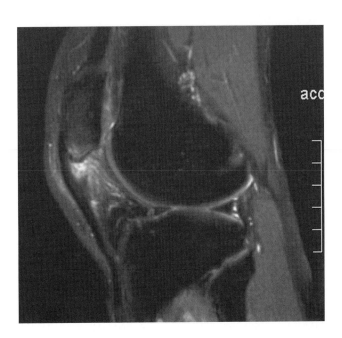

1. Is this condition an inflammatory process?

2. Who is at risk for developing this condition?

3. What is the most common clinical complaint?

4. What are some conditions that present with anterior knee pain?

Chronic Patellar Tendinosis (Jumper's Knee)

1. No, it is a degenerative process. There is a conspicuous absence of inflammatory cells when the abnormal tissue is evaluated microscopically.

2. Athletes who participate in activities that require repetitive, violent contraction of the quadriceps musculature such as basketball and volleyball.

3. Chronic anterior knee pain.

4. Chondromalacia, patellofemoral joint osteoarthritis, crystal deposition arthropathies, osteochondral defect, plica syndrome, Hoffa's syndrome, prepatellar bursitis, patellar contusion, and jumper's knee.

Reference

Yu JS, Popp JE, Kaeding CC, Lucas J: Correlation of MR imaging and pathologic findings in athletes undergoing surgery for chronic patellar tendinitis. *AJR Am J Roentgenol* 165:115–118, 1995.

Cross-Reference

Musculoskeletal Imaging: THE REQUISITES, 3rd ed, pp 240–242.

Comment

Patellar tendinosis is caused by repeated microtears occurring at the enthesis of the patellar tendon. Histologically, it is characterized by chronic degeneration, which disrupts the architecture of the tendon. The degree of hyaline degeneration corresponds roughly to the duration of patient's symptoms and represents an end-stage process. As the disease progresses, it becomes increasingly more difficult to attain pain relief and the patient experiences diminished athletic performance. Anterior knee pain is best evaluated with magnetic resonance imaging. Not only is patellar tendinosis easily diagnosed, but so are other conditions that have a similar clinical presentation. The characteristic MR appearance of patellar tendinosis is focal thickening involving the proximal one third of the patellar tendon. The degree of thickening is often two to four times that of normal. The posterior tendon margin is usually indistinct and it may be associated with edema in Hoffa's fat pad. Involvement of the anterior fibers does not occur and can be useful in discriminating tendinosis from acute tears of the proximal patellar tendon. The signal intensity of the tendon is altered with ill-defined areas of intermediate signal intensity on PD and T2W images. Occasionally, relatively hyperintense signal changes on T2W and inversion recovery images reflect cystic degeneration. Marrow edema in the inferior pole of the patella is an occasional finding. The preferred treatment is surgical with debridement of degenerated tissue and placement of multiple longitudinal tenotomies if the patient fails conservative management. The end stage of this condition is rupture of the tendon.

Notes

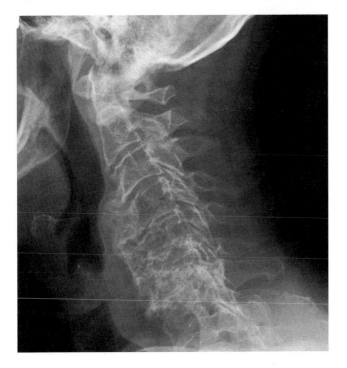 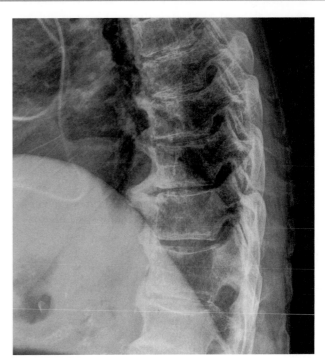

1. How do you think this patient presented clinically?

2. Why is ossification more pronounced on the right side of the spine?

3. Does the ossification progress as people age?

4. List some extraspinal manifestations of this condition.

Diffuse Idiopathic Skeletal Hyperostosis

1. With dysphagia from effacement of the esophagus.

2. The pulsating effect from the thoracic aorta inhibits soft tissue ossification.

3. Yes, there is an increasing prevalence with aging.

4. Enthesopathy and para-articular bony excrescences.

Reference

Resnick D, Niwayama G: Diffuse idiopathic skeletal hyperostosis (DISH): Ankylosing hyperostosis of Forestier and Rotes-Querol. In Resnick D (ed): *Diagnosis of Bone and Joint Disorders,* 4th ed. Philadelphia, WB Saunders, 2002, pp 1463–1495.

Cross-Reference

Musculoskeletal Imaging: THE REQUISITES, 3rd ed, pp 314–317.

Comment

Diffuse idiopathic skeletal hyperostosis is a common disorder of elderly people, characterized by undulating soft tissue calcification and hyperostosis along the anterolateral aspect of the spine involving at least four contiguous vertebral bodies. The soft tissues involved include the annular fibrosis, anterior longitudinal ligament, and paravertebral connective tissues. The clinical manifestations of this condition are generally mild, consisting of restricted motion and tendinitis from enthesopathy. The most common location affected is the thoracic spine. In isolated disease, the intervertebral discs do not undergo degeneration, thus the disc height is maintained. Laminated calcification and ossification develop along the spine, and the deposited bone may be variable in thickness ranging from 2 mm to 20 mm. It tends to have a wavy contour protruding at the disc space level due to the increased bone deposition at these levels. Radiolucent areas within the ossified mass at the level of the disk correspond to disc material that has extruded anteriorly, and characteristically terminate at the superior and inferior margins of the vertebra.

Enthesopathy is a common component of this condition. In the pelvis, ligament and tendinous calcification and ossification may occur in the iliac crest, ischium, and trochanteric regions of the femur. Iliolumbar, sacrotuberous, and sacroiliac ligament involvement is typical of advanced diffuse idiopathic skeletal hyperostosis.

Notes

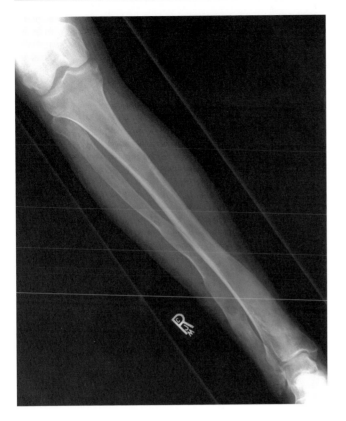 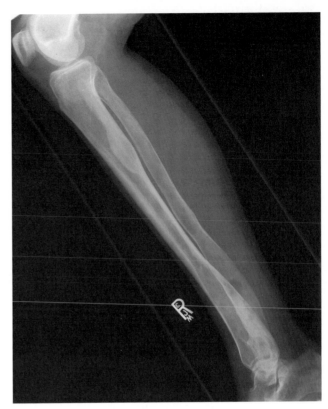

1. What is the diagnosis?

2. Can this condition undergo malignant transformation? If so, into what?

3. What is cherubism?

4. What is a characteristic of polyostotic disease?

Fibrous Dysplasia

1. Fibrous dysplasia.

2. Yes, in less than 1% of cases. Osteosarcomas, fibrosarcoma, and chondrosarcoma. One third of these patients have a previous history of radiation therapy.

3. Familial fibrous dysplasia characterized by bilateral expansile lesions in the mandible associated with multilocular cystic areas.

4. Ninety percent of cases involve only one limb.

References

Malloy PC, Scott WW Jr, Hruban RH: Fibrous dysplasia. *Skeletal Radiol* 22:66–69, 1993.

Shak ZK, Peh WC, Koh WL, Shek TW: Magnetic resonance imaging appearances of fibrous dysplasia. *Br J Radiol* 78:1104–1115, 2005.

Cross-Reference

Musculoskeletal Imaging: THE REQUISITES, 3rd ed, pp 460–465.

Comment

Fibrous dysplasia is a hamartomatous fibro-osseous metaplastic disorder caused by a defect in the germ plasm involving the proliferation and maturation of fibroblasts. The marrow becomes replaced by fibrous tissue. The variable amount of osteoid accounts for a wide range of radiographic densities in the bone. Clinically, patients are young and generally present in the first or second decade of life with pain or pathologic fractures. Patients with polyostotic disease frequently have cafe-au-lait spots (30% to 50%) and may present with endocrine dysfunction, particularly precocious puberty (referred to as McCune-Albright syndrome). About 90% of patients who have polyostotic disease have involvement in only one limb. The monostotic form has an affinity for the long bones and has a wide spectrum of radiographic appearances, ranging from fairly dense to relatively lytic.

The characteristic appearance is uniform ground-glass density seen centrally within the medullary cavity. The endosteal surface may be scalloped. Expansion of the bone is common as are bowing deformities. Lesions that have been present for a long period of time may demonstrate spotty calcification or a well-defined sclerotic rim. Pathologic fractures, due to weakening of the bone, can elicit a periosteal reaction but otherwise periostitis is not a typical feature of this condition. On magnetic resonance imaging, lesions are isointense with areas of hypointensity on T1W images and heterogeneously hyperintense on T2W images, and show a patchy enhancement pattern.

Notes

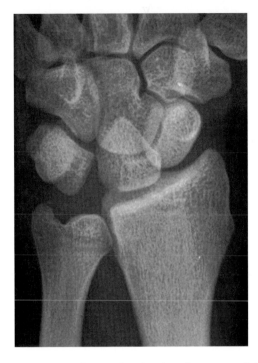 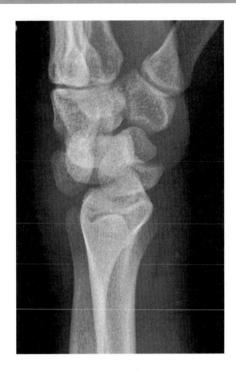

1. What radiographic landmarks are useful in assessing carpal stability?

2. What osseous injuries may occur in this injury?

3. Why is this not VISI (volar intercalated segmental instability)?

4. What would be an indication for magnetic resonance imaging? Computed tomography?

Midcarpal Dislocation

1. Intact proximal, middle, and distal carpal arcuate lines.

2. Fractures of the lunate and capitate.

3. The lunocapitate articulation is dislocated.

4. Occult fracture, triangular fibrocartilage tears, instability. Intra-articular entrapment of osseous fragments.

Reference

Yeager B, Dalinka M: Radiology of trauma to the wrist: Dislocations, fracture dislocations, and instability patterns. *Skeletal Radiol* 13:120–130, 1985.

Cross-Reference

Musculoskeletal Imaging: THE REQUISITES, 3rd ed, pp 147–150.

Comment

The most common mechanism of injury is a fall on the palm of the hand resulting in hyperextension of the wrist. In this position, the dorsal cortex of the distal radial articular surface fixes the lunate in place and apposes the scaphoid waist. Certain patterns of injury, referred to as *lesser arc injuries*, present a spectrum of injuries that reflect an increasing level of carpal instability. A stage 1 injury is referred to as scapholunate dissociation with rotatory subluxation of the scaphoid. Failure of the radiocapitate ligament causes perilunar instability, which leads to a stage 2 injury or perilunate dislocation. The capitate displaces dorsally, and the lunate may tilt volarly although remain articulated with the radius. Further disruption of the volar radiotriquetral ligament destabilizes the triquetrolunate joint resulting in a stage 3 injury or midcarpal dislocation. The lunate is volarly subluxed and the capitate is dorsally dislocated as seen in this patient. Complete disruption of the radiocarpal ligaments leads to a stage 4 injury or complete dislocation of the lunate. In this injury, the lunate is no longer articulated with either the radius or capitate and rotates volarly, but the latter two bones remain in linear alignment.

Notes

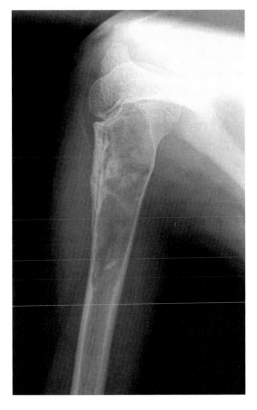

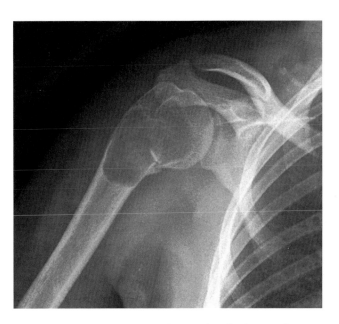

1. You are shown radiographs of two different patients with the same radiographic finding. What is it? Where is it most common?

2. What is meant by a pseudotrabeculated radiographic appearance?

3. At what age do most pathologic fractures that are related to this lesion occur?

4. When does this lesion stop growing?

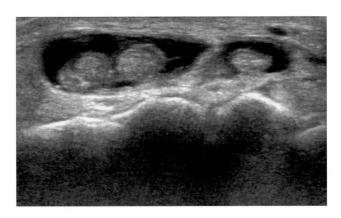

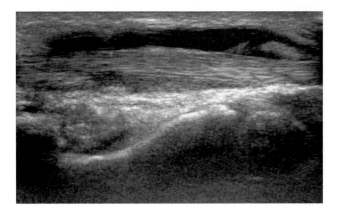

You are shown transverse (right side is radial) and longitudinal (right side is distal) sonograms of the dorsum of the wrist.

1. Which tendons are shown? Name two important landmarks and state whether you see them.

2. What is the observation and what does it mean?

3. What is de Quervain's stenosing tenosynovitis and which tendons are involved?

4. Which tendon lives in the sixth extensor compartment? What arthritic process frequently involves this compartment?

CASE 36

Simple Bone Cyst

1. The "fallen fragment" sign, a detached fragment of bone in the dependent portion of a cyst cavity. A simple bone cyst is most common in the proximal humerus.

2. Ridges between areas of endosteal scalloping give the appearance of coarsened trabeculation. There is no osseous matrix in the cyst itself.

3. The highest incidence occurs at about 10 years of age.

4. With epiphyseal closure.

References

Chigira M, Maehara S, Arita S, Udagawa E: The aetiology and treatment of simple bone cysts. *J Bone Joint Surg* 65[Br]:633–637, 1983.

Makley JT, Joyce MJ: Unicameral bone cyst (simple bone cyst). *Orthop Clin North Am* 20:407–415, 1989.

Cross-Reference

Musculoskeletal Imaging: THE REQUISITES, 3rd ed, pp 514–516.

Comment

A simple, or unicameral, bone cyst is common, and this lesion is a true fluid-filled cavity with a wall of fibrous tissue. Most of these cysts are discovered in people under the age of 20 years, either incidentally or because of a pathologic fracture. Males are twice as likely to have them. In adults, simple cysts have a predilection for the calcaneus and the innominate bones of the pelvis. In children and adolescents, 90% to 95% of cysts involve the long bones. The radiographic appearance is that of a lucent, well-demarcated geographic lesion that has its long axis parallel to the axis of the bone. It arises in the metaphysis but may migrate into the diaphysis with skeletal growth. The cyst is broader toward the metaphysis than toward the diaphysis. Abnormal remodeling of the bone is noticeable and the cortex occasionally appears expanded. A rim of sclerosis surrounding the lesion is variable in thickness but may be absent. Cortical disruption and periosteal reaction do not occur unless there is a pathologic fracture through the lesion. On magnetic resonance imaging, the typical features of a simple cyst are low signal intensity on T1W images and uniformly increased signal intensity on T2W images. Remember that hemorrhage in the cyst may alter its MR appearance. The "fallen fragment" sign represents a fracture fragment that has settled in the dependent portion of the fluid-filled cavity, revealing the true cystic nature of the lesion and that this finding is pathognomonic.

Notes

CASE 37

Extensor Digitorum Tenosynovitis

1. The extensor digitorum tendons. Extensor retinaculum (yes) and Lister's tubercle (no).

2. Anechoic fluid, with acoustic enhancement, distends the tendon sheath; tenosynovitis.

3. Idiopathic thickening of the tendon sheath of the first extensor compartment; extensor pollicis brevis and abductor pollicis longus.

4. Extensor carpi ulnaris tendon. Rheumatoid arthritis.

References

Gibbon WW: Applications of ultrasound in arthritis. *Semin Musculoskelet Radiol* 8:313–328, 2004.

Lee JC, Healy JC: Normal sonographic anatomy of the wrist and hand. *Radiographics* 25:1577–1590, 2005.

Cross-Reference

Musculoskeletal Imaging: THE REQUISITES, 3rd ed, pp 30–32.

Comment

Tenosynovitis is defined as inflammation of the tendon sheath. It is manifested by the presence of an abnormal amount of fluid within the tendon sheath. Tenosynovitis may result from generalized synovitis, such as rheumatoid arthritis, or may be localized owing to tendon degeneration, inflammation, tear, overuse, or tendon sheath trauma or infection. The wrist is a commonly affected area from both rheumatologic and traumatic causes, particularly the extensor compartments. Sonography is a rapid and accurate method for identifying this condition. Tendons have an echogenic appearance that consists of multiple parallel lines in the longitudinal plane and multiple dotlike echoes in the transverse plane. The extensor retinaculum, a fibrous band that extends obliquely across the dorsum of the wrist, appears as a thin hyperechoic structure that divides the dorsal surface into six compartments. Fluid in the tendon sheath produces posterior acoustic enhancement. Disorganization of the bundle architecture of the tendon may produce scattering of the ultrasound beam, producing a heterogeneous echotexture. Rheumatoid arthritis is a common cause of tenosynovitis, and the extensor carpi ulnaris is particularly prone to involvement. Other common sonographic manifestations of rheumatoid arthritis include widening of the tendon sheath, irregularity of the tendon margins, and synovial cyst formation.

Notes

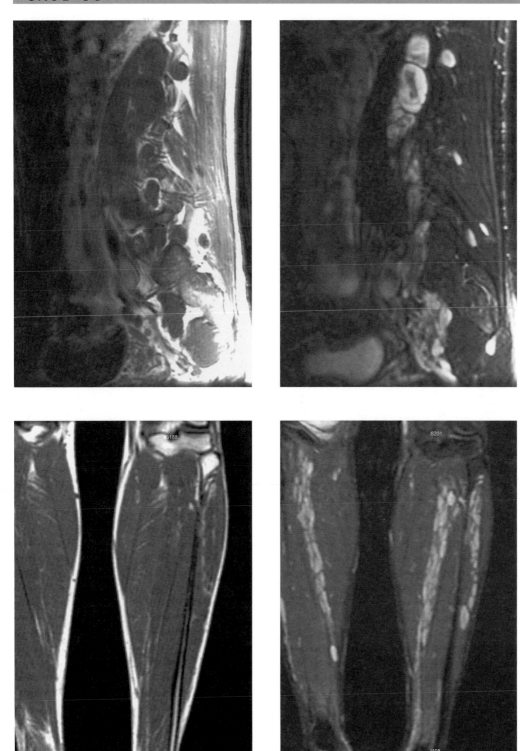

1. What is the most likely diagnosis?

2. A cystlike lesion in the mandible could represent what lesion?

3. What is the "fascicular" sign?

4. What is the "target" sign?

C A S E   3 8

Neurofibromatosis

1. Neurofibromatosis.

2. An intraosseous neurofibroma.

3. The small ringlike appearances of individual nerve fascicles in a neurofibroma.

4. Low signal intensity centrally with high signal intensity in the periphery on T2W images, most commonly seen with neurofibromas and occasionally seen with schwannomas.

References

Crawford AH, Schorry EK: Neurofibromatosis update. *J Pediatr Orthop* 26:413–423, 2006.

Lin DD, Barker PB: Neuroimaging of phakomatoses. *Semin Pediatr Neurol* 13:48–62, 2006.

Cross-Reference

Musculoskeletal Imaging: THE REQUISITES, 3rd ed, pp 500–503.

Comment

Neurofibromatosis is a hereditary dysplasia that affects all three germ layers. It is transmitted as an autosomal dominant trait although a family history is present in only 50% of cases. Other cases represent spontaneous mutations. Skin lesions are the most constant feature of neurofibromatosis with cafe-au-lait spots occurring in 90% of patients. An elevated epidermal mass, called *molluscum fibrosum*, is another common skin lesion. A flat or domelike nodule in the iris of the eye (Lisch nodule) is common in patients older than 5 years of age. The skeletal manifestations of neurofibromatosis are often the result of direct pressure from an adjacent tumor; however, dysplastic changes may involve the tibia, fibula, and clavicles, in the form of pseudoarthroses and bowing deformities. Acutely angled scoliosis, particularly when it involves the upper thoracic spine, is characteristic of this disorder. In the ribs, dysplastic changes may result in a ribbon-like deformity although intercostal neurofibromas may also produce similar erosive changes. Dumbbell-shaped neurofibromas exiting through the neural foramina can cause marked widening of the foramen. This abnormality can be very pronounced in the cervical spine. Cystic lesions in the bones can be caused by periosteal neurofibromas. Eccentrically located lytic lesions within the bone that have a sclerotic border may represent an intraosseous neurofibroma. It is most commonly seen in the mandible.

Notes

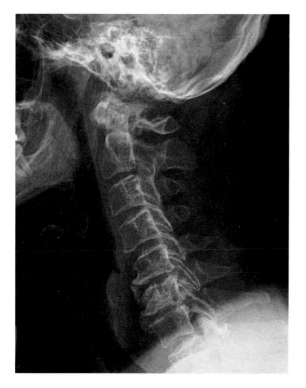 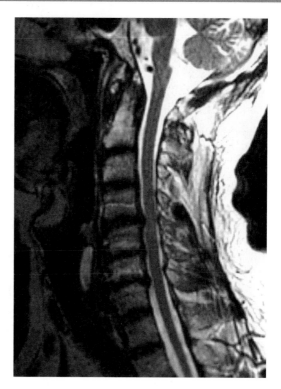

1. What is the major observation in this patient?

2. Name the joints that can encroach upon the cervical canal if degenerated.

3. When patients with congenital stenosis develop spondylosis, what should be kept in mind?

4. What are common symptoms?

Congenital Spinal Stenosis

1. Diffuse congenital spinal stenosis and degenerative changes of the disks with protrusion at C4-C5, C5-C6, and C6-C7.

2. Disk, apophyseal joint, and uncovertebral joint of Luschka.

3. They become more vulnerable to cord injury since spondylosis further compromises a canal that is already too small.

4. Parasthesia, weakness, and occasionally paralysis.

Reference

Pavlov H, Torg JS, Robie B, Jahre C: Cervical spinal stenosis: Determination with vertebral body ratio method. *Radiology* 164:771–775, 1987.

Cross-Reference

Musculoskeletal Imaging: THE REQUISITES, 3rd ed, pp 154–165.

Comment

Congenital spinal stenosis of the cervical spine is an important radiographic finding. Frequently, patients with a narrow canal present after trauma with transient sensory and motor symptoms in the arms, legs, or all four extremities. Sensory changes may include numbness, burning, tingling, and parasthesia. Motor symptoms may include weakness and paralysis. When the injury is relatively minor, the neurologic symptoms are transient and may last for a duration ranging from a few seconds to several minutes.

When the injury is more severe and involves significant axial loading, hyperextension, or hyperflexion, the symptoms may be permanent. The caliber of the cervical canal can be assessed by two methods on a lateral radiograph. In one method, the canal is measured from the posterior cortex of the vertebral body to the spinolaminar line. Symptoms of cord compression occur when the measurement is less than 10 mm. This technique does not correct for magnification, rotation, or variability in body size. A more useful technique is called the Pavlov ratio. In this method, the sagittal diameter of the spinal canal is divided by the sagittal diameter of the corresponding vertebral body. A ratio of 0.8 or less is considered significant and highly suggestive of congenital cervical spine stenosis.

Notes

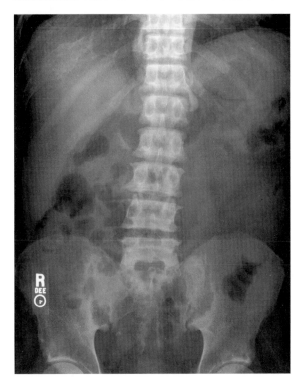

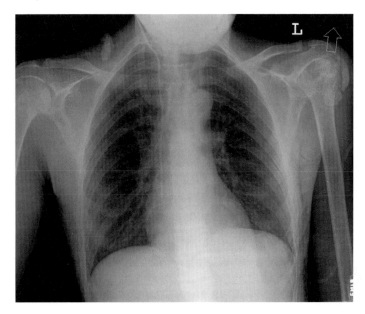

1. These two patients have the same disease. What is the diagnosis?

2. What are the primary causes of this disease and their relative incidence?

3. What is the radiologic hallmark of this disease?

4. What would you consider a good screening radiographic series for this disorder?

C A S E 4 0

Hyperparathyroidism

1. Hyperparathyroidism.

2. Single parathyroid adenoma (50% to 80%), multiple adenomas (10%), parathyroid hyperplasia (10% to 40%), and carcinoma (rare).

3. Bone resorption.

4. Radiographs of the hand, pelvis, and shoulders.

Reference

Pugh DG: Subperiosteal resorption of bone: A roentgenologic manifestation of primary hyperparathyroidism and renal osteodystrophy. *AJR* 66:577–586, 1951.

Cross-Reference

Musculoskeletal Imaging: THE REQUISITES, 3rd ed, pp 374–376 and 381–385.

Comment

Hyperparathyroidism refers to a group of disorders that are characterized by the presence of increased circulating parathyroid hormone (PTH). The presence of excess PTH results in increased osteoclastic resorption of the bone. Osteocytic osteolysis is responsible for the initial calcium release from the bone. In primary hyperparathyroidism, the parathyroid gland overproduces PTH. Patients present with weakness, lethargy, bone pain, polydypsia, and polyuria. Other associated abnormalities include nephrolithiasis, gastrointestinal ulcers, and pancreatitis. Common causes of the primary form of the disease include an adenoma, hyperplasia of the gland, parathyroid carcinoma, tumors that secrete PTH-like substances, and type 2 multiple endocrine neoplasia. Secondary hyperparathyroidism occurs in response to chronic hypocalcemia, usually from renal glomerular disease and, sometimes, malabsorption. Tertiary hyperparathyroidism refers to an autonomous gland that has escaped the regulatory effects of serum calcium after a prolonged period of stimulation, typically occurring in patients on chronic hemodialysis.

Bone resorption (particularly subperiosteal) is the radiologic hallmark of hyperparathyroidism. Both patients have secondary hyperparathyroidism from chronic renal failure induced by diabetes mellitus. The first patient demonstrates classic findings of subchondral bone resorption of the sacroiliac joints. Did you notice the brown tumor in the right 10th rib? The second patient shows classic distal clavicular resorption and tumoral calcinosis in the left shoulder. Other common preferred sites of bone resorption are the medial metaphyseal surfaces of the proximal femur, humerus, and tibia; distal metaphysis of the radius and ulna; symphysis pubis; the radial aspect of the middle phalanges; and distal acro-osteolysis.

Notes

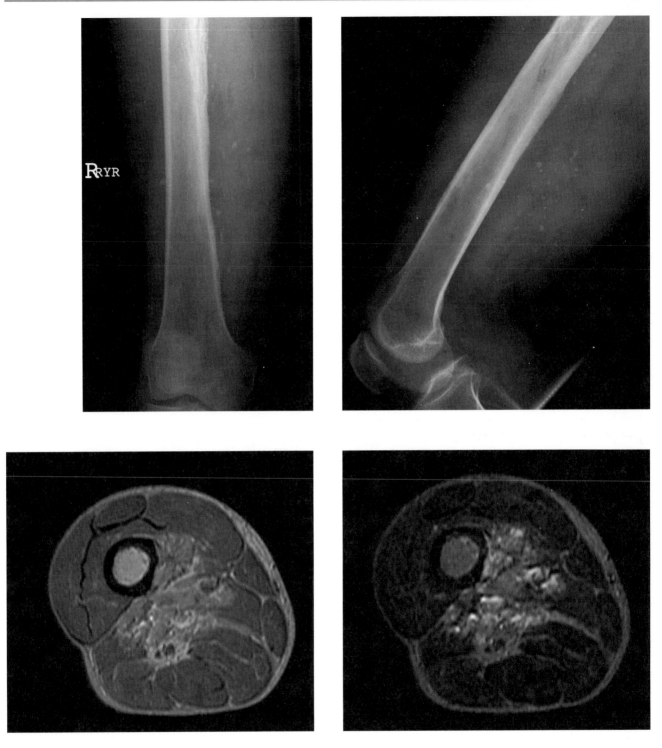

1. What is the likely diagnosis?

2. How do you think this patient presented?

3. What are the calcifications that you see on the radiographs?

4. What do they tell you about the lesion?

Soft Tissue Hemangioma

1. Soft tissue hemangioma.

2. Painful mass.

3. Phleboliths.

4. It is most likely a cavernous hemangioma.

Reference

Murphey MD, Fairbairn KJ, Parman LM, et al: Musculoskeletal angiomatous lesions: Radiologic-pathologic correlation. *Radiographics* 15:893–917, 1995.

Cross-Reference

Musculoskeletal Imaging: THE REQUISITES, 3rd ed, pp 478–479 and 485–487.

Comment

A hemangioma is a benign vascular lesion and is divided into either capillary or cavernous types and arteriovenous or venous, depending on its predominant composition. It is one of the most common soft tissue tumors, accounting for 7% of all benign tumors. Clinically, these lesions may change in size and are painful. They are generally more common in women and may increase in size with pregnancy. Cavernous hemangiomas are composed of large, dilated, blood-filled spaces lined by flattened endothelium and are less common than capillary types. They are usually intra-muscular, and these types do not involute and may require surgical resection. Calcifications in the form of phlebolith are characteristic, but nonspecific curvilinear calcification may also occur. Reactive changes to the adjacent bone may cause overgrowth or periosteal reaction. On magnetic resonance imaging, a lesion demonstrates low to intermediate signal intensity on T1W images. Overgrowth of adipose tissue is a reactive phenomenon most frequently associated with hemangiomas and may be seen as areas of higher signal intensity on T1W images. On T2W images, very high signal intensity owing to vascular tissue mixed with lower signal intensity from fat is notable. Contrast administration enhances the lesion and feeding vessels. Phleboliths appear as circular areas of low signal intensity.

Notes

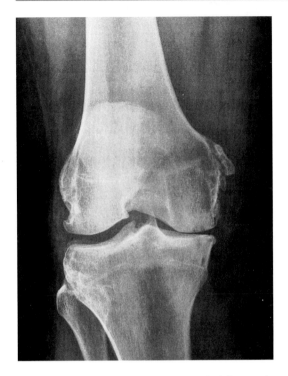 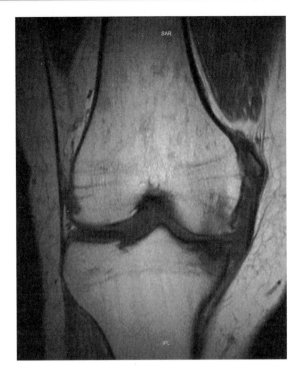

1. What is the finding in the medial femoral metaphysics and what does it represent?

2. What are the layers of the medial collateral ligament (MCL)? What separates these layers?

3. What was the mechanism of injury?

4. What would you expect to see in the acute phase of the injury on magnetic resonance imaging?

Pellegrini-Stieda Lesion

1. Pellegrini-Stieda lesion; post-traumatic calcification/ossification of the proximal attachment of the medial collateral ligament (MCL) representing a remote injury.

2. There are two layers: the tibiocollateral ligament (superficial layer) and the meniscofemoral and meniscotibial ligaments (deep layer). A small bursa.

3. Valgus injury to a flexed knee.

4. Thickening of the proximal anterior fibers of the MCL with or without interstitial edema, with surrounding perifascicular edema.

Reference

Mendes LF, Pretterklieber ML, Cho JH, et al: Pellegrini-Stieda disease: A heterogeneous disorder not synonymous with ossification/calcification of the tibial collateral ligament—anatomic and imaging investigation. *Skeletal Radiol* 35:916–922, 2006.

Cross-Reference

Musculoskeletal Imaging: THE REQUISITES, 3rd ed, pp 239 and 241.

Comment

A Pellegrini-Stieda lesion represents post-traumatic calcification or ossification around the origin of the MCL. It may be caused by a remote tear with ossification of a hematoma in or around the proximal fibers or from an avulsion fracture at the insertion of the MCL (Stieda fracture). The MCL comprises two layers of connective tissue separated by a small bursa. The fibers of the MCL are taut when the knee is extended and help prevent hyperextension. The MCL remains taut throughout flexion, helping prevent valgus angulation when the knee is flexed. Most injuries occur when the knee is flexed and a valgus stress is applied to the knee. The radiographic appearance is characteristic, with a crescent shaped ossification arising from the anterior and superior margin of the medial femoral condyle. On magnetic resonance imaging, a Pellegrini-Stieda lesion appears as an ossicle or enthesophyte with characteristic fat containing marrow within the proximal fibers of the MCL. The ligament is typically thickened and may be stripped from the epicondylar portion of the medial femoral condyle.

Notes

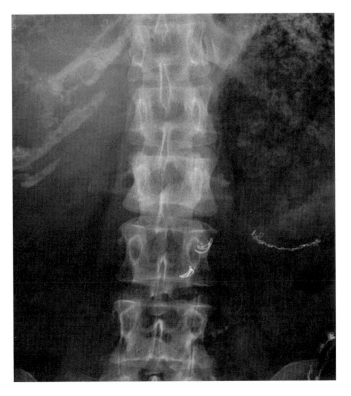

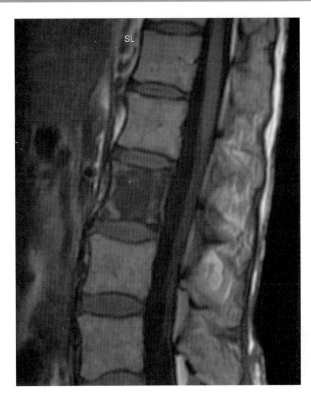

1. List your differential considerations.

2. What neoplasms can cause osteoblastic metastasis?

3. Which disease is associated with the "sandwich vertebra" sign?

4. How is fluorosis different radiographically from the other conditions that depict diffusely increased bone density?

Ivory Vertebra

1. Osteoblastic metastasis, lymphoma, chronic infection, and occasionally osteosarcoma. Paget's disease would be a consideration if the vertebra was enlarged or if the anterior curvature was filled in.

2. Pure osteoblastic lesions—prostate carcinoma; common osteoblastic lesions—bronchial carcinoid tumor and carcinomas of the breast, bladder, nasopharynx, and stomach; medulloblastoma; and neuroblastoma. Occasional osteoblastic lesions—chordoma, lymphoma, and multiple myeloma.

3. Osteopetrosis tarda; refers to increased density occurring at the endplates.

4. Development of prominent densely sclerotic osteophytes, which project into the paravertebral soft tissues, at the attachment of ligaments, tendons, and muscle.

Reference

Silverman IE, Flynn JA: Images in clinical medicine. Ivory vertebra. *N Engl J Med* 338:100, 1998.

Cross-Reference

Musculoskeletal Imaging: THE REQUISITES, 3rd ed, p 497.

Comment

Metastasis is the most common tumor of the spine. Metastasis to the axial skeleton occurs in nearly one half of patients who have been discovered to have osseous metastasis on bone scintigraphy, most frequently involving the thoracic and lumbar vertebral bodies. When a vertebral body is heterogeneously or homogenously sclerotic, it is referred to as an ivory vertebra. When the process is more diffuse, affecting numerous vertebral bodies, other conditions such as mastocytosis, tuberous sclerosis, myelofibrosis, renal osteodystrophy, fluorosis, and osteopetrosis should be considered.

Notes

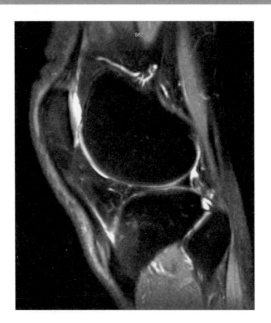

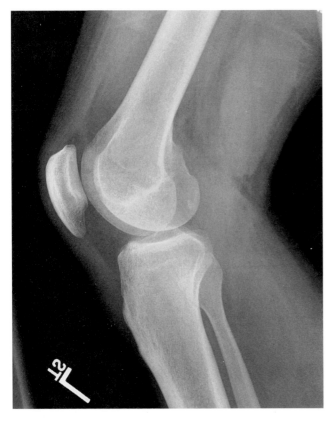

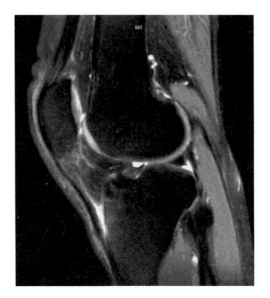

1. What is the diagnosis?

2. What is its etiology?

3. What is the essential clinical and radiographic finding of this condition?

4. List some potential complications of this disease.

Osgood-Schlatter Disease

1. Osgood-Schlatter disease.

2. Osteochondrosis of the tibial tuberosity.

3. Soft tissue swelling in the anterior knee.

4. Nonunion of the bone fragment, patellar subluxation, chondromalacia, avulsion of the patellar tendon, and genu recurvatum.

Reference

Rosenberg ZS, Kawelblum M, Cheung YY, et al: Osgood-Schlatter lesion: Fracture or tendinitis? Scintigraphic, CT, and MR imaging features. *Radiology* 185:853–858, 1992.

Cross-Reference

Musculoskeletal Imaging: THE REQUISITES, 3rd ed, p 219.

Comment

Osgood-Schlatter disease, an osteochondrosis of the tibial tuberosity, is a disease of adolescents, most commonly affecting boys between the ages of 10 and 15 years, although occasionally it affects adults. Patients present with pain, soft tissue swelling, and tenderness in the anterior knee in the proximity of the tibial tuberosity. A history of recent athletic activity that includes kicking, jumping, and squatting is characteristic of this disorder, and typical patients recall a recent growth spurt. The diagnosis of acute Osgood-Schlatter disease is based on the observations of soft tissue swelling anterior to the tuberosity and loss of the sharp margination of the patellar tendon. Fragmentation of the tibial tuberosity becomes apparent after 3 to 4 weeks. After the acute stage, a persistent ossific fragment or fragments in a thickened patellar tendon mark the site of previous disease. The diagnosis is made with relative ease on magnetic resonance imaging. Variable thickening of the distal patellar tendon, anterior subcutaneous edema, edema in Hoffa's fat pad, and distension of the deep infrapatellar bursa often accompany or precede the fragmentation of the tibial tuberosity. Bone marrow edema manifested as areas of low signal intensity on T1W and high signal intensity on T2W images may be evident in the anterior aspect of the tibial metaphysis and epiphysis.

Notes

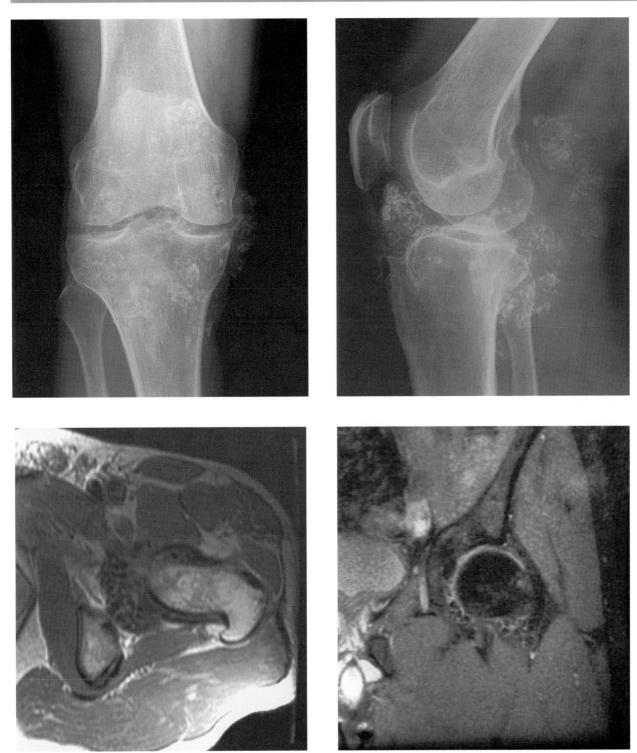

1. The radiographs are of one patient while the magnetic resonance images are of another. What disorder is shown in both joints?

2. What is the differential diagnosis?

3. Is this process polyarticular or monoarticular?

4. How is it treated? Does it recur?

Synovial Chondromatosis

1. Synovial chondromatosis.

2. Osteoarthritis with intra-articular bodies, osteochondritis dissecans, infection by low virulence organisms such as *Mycobacterium tuberculosis*, and trauma. If nodules are small, rice bodies of rheumatoid arthritis may be considered.

3. Monoarticular.

4. Synovectomy. It is not uncommon for these to recur.

References

Crotty JM, Monu JU, Pope TL, Jr: Synovial osteochondromatosis. *Radiol Clin North Am* 34:327–342, 1996.

Narvaez JA, Narvaez J, Aguilera C, et al: MR imaging of synovial tumors and tumor-like lesions. *Eur Radiol* 11:2549–2560, 2001.

Cross-Reference

Musculoskeletal Imaging: THE REQUISITES, 3rd ed, pp 355–356.

Comment

Synovial chondromatosis is a synovial metaplastic disorder of unknown etiology characterized by the formation of numerous intra-articular cartilaginous nodules. It is a monoarticular disorder with a chronic progressive course that leads to osteoarthritis owing to joint damage. The knee, hip, elbow, and shoulder are the joints most frequently affected. The diagnosis becomes evident by the third to fifth decades of life, and is more predominant in males. The disease is caused by villous or nodular cartilage metaplasia of the synovium. The cartilage nodules grow to a size no bigger than 2 cm, then break off, becoming loose in the joint. Microscopically, considerable peripheral cellular proliferation with atypical nuclei may be mistaken for neoplasia, although this is a benign process. These two patients show characteristic imaging appearances. Radiographically, numerous uniform-sized intra- and juxta-articular bodies with variable mineralization are a primary feature. On magnetic resonance imaging, more numerous intra-articular bodies are notable since this modality is sensitive to nonmineralized nodules. The round nodules usually show intermediate to low signal intensity on all sequences and may be associated with osseous erosion.

Notes

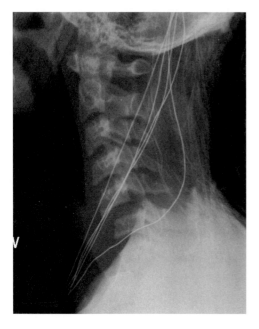
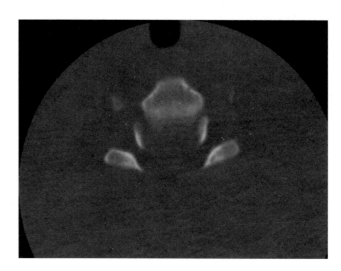

1. What is the diagnosis and is this considered a stable or unstable abnormality?
2. What ligaments do you think are involved?
3. What percentage of patients present with neurologic symptoms?
4. What are some potential associated injuries?

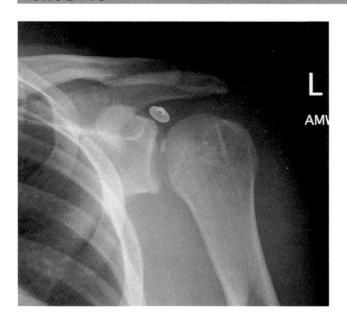
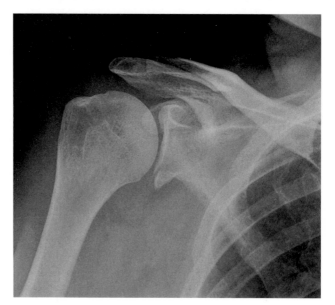

You are shown radiographs from two different patients.

1. What is the main finding on the first radiograph and what does it mean?
2. What is the injury mechanism?
3. The second radiograph is a different patient with the same injury mechanism. What is the finding?
4. What other osseous lesions should you look for?

CASE 47

Flexion Injury—Bilateral Jumped Facets

1. Hyperflexion injury with bilaterally dislocated facet joints at C5-C6; unstable.

2. Rupture of posterior annulus fibrosus, posterior longitudinal ligament, and capsular, interspinous, and supraspinous ligaments, as well as stripped anterior longitudinal ligament.

3. Seventy-five percent.

4. Vascular injury to vertebral artery and disc herniation.

Reference

Berquist TH: Imaging of adult cervical spine trauma. *Radiographics* 8:667–694, 1988.

Cross-Reference

Musculoskeletal Imaging: THE REQUISITES, 3rd ed, pp 172–174.

Comment

Hyperflexion injuries of the cervical spine are the most common injury mechanisms affecting the cervical spine. Many are caused by a direct blow against the top of the skull resulting in forward arching of the head. A hyperflexion sprain disrupts the ligaments of the posterior column, and, in severe cases, the posterior longitudinal ligament and posterior portion of the annulus fibrosus in the middle column of the spine. The injury typically occurs in the absence of any fracture, although minor wedgelike compressions of the anterior portions of the vertebral body exist. Focal kyphosis measuring 11 degrees greater than at adjacent levels is indicative of posterior ligament damage. When the injury is severe, the facet joints can become dislocated and "locked" end to end. Ligament damage is much more extensive when there are jumped facet joints owing to complete disruption in the posterior and middle columns and variable disruption of the ligaments in the anterior column. The lateral radiograph is characteristic. There is severe malalignment with anterior displacement of C5 and a marked focal kyphosis. The inferior edge of the superior facet is perched against the superior edge of the inferior facet. The axial computed tomography image shows bilateral "naked" or disarticulated facets. The lateral radiograph also shows disproportionate widening of the interspinous distance, anterior narrowing of the C5-C6 disc, and compromise of the spinal canal.

Notes

CASE 48

Anterior Shoulder Dislocation (Osseous)

1. Hill-Sachs lesion; prior anterior glenohumeral joint dislocation.

2. Hyperabduction of an externally rotated and extended arm.

3. An osseous Bankart lesion.

4. A fracture of the greater tuberosity.

Reference

Richards RD, Sartoris DJ, Pathria MN, Resnick D: Hill-Sachs lesion and normal humeral groove: MR imaging features allowing their differentiation. *Radiology* 190:665–668, 1994.

Cross-Reference

Musculoskeletal Imaging: THE REQUISITES, 3rd ed, pp 77–85 and 98–105.

Comment

Approximately 50% of all dislocations in the human body involve the glenohumeral joint. Nearly 95% result in anterior displacement of the humeral head with respect to the glenoid fossa. An indirect force, such as a fall on an outstretched arm, is the most common mechanism of injury. The main factor that determines a patient's risk for recurrence is the age of the patient during the initial dislocation. Four types of anterior dislocations have been described: subcoracoid, subclavicular, subacromial, and intrathoracic. The shoulder must be closely scrutinized for associated injuries after establishing a diagnosis of a dislocation. An impaction fracture of the posterolateral aspect of the humeral head (Hill-Sachs lesion), fracture of the glenoid rim (osseous Bankart lesion), and greater tuberosity fractures are important observations that may be detected on the initial radiographs. Computed tomography may be useful in confirming fractures and quantifying the size and displacement, particularly with glenoid rim fractures. Soft tissue injuries to the labrum, anterior capsule, and the subscapularis tendon are deferred to magnetic resonance imaging. It has been speculated that the size of a Hill-Sachs lesion may be proportional to the length of time that the head has been dislocated and/or with the number of recurrences although there is debate regarding this issue. Remember, the physiologic trough can mimic a Hill-Sachs lesion on cross-sectional imaging; however, the physiologic trough does not extend to the superior-most centimeter of the humeral head, that is, the initial three or four axial images of the humerus.

Notes

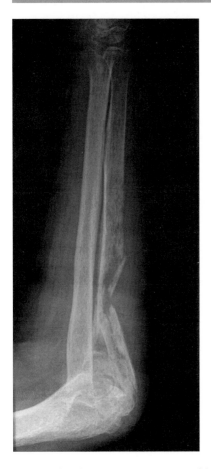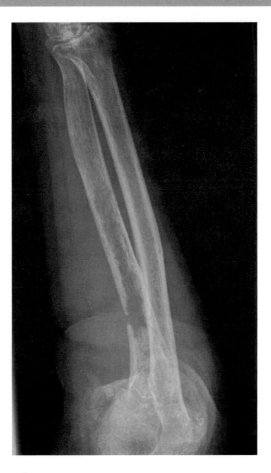

1. List the three main patterns of bone destruction.

2. What is the dominant pattern shown in this patient? What are processes that can cause this particular pattern of bone destruction?

3. What mechanisms allow the spread of tumor to bone?

4. List the most common tumor of origin for bone metastasis in adult men, adult women, and children.

Permeative Bone Destruction

1. Geographic, moth-eaten, and permeative.

2. Permeative pattern. Metastasis, primary bone tumors (i.e., Ewing's sarcoma), multiple myeloma, leukemia, eosinophilic granuloma, and osteomyelitis.

3. Direct extension, lymphatic spread, hematogenous spread, and intraspinal spread.

4. Adult men: prostate, lung, and bladder; adult women: breast and uterus; children: neuroblastoma, Ewing's sarcoma, osteosarcoma, and soft tissue tumors.

Reference

Enneking WF: Staging of musculoskeletal neoplasms. *Skeletal Radiol* 1985; 13:183–194.

Cross-Reference

Musculoskeletal Imaging: THE REQUISITES, 3rd ed, pp 407–409.

Comment

There are three basic patterns of bone destruction: geographic, a marginated or circumscribed solitary area of bone lysis; moth-eaten, caused by numerous smaller osteolytic lesions and endosteal excavations generally indicating a more aggressive lesion; and permeative, an aggressive infiltrative process that causes cortical tunneling, and numerous tiny and indistinct osteolytic lesions with poor margination between abnormal and normal bone. This patient has lung cancer and demonstrates a good example of a permeative pattern of bone destruction from an osseous metastasis. There is a pathologic fracture that contributed to the development of periosteal reaction. There are many etiologies of a permeative pattern of bone destruction including both benign and malignant processes, so it is important to search for other clues that can aid in narrowing the differential diagnosis such as the age of the patient, presence of other lesions, soft tissue involvement, underlying systemic disease, and constitutional signs (e.g., fever, elevated white blood cell count).

Notes

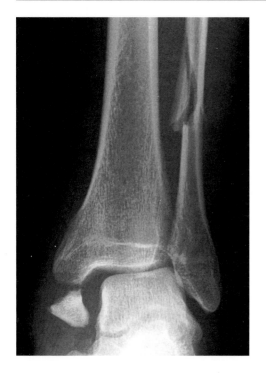
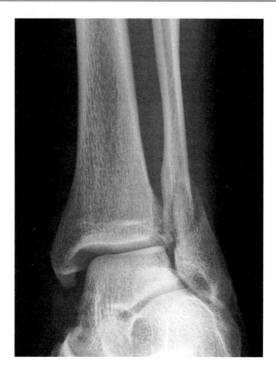
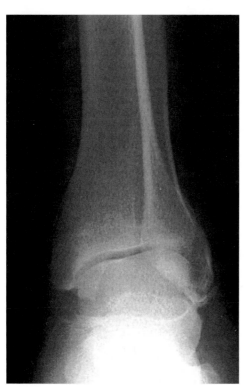

1. These three patients have different ankle fractures. Classify them using the Weber classification.

2. What is the Weber classification based on?

3. What is a Maisonneuve fracture? Does it fit in the Weber classification?

4. In what view(s) is/are a posterior tibiofibular ligament avulsion best seen?

C A S E 5 0

Weber Classification

1. Weber C2, Weber B2, and Weber A1.

2. The level of fibular fracture and integrity of the syndesmotic ligaments.

3. It is a fracture of the proximal fibula (often the neck) with either a fracture of the medial malleolus or a deltoid ligament injury and rupture of the syndesmotic ligaments. Yes, Weber C3.

4. Lateral view, but occasionally the mortise (oblique) view.

Reference

Hall H: A simplified workable classification of ankle fractures. *Foot Ankle* 1:5–10, 1980.

Cross-Reference

Musculoskeletal Imaging: THE REQUISITES, 3rd ed, pp 252–255.

Comment

Ankle fractures are frequently complex. Osseous injuries are related to the position of the foot when it is injured and also on the direction of the injury force. The Weber classification identifies three injury patterns based on the level of a fibular fracture (which is predictive of a syndesmotic injury) and the degree of displacement of the ankle mortise. In type A injuries, fractures occur below the tibiotalar joint and do not involve the distal tibiofibular syndesmosis. In type B injuries, the fibular fracture occurs at the level of the joint and has an oblique orientation. This injury produces partial disruption of the syndesmosis. Types A and B are further subclassified into subtypes 1 (isolated), 2 (with medial malleolus or deltoid ligament injury), and 3 (with posterior tibial injury). There are three type C fractures. Type C1 is characterized by an oblique fibular fracture above the level of the distal tibiofibular ligaments. Type C2 lesions are characterized by an even more proximal fibular fracture, reflecting an extensive rupture of the syndesmosis, while a C3 is a Maisonneuve fracture. These injuries are associated with extensive tears of the tibiofibular ligaments and variably sized tears of the interosseous ligament. The Weber classification correlates well with prognosis and is useful for treatment.

Notes

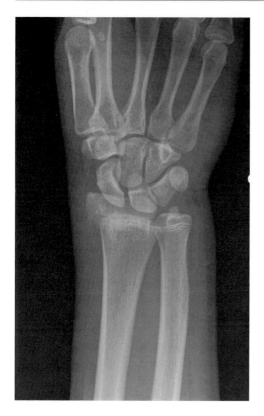 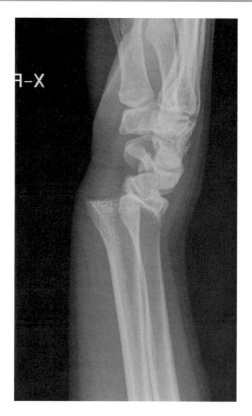

1. List the types of pediatric fractures. Which is shown?

2. In the wrist, the fracture produced is age dependent. List the type of fracture one would expect in patients whose ages are 5, 15, 25, and 45 years.

3. What forces are required to generate a lead-pipe fracture? How does this fracture appear radiographically?

4. Can a buckle fracture occur in adults?

Salter Fracture

1. Torus, greenstick, lead-pipe, plastic, and physeal (growth plate) fractures. Physeal plate.

2. At age 5, torus fracture of the radius/ulna; age 15, Salter-Harris injury of distal radius; age 25, scaphoid fracture; and age 45, Colles fracture.

3. Requires a combination of compressive and angular forces. Torus fracture on the compressive side and greenstick fracture on the tensile side.

4. Yes, in osteoporotic people.

References

Van Herpe LB: Fractures of the forearm and wrist. *Orthop Clin North Am* 7:543–556, 1976.

Wood VE: Fractures of the hand in children. *Orthop Clin North Am* 7:527–542, 1976.

Cross-Reference

Musculoskeletal Imaging: THE REQUISITES, 3rd ed, pp 49–53.

Comment

Pediatric fractures often appear different from those that occur in adults because these fractures may not entirely penetrate the shaft of the bone. A torus fracture, for instance, occurs when the injury is not of sufficient force to completely disrupt the bone but is sufficient to cause buckling of the cortex. The force is often a longitudinal load such as a fall on an outstretched hand, which causes compression of the bone. The location that is most susceptible to this type of injury is the metaphyseal region of a long bone. The characteristic appearance of this fracture is bulging of the cortex when viewed tangentially, and a transverse band of increased density from the impacted bone when viewed *en face*. Greenstick fractures are caused by an angular force and may convert into a complete fracture as the bone continues to grow. The bone breaks at the side subjected to tensile forces. A plastic fracture is caused by longitudinal stresses on the bone, which causes the bone to bow due to compressive forces. Initially, the bowing deformity is reversible. With a greater force, an irreversible bowing deformity occurs. With an even further increase in force, the bone ultimately breaks completely.

Physeal fractures account for 15% of pediatric fractures and are often characterized using the Salter-Harris classification. In a type 1 fracture, only the physis is involved. A type 2 fracture involves the physis and metaphysis, as in this patient—did you notice the small triangular metaphyseal fragment dorsally? It is the most common of the physeal injuries. A type 3 fracture involves the physis and epiphysis. In a type 4 fracture, the injury involves the epiphysis, physis, and metaphysis. A type 5 fracture is a compression injury of the physis.

Notes

Fair Game

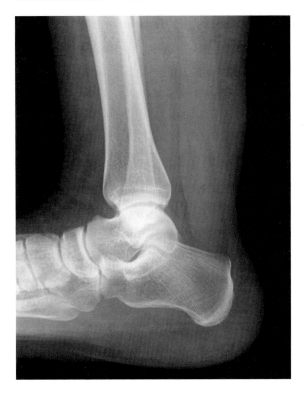
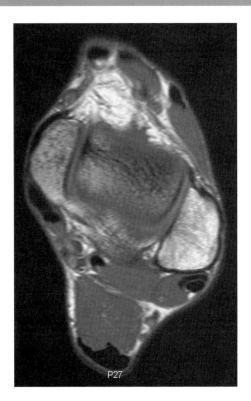

1. What is your diagnosis?

2. What is the classic presentation?

3. When patients present with exercise-induced claudication, what is the preferred treatment?

4. What muscle can present with tarsal tunnel syndrome?

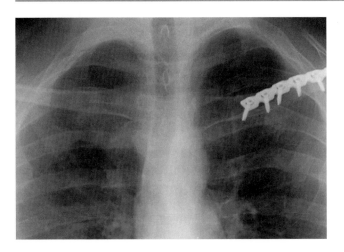
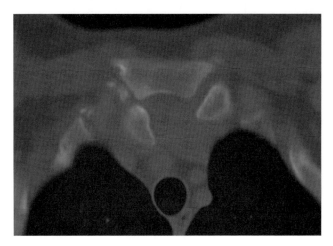

1. What is the single most important observation on the close-up view of the chest radiograph?

2. What are some potential injuries that this patient may have had?

3. How often do these complications occur?

4. How are most of these injuries treated?

Accessory Soleus Muscle

1. Accessory soleus muscle.

2. Adolescent presents with a painless mass, soft tissue swelling, or claudication.

3. Fasciotomy.

4. Accessory flexor digitorum longus.

Reference

Yu JS, Resnick D: MR imaging of the accessory soleus muscle. *Skeletal Radiol* 23:525–528, 1994.

Cross-Reference

Musculoskeletal Imaging: THE REQUISITES, 3rd ed, p 267.

Comment

This patient has an accessory soleus muscle. At the level of the tibiotalar joint, only two muscles should be visualized, the flexor hallucis longus and peroneus brevis muscles. Posterior to these muscles is a large fat pad, called *Kager's pad*, which has the appearance of a large triangular radiolucency with the Achilles tendon marking its posterior border and the calcaneus marking its inferior border. When a soft tissue mass is detected in Kager's pad, you should consider the possibility of an anomalous muscle. An accessory soleus muscle is best depicted on magnetic resonance imaging. On sagittal images, it characteristically appears as a fusiform-shaped soft tissue mass demonstrating T1 and T2 values identical to those of normal muscle. On transaxial images, the muscle appears as a sharply marginated, ovoid mass seen at the level of the tibiotalar joint. This muscle is enveloped by its own fascia, deriving its blood supply from the posterior tibial artery and innervation from the posterior tibial nerve. It arises from either the anterior surface of the soleus muscle or from the soleal line of the tibia and fibula. It may insert into the Achilles tendon, the upper surface of the calcaneus, or the medial aspect of the calcaneus. Other commonly seen anomalous muscles in the posterior ankle include an accessory flexor digitorum longus and peroneus quartus muscles.

Notes

Posterior Sternoclavicular Joint Dislocation

1. Asymmetry of the height of the clavicular heads.

2. Laceration of the superior vena cava, thoracic outlet syndrome from venous compression, compression of the recurrent laryngeal nerve, rupture or compression of the trachea, pneumothorax, esophageal rupture, or injury to the subclavian or carotid artery.

3. In about 25% of posterior dislocations.

4. Conservatively.

References

Ferrera PC, Wheeling HM: Sternoclavicular joint injuries. *Am J Emerg Med* 18:58–61, 2000.

Habib PA, Huang GS, Mendiola JA, Yu JS: Anterior chest pain: Musculoskeletal considerations. *Emerg Radiol* 11:37–45, 2004.

Cross-Reference

Musculoskeletal Imaging: THE REQUISITES, 3rd ed, pp 75–76.

Comment

Sternoclavicular joint dislocations are rare injuries. Many dislocations of this joint are caused by an indirect force that is transmitted along the longitudinal axis of the clavicle while others are caused by massive direct trauma to the anterior surface of the chest. The diagnosis of a sternoclavicular joint dislocation is difficult radiographically. Detection requires asymmetry of the position of the medial ends of the clavicle on a frontal radiograph, yet the limitation of radiographs is that anterior and posterior subluxation is impossible to identify in many instances. The imaging modality of choice is computed tomography, which displays not only the direction of the dislocation and degree of displacement but also any potential complication to the adjacent structures, such as an injury to the great vessels.

The majority of complications associated with sternoclavicular dislocations occur with posterior dislocations. Approximately 25% of these dislocations are associated with a laceration of the superior vena cava, thoracic outlet syndrome from venous compression, compression of the recurrent laryngeal nerve, rupture or compression of the trachea, pneumothorax, esophageal rupture, or injury to the subclavian or carotid artery. Closed reduction and immobilization of the arm with a sling is the treatment of choice in the majority of situations.

Notes

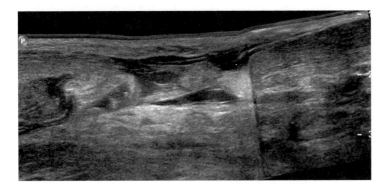

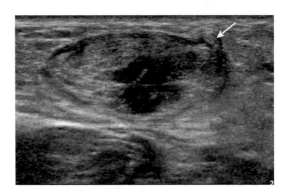

You are shown longitudinal (right side is distal) and transverse (right side is medial) sonograms of the Achilles tendon.

1. What is the diagnosis? Is this a common location?

2. What do the anechoic areas around the tendon represent? Acoustic shadowing may be indicative of what process?

3. What does the arrow show on the transverse image?

4. What is the Thompson test? How accurate is physical examination?

CASE 54

Achilles Tendon Rupture

1. Rupture of the Achilles tendon with retraction. Yes, most occur approximately 2 to 6 cm above the insertion.

2. Interposed hemorrhage. Sound-beam refraction at the frayed ends of a full thickness tear and occasionally calcification.

3. Plantaris tendon.

4. Squeezing the gastrocnemius muscle (patient in prone position) does not produce normal plantar flexion. Accuracy is 75%.

References

Fessel DP, van Holsbeeck MT: Ultrasound of the foot and ankle. *Semin Musculoskelet Radiol* 2:271–282, 1998.

Hartgerink P, Fessel DP, Jacobson JA, van Holsbeeck MT: Full- versus partial-thickness Achilles tendon tears: Sonographic accuracy and characterization in 26 cases with surgical correlation. *Radiology* 220: 406–412, 2001.

Cross-Reference

Musculoskeletal Imaging: THE REQUISITES, 3rd ed, pp 258–263.

Comment

The Achilles tendon is the largest tendon in the ankle, originating from the union of the gastrocnemius and soleus tendons and inserting on the posterior surface of the calcaneus. A rupture of this tendon is a severe injury, and is caused by indirect trauma related to strenuous tensile forces. The majority of injuries are "pushing off" injuries with the foot in plantar flexion and the knee in extension, although a fall on the forefoot causing forced dorsiflexion of the foot can also injure the tendon. When a rupture occurs spontaneously, it tends to affect middle-age people who have an underlying systemic disorder such as gout, chronic renal failure, diabetes mellitus, hyperparathyroidism, rheumatoid arthritis, and systemic lupus erythematosis. Patients present with acute onset pain, ankle swelling, and an inability to rise on their toes.

On sonography, a complete tear is depicted by disruption of all of the tendon fibers, commonly with distraction measuring 2 cm. Acoustic shadowing related to sound-beam refraction correlates with a full thickness tear, although it may occasionally be due to calcifications. Fat herniation into the defect is common, and in full tears, visualization of the plantaris tendon is fairly common as in this case. A partial tear or tendinosis is depicted by thickening of the tendon in the anteroposterior dimension, often greater than 10 mm. Abnormal echogenicity is often present. Sonography has a reported accuracy above 90%, with a sensitivity of 100% and a specificity of 83%.

Notes

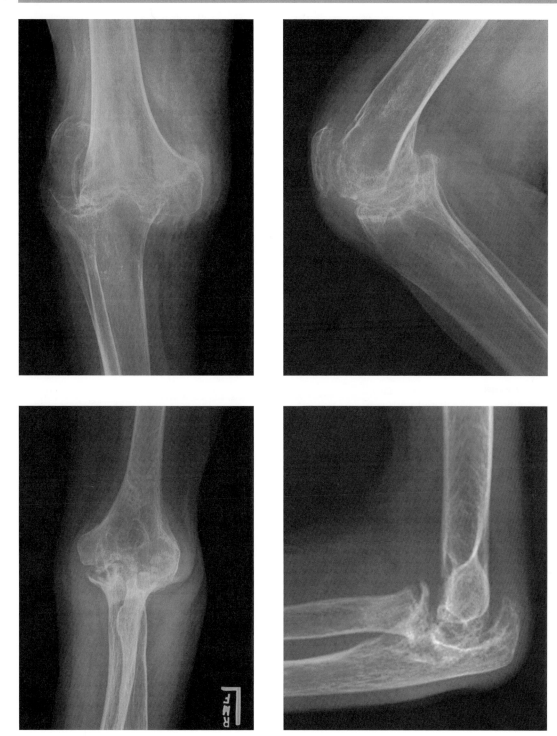

1. Does this patient have active disease? How do you know?

2. What is the differential diagnosis for para-articular soft tissue nodules/masses?

3. What conditions can produce marked asymmetric skeletal involvement in this disease process?

4. What is Felty's syndrome?

Rheumatoid Arthritis

1. Yes. Soft tissue swelling and effusions suggest active synovitis.

2. Rheumatoid arthritis, rheumatic fever, collagen-vascular diseases, sarcoidosis, Weber-Christian disease, gout, xanthomatosis, and infection.

3. Unilateral neurologic deficits such as hemiparalysis or marked asymmetric muscular weakness, which protect the ipsilateral side from the effects of rheumatoid arthritis.

4. Rheumatoid arthritis, splenomegaly, and leukopenia.

Reference

Britton CA, Wasko MC: Rheumatoid arthritis. *Semin Roentgenol* 31:198–207, 1996.

Cross-Reference

Musculoskeletal Imaging: THE REQUISITES, 3rd ed, pp 290–298.

Comment

The earliest pathologic abnormality of rheumatoid arthritis is acute synovitis, which is associated with synovial congestion and edema that cause hypertrophy and villous transformation of the synovium. Villous hypertrophy form papillary fronds measuring 1 to 2 mm, and this may be evident on magnetic resonance imaging. The irregularity of the synovial tissue is most prominent at the edges of the articular cartilage. Pannus and toxic debris in the synovial fluid cause cartilaginous and osseous destruction. Histologically, cellular infiltration occurring diffusely or in small nodular aggregates, called Allison-Ghormley nodules, may be evident in the superficial portion of the synovium.

The characteristic radiographic features of rheumatoid arthritis include soft tissue swelling, periarticular osteoporosis, early joint space narrowing, articular erosions, and marginal erosions caused by the extension of pannus into synovial pockets that expose regions that do not contain a protective cartilaginous layer (bare areas). An important observation in this patient is the lack of reactive bone changes despite marked joint narrowing. Although symmetry is the hallmark of rheumatoid arthritis, several exceptions are notable. Early in the disease process, involvement may be monoarticular or pauciarticular in 5% to 20% of patients. Stroke or other neurologic conditions that affect only one side of the body can cause asymmetric joint involvement. And remember, in larger joints, involvement occasionally is asymmetric as well.

Notes

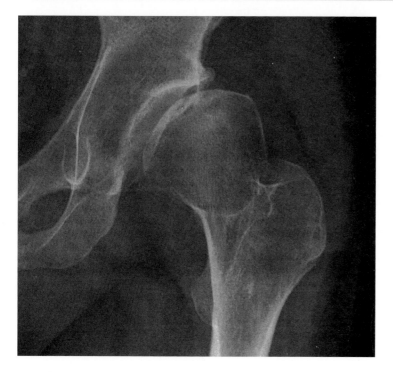

1. What does this patient have?
2. Why is the left side more frequently affected?
3. Explain why the changes in the acetabulum occur.
4. What is a "pulvinar"?

C A S E 5 6

Developmental Dysplasia of the Hip

1. Developmental dysplasia of the hip (DDH).

2. The fetal spine is usually to the maternal left in a fetal vertex presentation and the left knee is constricted.

3. Ligamentous laxity allows extra mobility of the femoral head. The acetabulum compensates by becoming wider and shallower, which then allows more head mobility.

4. The fibrofatty tissue that accumulates to fill in the acetabulum in DDH.

References

Broughton NS, Brougham DI, Cole WG, Menelaus MB: Reliability of radiological measurements in the assessment of the child's hip. *J Bone Joint Surg* 71-B:6–8, 1989.

Harcke HT: Screening newborns for developmental dysplasia of the hip: The role of sonography. *AJR Am J Roentgenol* 162:395–397, 1994.

Cross-Reference

Musculoskeletal Imaging: THE REQUISITES, 3rd ed, pp 597–606.

Comment

Developmental dysplasia of the hip (DDH), also known as congenital hip dysplasia or dislocation, represents a spectrum of congenital hip conditions that have in common the potential for development of acetabular dysplasia in infancy and childhood. It can occur in association with other congenital defects, such as Chiari II malformation, or in isolation owing to severe hip laxity. It has an incidence of 1 per 1000 live births and is six times more prevalent in girls. When intermittent hip dislocations occur they are easily reduced. This disease is progressive and may lead to osteoarthritis.

Ultrasonography is the modality of choice in neonates since it allows visualization of the cartilaginous femoral head and unossified acetabulum. The osseous portion of the superior acetabulum should cover at least half of the cartilaginous femoral head. The alpha angle should be less than 60 degrees. Radiography is useful in infants older than 3 months and the preferred modality after 6 months. The ossification center of the femoral head should lie inferior to Hilgenreiner's line and medial to Perkin's line. The acetabular index should be less than 30 degrees. In older children, sequential measurements are more reliable than a single evaluation and the most helpful measurements include the acetabular index, center-edge angle, and the c/b ratio. Magnetic resonance imaging is useful as it depicts the femoral head and acetabular cartilage, and potential soft tissue impediments such as pulvinar, inverted limbus, tight psoas tendon, and redundant ligamentum teres.

Notes

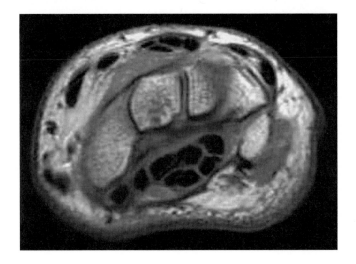 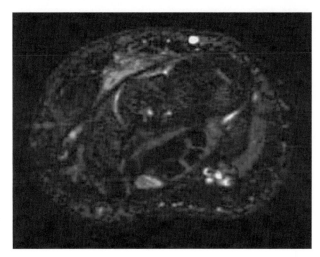

1. List the clinical manifestations of this condition.

2. What is a positive Tinel's sign? What is a Phalen's test?

3. List some magnetic resonance imaging findings.

4. Which observation on magnetic resonance imaging is most specific?

Carpal Tunnel Syndrome

1. Noctural hand discomfort, paresthesia in the thumb and second, third, and radial side of the fourth fingers, and weakness and atrophy of the thenar musculature.

2. Tingling in the digits supplied by the median nerve. Flex both wrists for 60 seconds—numbness in the median nerve distribution should occur within 60 seconds in the presence of carpal tunnel syndrome.

3. Compression, diffuse flattening, or an abrupt change in the morphology of the median nerve, edema of the nerve, or enhancement with gadolinium administration.

4. Abrupt change in morphology.

References

Andreisek G, Crook DW, Burg D, et al: Peripheral neuropathies of the median, radial, and ulnar nerves: MR imaging features. *Radiographics* 26:1267–1287, 2006.
Yu JS: Magnetic resonance imaging of the wrist. *Orthopedics* 17:1041–1048, 1994.

Cross-Reference

Musculoskeletal Imaging: THE REQUISITES, 3rd ed, p 157.

Comment

Carpal tunnel syndrome is a common neuropathy of the upper extremity caused by compression of the median nerve in the carpal tunnel. It typically involves middle-age women and presents as a bilateral condition in nearly one half of those affected. Several common causes of carpal tunnel syndrome include tenosynovitis, masses (ganglion or neuroma), synovial proliferation, and diminished girth of the carpal channel from post-traumatic osseous changes and fibrosis. Chronic hypoxia has also been suggested as a potential precipitating event. Most cases of carpal tunnel syndrome, however, are idiopathic and are likely the result of a normal aging process. Magnetic resonance imaging is useful for confirming the diagnosis of carpal tunnel syndrome in patients exhibiting symptoms. Characteristic findings are depicted on true transaxial images of the wrist. Observations diagnostic of this condition include compression and flattening of the median nerve, increased signal intensity in the median nerve on T2W images (as seen in this patient), bowing of the flexor retinaculum, loss of the normal fat between the carpal bones and the tendons, and/or an abrupt change of the diameter of the median nerve.

Notes

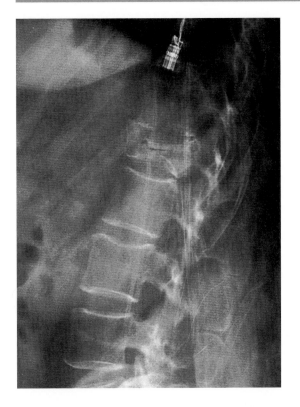

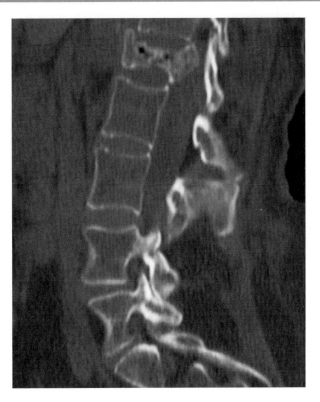

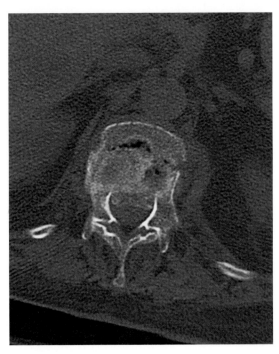

1. What is the main finding?

2. What does this mean and is it benign or aggressive?

3. What is the likelihood of a gas-forming infection?

4. What must be seen on magnetic resonance imaging to make this diagnosis?

Kummell's Disease

1. A vacuum phenomenon in a vertebral cleft.

2. It indicates avascular necrosis of L1; benign.

3. None.

4. Either low signal intensity gas on all pulse sequences or the "double-line" sign.

References

Bhalla S, Reinus WR: The linear intravertebral vacuum: A sign of benign vertebral collapse. *AJR Am J Roentgenol* 170:1563–1569, 1998.

Naul LG, Peet GJ, Maupin WB: Avascular necrosis of the vertebral body: MR imaging. *Radiology* 172:219–222, 1989.

Cross-Reference

Musculoskeletal Imaging: THE REQUISITES, 3rd ed, pp 349 and 352.

Comment

Kummell's disease is an uncommon spinal disorder characterized by avascular necrosis of a vertebral body, typically occurring in a delayed fashion after minor trauma. The initial force must be sufficient to cause trabecular or endplate injury but is not detected. The interaction between vertebral microtrauma and processes that interfere with osseous repair predispose to this disorder. The radiographic imaging of avascular necrosis of the spine is nonspecific. The vertebral body appears diminished in height, may be increased in density, and contains gas within the body. The gas is believed to represent a vacuum phenomenon, similar to gas in healthy joints, which fill in low pressure intravertebral clefts. On magnetic resonance imaging, the gaseous space is very low in signal intensity on all pulse sequences, but may eventually fill with fluid or granulation tissue. A "double-line" sign may be present on T2W images. Many patients who develop Kummell's disease have received corticosteroid therapy; however, alcoholism, radiation therapy, and other typical etiologies of osteonecrosis are also major considerations. The observation of intravertebral vacuum clefts excludes acute fracture, infection, or a neoplastic process.

Notes

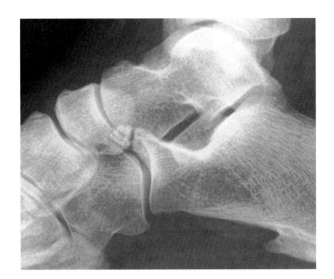

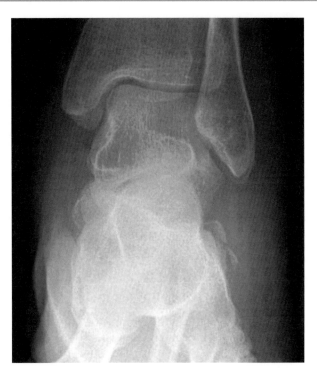

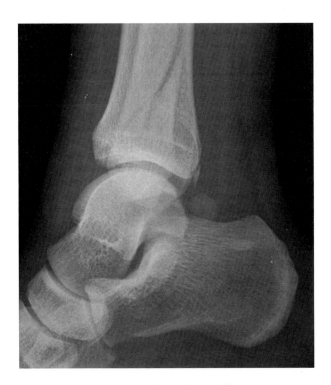

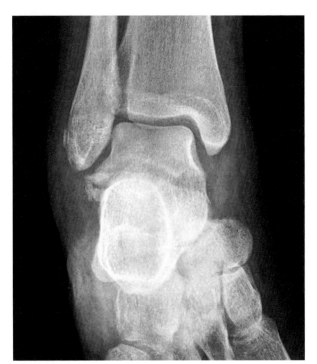

You are shown images from four different patients.

1. This patient has ankle pain. What is the injury?
2. This patient has ankle pain. What is the injury?
3. This patient has ankle pain. What is the injury?
4. This patient has ankle pain. What is the injury?

Subtle Ankle Fractures

1. Fracture of the anterior calcaneal process.

2. Avulsion fracture of the calcaneus at the attachment of the extensor digitorum brevis muscle.

3. Posterior tibial malleolus fracture. (Did you notice the fibular fracture also?)

4. Fracture of the lateral talus process.

Reference

Long D, Yu JS, Vitellas K: The ankle joint: Imaging strategies in the evaluation of ligamentous injuries. *Crit Rev Diagn Imagin* 39:393–445, 1998.

Cross-Reference

Musculoskeletal Imaging: THE REQUISITES, 3rd ed, pp 252–258.

Comment

Ankle sprains are one of the most common injuries seen in emergency departments. As many as 37 per 1000 people seek emergent medical care for this injury. Twenty-five percent of all athletic injuries are related to the ankle joint, although these figures do not reflect the true incidence of ankle sprains since many injuries are never brought to medical attention. When presented with a patient who has sustained an ankle injury, it is important to establish the correct diagnosis. The management may be conservative or surgical, but it relies on the accuracy of the initial diagnosis and precise identification of the severity of the injury. About 98% of ankle fractures occur in these seven locations, so you should look carefully at these areas in the ankle in every radiographic study, regardless of the mechanism of injury. Some are more difficult to detect unless you carefully inspect the films. They include: (1) medial and lateral malleolus, (2) posterior tibial malleolus, (3) talar dome, (4) fifth metatarsal base, (5) anterior calcaneal process, (6) lateral talar process, and (7) the lateral calcaneus at the attachment of the extensor digitorum brevis muscle. Remember to use soft tissue swelling as an indicator of fracture location.

Notes

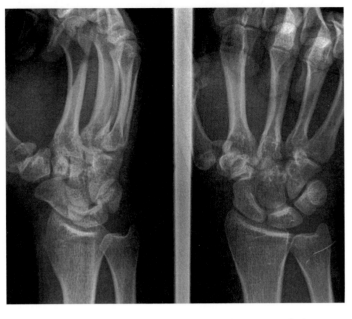 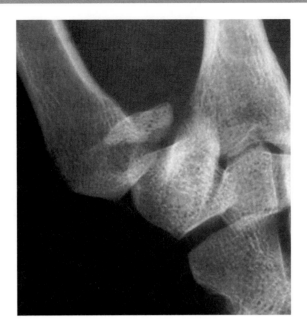

1. What is the diagnosis and what would you include in your final report?

2. What is the treatment of choice? Why?

3. What makes this fracture unstable?

4. What structure stabilizes the triangular fragment of bone that is not displaced?

Bennett Fracture

1. Bennett fracture. Identify the number of fragments, metacarpal bone displacement, size and position of the volar fragment, and fracture gaps that exceed 3 mm.

2. Surgery. Marked displacement of fracture fragments and angular deformity of articular surface.

3. Action of the abductor pollicis longus muscle produces distraction, but the pull of the adductor pollicis longus and flexor pollicis brevis, by their more distal attachment, augments the displacement.

4. Deep anterior oblique ligament, also known as the volar beak ligament.

References

Breen TF, Gelberman RH, Jupiter JB: Intra-articular fractures of the basilar joint of the thumb. *Hand Clin* 4:491–501, 1988.

Peterson JJ, Bancroft LW: Injuries of the fingers and thumb in the athlete. *Clin Sports Med* 25:527–542, 2006.

Cross-Reference

Musculoskeletal Imaging: THE REQUISITES, 3rd ed, pp 159–160.

Comment

Fractures of the first metacarpal bone are the second most frequently fractured metacarpal bone after the fifth metacarpal. Nearly 80% of fractures of this bone involve the base. Basilar fractures can be divided into four types: epibasal, Bennett, Rolando, and comminuted. Epibasal fractures are extra-articular fractures through the first metacarpal base and can be transversely or obliquely oriented. Comminuted fractures result in numerous bone fragments and frequently have more than one intra-articular fracture extension. A Bennett fracture is defined as an intra-articular two-part fracture of the base of the first metacarpal. It is the most common thumb fracture, accounting for about one third of all fractures of the first metacarpal bone. A Rolando fracture is a similar fracture but it produces a three-part fracture. When evaluating radiographs of the first metacarpal, recall the anatomy of the first carpometacarpal joint. The deep anterior oblique ligament, which is intracapsular in location, is the most important stabilizer of this joint. It inserts on the ulnar articular margin of the medial volar beak of the first metacarpal base. When a Bennett or Rolando fracture occurs, the medial volar beak remains attached to this ligament while the rest of the metacarpal base becomes displaced radially due to the pull of the abductor pollicis longus muscle.

Notes

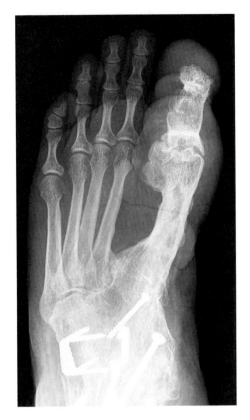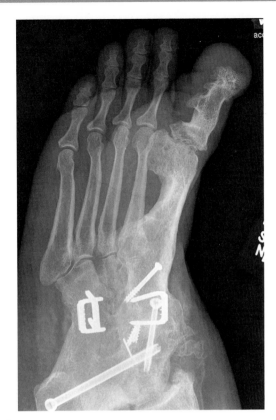

1. What is the most likely cause of the deformity that you see?

2. When does it become clinically evident?

3. Is the trabecular architecture normal?

4. When the upper extremity is involved, what is the most frequent distribution?

C A S E 6 1

Macrodystrophia Lipomatosa

1. Macrodystrophia lipomatosa. Vascular lesions, Klippel-Trenaunay-Weber syndrome, and neurofibromatosis can also cause localized gigantism.

2. Most are obvious by childhood.

3. Yes.

4. Distribution of the median nerve.

References

Goldman AB, Kaye JJ: Macrodystrophia lipomatosa: Radiographic diagnosis. *AJR Am J Roentgenol* 128: 101–105, 1977.

Gupta SK, Sharma OP, Sharma SV, et al: Macrodystrophia lipomatosa: Radiographic observations. *Br J Radiol* 65:769–773, 1992.

Cross-Reference

Musculoskeletal Imaging: THE REQUISITES, 3rd ed, pp 475 and 480.

Comment

Macrodystrophia lipomatosa is a rare, localized form of gigantism with overgrowth of fibroadipose tissue and associated increased blood flow resulting in enlargement of the bones and soft tissues usually in the hand or foot. Radiographically, it appears as hypertrophy of the osseous structures and soft tissue elements of the affected digit, with lucencies in the soft tissues characteristic of fat. The osseous enlargement is in both length and transverse diameter but the trabecular pattern is usually normal. Slanting of the articular surfaces of joints is common. Pathologically, there is proliferation of all mesenchymal components with disproportionate increase in adipose tissue. The disorder becomes evident in childhood although it may be recognized at birth or in the neonatal period. The most frequent distribution in the upper extremity follows the distribution of the median nerve and the plantar nerves in the lower extremity. As the patient grows, the deformity begins to mechanically interfere with joint function, vascular supply, and innervation. Other features of this disorder include early maturation of the growth plates, syndactyly, brachydactyly, and symphalangism.

Notes

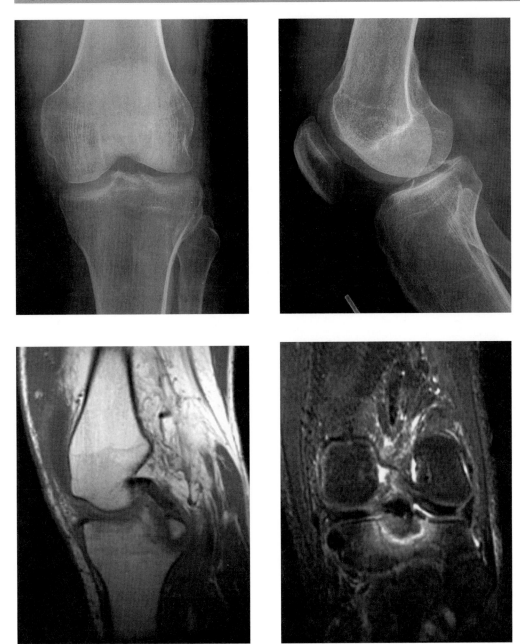

1. How would you classify the injury, low or high velocity?
2. What was the likely mechanism of injury?
3. Where do ruptures of this ligament commonly occur?
4. What two structures may be found adjacent to this ligament?

Posterior Cruciate Ligament Osseous Avulsion

1. Osseous avulsions of the cruciate ligaments are considered high velocity injuries.

2. Dashboard injury, direct impaction on the anterior tibia with the knee flexed.

3. Occurrence: 50% to 75% midsubstance, 30% to 35% femur avulsion, and 20% to 30% tibia avulsion.

4. The meniscofemoral ligaments of Humphrey (anterior) and Wrisberg (posterior).

References

Griffith JF, Antonio GE, Tong CW, Ming CK: Cruciate ligament avulsion fractures. *Arthroscopy* 20:803–812, 2004.

Grover JS, Bassett LW, Gross ML, et al: Posterior cruciate ligament: MR imaging. *Radiology* 174:527–530, 1990.

Cross-Reference

Musculoskeletal Imaging: THE REQUISITES, 3rd ed, pp 237–239.

Comment

The posterior cruciate ligament (PCL) is the primary stabilizer of the knee joint against posterior translation of the tibia or excessive external rotation of the femur. It attaches proximally to the lateral aspect of the medial femoral condyle and courses in a posterior direction to attach distally in the posterior tibia near its cortex. It comprises two paired bands: the anterolateral bands that tighten when the knee flexes and the posteromedial bands that tighten when the knee extends. On magnetic resonance imaging, the appearance of the PCL is a tubular arc of uniform low signal intensity with a cross-sectional diameter measuring 1 cm. When examining the PCL, one must scrutinize both the morphology and signal intensity of this ligament as well as its point of attachments. Acute tears may either disrupt the morphology, resulting in surface irregularities, gaps with frayed ends, focal thickening or attenuation, or avulse a piece of its bony attachment. Acutely, the change in morphology is associated with interstitial edema and hemorrhage, seen as areas of high signal intensity on T2W images, and occasionally marrow edema when the bone attachment has been avulsed. Radiographically, this injury is extremely difficult to visualize due to overlapping osseous structures but you should always look for it when there is a traumatic effusion.

Notes

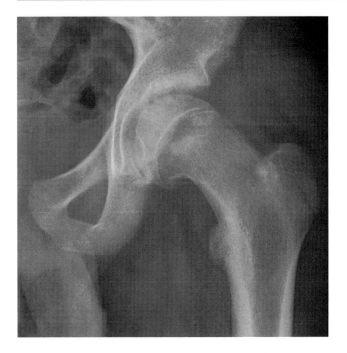 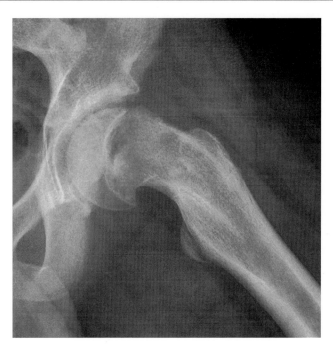

1. What is your diagnosis?

2. What are key factors that allow this condition to develop?

3. Although the etiology is unknown, what are several predisposing conditions?

4. What is the aim of treatment? What is considered the treatment of choice?

Slipped Capital Femoral Epiphysis

1. Slipped capital femoral epiphysis (SCFE) of the left hip.

2. Between the ages of 10 and 16 years, the skeleton undergoes rapid development, muscle strength increases, and the femoral neck develops greater varus.

3. Trauma, obesity, hormonal abnormalities such as hypothyroidism, rapid growth spurts, renal osteodystrophy, and poor nutrition.

4. Restoring fusion of the growth plate. Pinning the epiphysis with minimal reduction.

Reference

Reynolds RA: Diagnosis and treatment of slipped capital femoral epiphysis. *Curr Opin Pediatr* 11:80–83, 1999.

Cross-Reference

Musculoskeletal Imaging: THE REQUISITES, 3rd ed, pp 200–201.

Comment

SCFE is a childhood disorder of the hip characterized by posterior and inferior displacement of the proximal femoral epiphysis. It is usually a unilateral process, although 20% to 30% of cases are bilateral. Histologically, the abnormality occurs through the zone of hypertrophy in the growth plate. Clinically, patients present with poorly localized pain and a limp. The key to making the diagnosis is having both anteroposterior and frog-leg lateral radiographs available. A line drawn tangent to the lateral femoral neck cortex should intersect the femoral epiphysis laterally. This patient demonstrates classic findings. The cartilagenous growth plate is widened and there is irregularity and rarefaction of the metaphysis. Close scrutiny of the frog-leg lateral projection reveals posterior slippage of the epiphysis. As slippage progressed, the femoral epiphysis displaced medially, concomitantly widening the growth plate. SCFE may be classified according to the duration of symptoms or the degree of slippage. Patients are considered to have acute slips when symptoms have been present for less than 3 weeks. When symptoms last more than 3 weeks, it indicates a more chronic condition, associated with the development of characteristic radiographic abnormalities. The most severe consequence of SCFE is chondrolysis caused by pannus-like granulation tissue that erodes the articular cartilage. This complication predisposes the patient to secondary osteoarthritis.

Notes

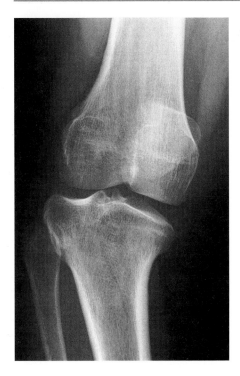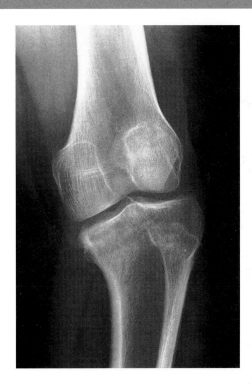

1. You are shown bilateral knee radiographs. What is the disorder and what is the most common type?

2. Which type is bilateral?

3. Which type causes pain?

4. Which type is characterized by a large bony outgrowth from the medial metaphysis?

Blount's Disease

1. Adolescent type of Blount's disease; infantile type is more common than adolescent.

2. Infantile in 50% to 75% of cases. Adolescent type is bilateral in 10% of cases.

3. Adolescent type.

4. Infantile type.

Reference

Cheema JI, Grissom LE, Harcke HT: Radiographic characteristics of lower-extremity bowing in children. *Radiographics* 23:871–880, 2003.

Cross-Reference

Musculoskeletal Imaging: THE REQUISITES, 3rd ed, p 357.

Comment

Blount's disease, also known as tibia vara, is the result of an insult to the growth of the medial aspect of the proximal tibial epiphysis either from trauma or dysplasia. Two types are well known: an infantile type with deformity occurring in the first few years of life, and an adolescent type in which the deformity occurs in children between the ages of 8 and 15 years. The infantile type is eight times more common. The infantile type is bilateral in 50% to 75% of cases, and patients tend to be obese and early walkers. There is no sexual predilection. The disorder does not cause pain and is characterized by increasing deformity and shortening of the leg. The classic radiographic presentation is varus deformity of the tibia owing to the angulation of the metaphysis and the tibial shaft is adducted without intrinsic curvature. A depressed medial tibial metaphysis with an osseous excrescence is seen. The adolescent variety is unilateral in over 90% of cases, does cause pain, and produces less pronounced deformity. It is likely post-traumatic resulting in growth arrest of the tibia. Sclerosis in the growth plate of the medial tibial metaphysis is common.

Notes

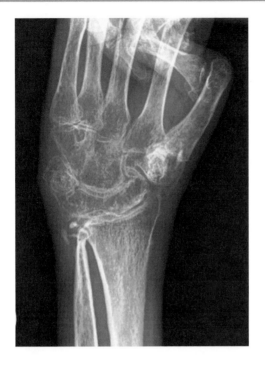
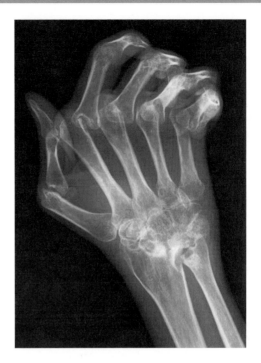
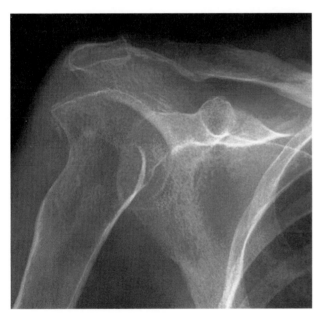
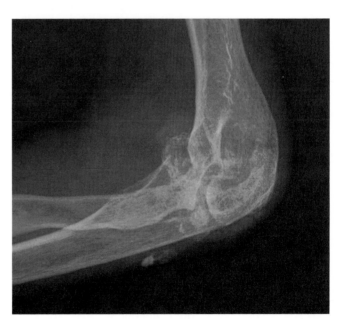

1. What is the most likely diagnosis?
2. What is distinctive about the hands?
3. What is CREST syndrome?
4. List the target organs in patients with this disease.

Scleroderma

1. Scleroderma.

2. Resorption of bone in both first carpometacarpal joints and joint erosions associated with capsular and subcutaneous calcifications.

3. Calcinosis, Raynaud's phenomenon, esophageal abnormalities, sclerodactyly, and telangiectasia.

4. The skin, gastrointestinal tract, lungs, kidneys, heart, and structures of the musculoskeletal system.

References

Gold RH, Bassett LW, Seeger LL: The other arthritides: Roentgenologic features of osteoarthritis, erosive osteoarthritis, ankylosing spondylitis, psoriatic arthritis, Reiter's disease, multicentric reticulohistiocytosis, and progressive systemic sclerosis. *Radiol Clin North Am* 26:1195–1212, 1988.

Hanlon R, King S: Overview of the radiology of connective tissue disorders in children. *Eur J Radiol* 33:74–84, 2000.

Cross-Reference

Musculoskeletal Imaging: THE REQUISITES, 3rd ed, pp 329–331.

Comment

Scleroderma is an autoimmune disorder of unknown etiology that is characterized by small vessel disease and fibrosis in several organ systems. It has a female predominance by a ratio of 3:1. The disorder becomes clinically evident by the third to fifth decades of life but it can present in children. A common presentation is Raynaud's phenomenon but other early manifestations include thickening of the skin and edema of the extremities. Pain and stiffness involving the small joints of the hands and knees, and dysphagia also are typical presenting complaints. With progression of the disease, skin changes in the fingers, face, and feet become predominant features appearing taut, shiny, and atrophic. The soft tissues of the distal fingers become tapered, and ulcerated subcutaneous calcific deposits develop in more extensive disease.

Radiographically, abnormalities of the hands are characterized by resorption of the soft tissues often producing a conical shape to the ends of the digits and acro-osteolysis. About 25% of patients exhibit calcifications, occurring in the subcutaneous tissues or in the joint capsule. Erosions similar to those in rheumatoid arthritis are common and may occur in 40% to 80% of patients affected. A distinctive feature of these erosions is their predilection for the interphalangeal joints.

Severe resorption of the first carpometacarpal joint with radial subluxation of the first metacarpal bone is nearly pathognomonic of scleroderma.

Notes

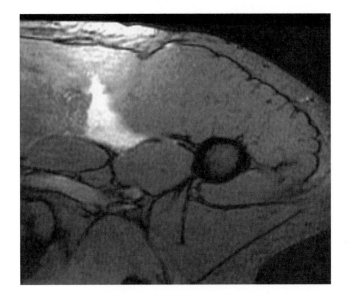
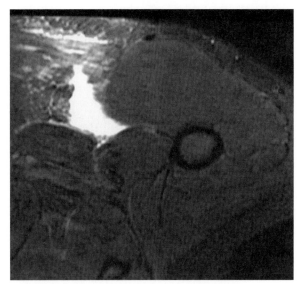
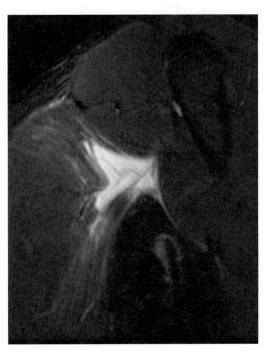
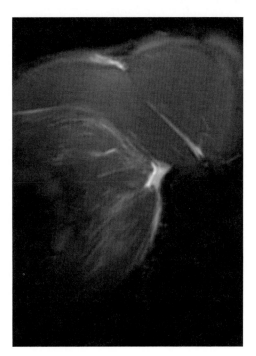

1. What are the diagnosis and pertinent findings?

2. Where is the point of failure?

3. How did this injury most likely occur?

4. What determines the treatment of choice?

Pectoralis Major Muscle Tear

1. There is a tear of the pectoralis major muscle with retraction of the muscle, interstitial edema, and early formation of a hematoma.

2. At the myotendinous junction. Note that on the gradient echo axial image, the tendon is still attached to the humerus.

3. The patient is a weightlifter and was in the act of benching 600 pounds.

4. The location of the tear.

Reference

Yu JS, Habib PA: Common injuries related to weightlifting: MR imaging perspective. *Semin Musculoskelet Radiol* 9:289–301, 2005.

Cross-Reference

Musculoskeletal Imaging: THE REQUISITES, 3rd ed, pp 68-70.

Comment

This case is straightforward. The most important aspect of this case is identifying the location of the tear. Failure of the pectoralis muscle can occur in the muscle, at the myotendinous junction, or in the tendinous insertion. A rupture of the pectoralis muscle is a well-known injury among weightlifters. The pectoralis major muscle is fan-shaped with two origins, from the medial two thirds of the clavicle and from the anterior surface of the manubrium and sternal body. These muscle fibers converge just proximal to its insertion of the lateral lip of the bicipital groove of the humerus. Magnetic resonance imaging is useful in determining the location and extent of the injury. The location of a tear dictates whether surgery should be performed. Tendon avulsion from the humerus is generally surgically repaired, whereas muscle or myotendinous junction tears are treated conservatively. The majority of tears are partial tears at the myotendinous junction, whereas complete tears involving the insertion occur 20% of the time. In acute tendinous avulsions, retraction of the muscle can retract as much as 13 cm.

Notes

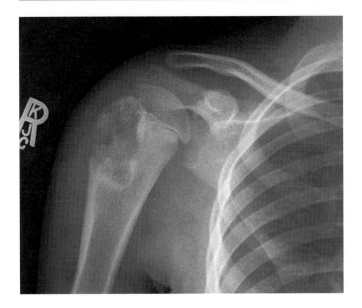 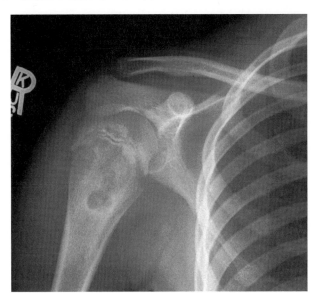

1. What is the most likely diagnosis? Is it benign or malignant?

2. Is matrix calcification a common finding?

3. Histologically, are hemorrhagic cysts associated with this lesion?

4. What is a characteristic observation on magnetic resonance imaging?

Chondroblastoma

1. A chondroblastoma. Benign.

2. Yes, it may be seen in 30% to 50% of cases.

3. Yes, it may even resemble an aneurysmal bone cyst in 10% of cases.

4. Identification of peritumoral edema is very common owing to the hypervascularity associated with this lesion.

Reference

Weatherall PT, Maale GE, Mendelsohn DB, et al: Chondroblastoma: Classic and confusing appearance at MR imaging. *Radiology* 190:467–474, 1994.

Cross-Reference

Musculoskeletal Imaging: THE REQUISITES, 3rd ed, pp 452–455.

Comment

Chondroblastoma is a benign tumor of bone characterized by chondroblasts and multinucleated giant cells. Nearly 90% of patients present between the ages of 5 and 25 years, and there is a twofold male predilection. The most common complaint is pain referring to a joint. Tenderness, swelling, decreased range of motion, numbness, muscle atrophy, and weakness may be discovered on physical inspection. The femur (33%), humerus (20%), and tibia (20%) are preferred sites of involvement although about 10% of chondroblastomas occur in the bones of the hands and feet, especially in the talus and calcaneus. The radiographic hallmark of this tumor is a well-defined osteolytic lesion that is centrally or eccentrically located within the epiphysis or apophysis of a bone. Remember that the tuberosities of the humerus are apophyseal regions. A thin sclerotic rim surrounds the lesion separating it from the normal marrow. Calcifications may be evident in 30% to 50% of cases. Periostitis is notable in one third of all cases. Aggressive features, such as joint invasion and extension into the adjacent soft tissue and bones and marked enhancement, are not uncommon. The differential diagnosis includes infection and eosinophilic granuloma although these lesions have their epicenters in the metaphysis of the bone. A giant cell tumor generally occurs in the epiphysis of a bone, but lacks matrix calcification or a sclerotic rim.

Notes

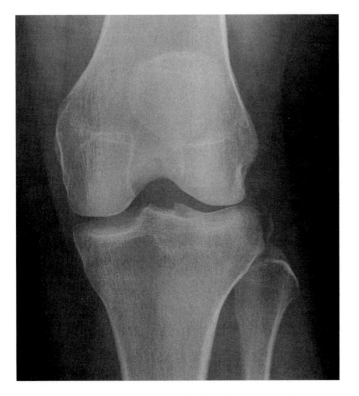
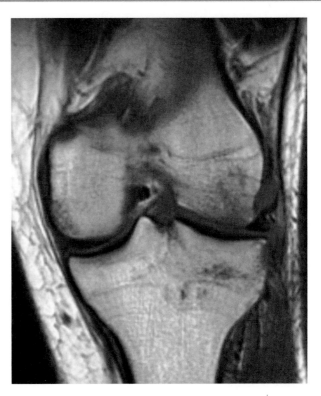

1. What is your diagnosis and what does it imply?

2. What structures are involved in this injury?

3. Marrow edema in the medial femoral condyle and posteromedial tibia suggest what mechanism of injury?

4. What injuries would you expect to find on a magnetic resonance imaging examination?

Segond Fracture

1. Segond fracture; an anterior cruciate ligament tear.

2. Iliotibial band and the anterior oblique band of the fibulocollateral ligament. The lateral capsular ligament is no longer considered the primary structure responsible for this injury.

3. Internal rotation of the femur on a fixed tibia with varus angulation.

4. Injuries to the anterior cruciate ligament (80% to 100%), medial collateral ligament (80% to 90%), meniscus (50%), and articular cartilage (25%).

References

Campos JC, Chung CB, Lektrakul N, et al: Pathogenesis of the Segond fracture: Anatomic and MR imaging evidence of an iliotibial tract or anterior oblique band avulsion. *Radiology* 219:381–386, 2001.

Dietz GW, Wilcox DM, Montgomery JB: Segond tibial condyle fracture: Lateral capsular ligament avulsion. *Radiology* 159:467–469, 1986.

Cross-Reference

Musculoskeletal Imaging: THE REQUISITES, 3rd ed, pp 217–220.

Comment

This lesion was initially described in 1879 when Segond demonstrated that internal rotation of the tibia with the knee in flexion resulted in tension of the lateral joint capsule. When the tension exceeded the strength of the bone, a small avulsion fracture occurred in the lateral tibia about 4 mm distal to the lateral joint line. Radiographically, the abnormality ranges from a small vertical sliver of bone to a sizeable bone fragment. The importance of this fracture is that it has a strong association with a rupture of the anterior cruciate ligament. The Segond fracture can sometimes be mistaken for other injuries in the lateral aspect of the knee because this fracture is not apparent on lateral radiographs. An avulsion of the lateral collateral ligament may simulate a Segond fracture but the bone fragment tends to be displaced more proximally and posteriorly than the Segond fracture. You should look for a concomitant abnormality in the fibular head when you suspect this injury. Recent studies suggest that an avulsion of the iliotibial band or oblique band of the lateral collateral ligament constitutes the true source of the Segond injury.

Notes

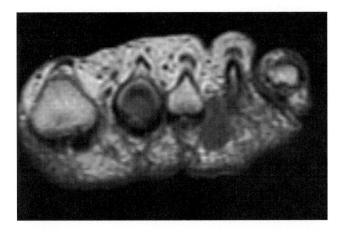

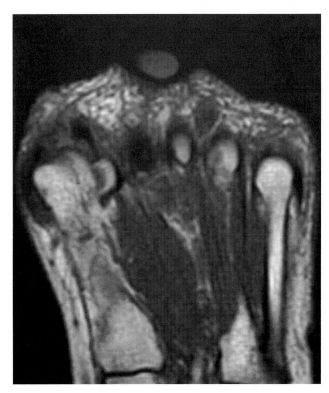

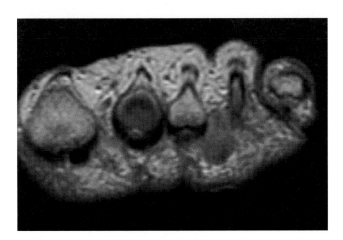

1. What is the diagnosis?

2. What are some contributing factors that allow this lesion to develop?

3. Is there a critical size for the lesion to be considered symptomatic?

4. Is this lesion vascular?

Morton's Neuroma

1. Morton's neuroma.

2. Excessive motion of the third and fourth metatarsal heads, rigid intermetatarsal ligament, and increased stress on the nerve.

3. Yes, some believe that the transverse diameter should be at least 5 mm.

4. Yes, that is why it enhances intensely on contrast-enhanced magnetic resonance imaging.

References

Ashman CJ, Klecker RJ, Yu JS: Forefoot pain involving the metatarsal region: Differential diagnosis with MR imaging. *Radiographics* 21:1425–1440, 2001.

Yu JS, Tanner JR: Considerations in metatarsalgia and midfoot pain: An MR imaging perspective. *Semin Musculoskelet Radiol* 6:91–104, 2002.

Cross-Reference

Musculoskeletal Imaging: THE REQUISITES, 3rd ed, pp 502–505.

Comment

A Morton's neuroma, a neuroma of the interdigital nerve, is one of the most common nerve problems affecting the foot. It is a mechanically induced degenerative neuropathy, which has a strong predilection for the third common digital nerve. It is particularly common in middle-aged women. The excessive motion between the third and fourth metatarsal heads flanking the third common digital nerve, the stout third transverse intermetatarsal ligament overlying this nerve, and excessive weight-bearing stress on the foot, such as occurs with wearing pointed and high-heeled shoes, collectively produce microdamage to the third common digital nerve. If allowed to continue for a long period of time, this can lead to nerve fiber degeneration and excessive intraneural and juxtaneural reparative fibrous tissue formation resulting in a masslike enlargement of the nerve. Such enlargement can then create further trauma and increased symptoms. Sonography and magnetic resonance imaging (MRI) are able to demonstrate the lesion, but MRI has the added advantage of excluding other causes of metatarsalgia, such as stress fractures. This patient shows the classic finding of a teardrop-shaped mass between the metatarsal head depicting isointense signal intensity to muscle on T1W images, and enhancement after administration of intravenous gadolinium solution (lower left image). Surgical resection is advocated when conservative measures fail.

Notes

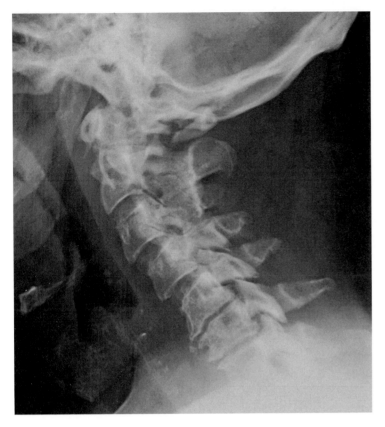

1. What is the cause of this patient's acute symptoms?

2. Is it stable?

3. Are these frequently bilateral or unilateral?

4. What is causing the distraction and angulation?

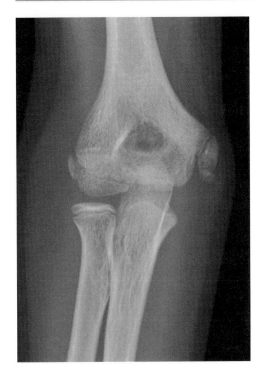 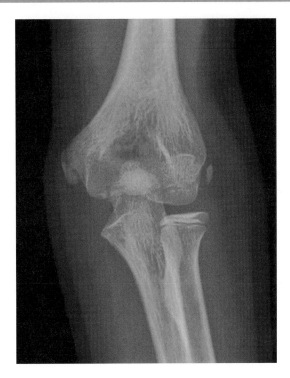

1. You are shown bilateral radiographs of the elbow in a patient with right elbow pain. What is the diagnosis?

2. What is the mechanism of injury?

3. What fractures are commonly associated with elbow dislocations? How often do they occur?

4. In the pediatric patient, what can happen if the elbow dislocates? What is the most serious complication?

Medial Epicondyle Apophysitis

1. Medial epicondyle apophysitis (little leaguer's elbow).

2. Repeated valgus stress on the elbow. He is probably a throwing athlete.

3. Fractures of the coronoid process, humeral epicondyles, and radial head. Twenty-five percent of cases.

4. Avulsion of the medial epicondylar ossification center. Entrapment in the joint.

References

Adirim TA, Cheng TL: Overview of injuries in the young athlete. *Sports Med* 33:75–81, 2003.

Cassas KJ, Cassettari-Wayhs A: Childhood and adolescent sports-related overuse injuries. *Am Fam Physician* 73:1014–1022, 2006.

Cross-Reference

Musculoskeletal Imaging: THE REQUISITES, 3rd ed, pp 118–121.

Comment

The elbow is a commonly traumatized joint in skeletally immature athletes. Medial epicondyle avulsion and apophysitis are common disorders in throwing athletes. For instance, more than half of adolescent baseball pitchers experience some type of elbow injury during a season. The medial apophyseal plate is biomechanically weaker than the anterior band of the ulnar collateral ligament and is susceptible to injury when a valgus force generated during throwing overwhelms the growth plate. Additionally, the flexor pronator group of muscles exerts traction on the weak physeal plate during the act of throwing. This combination is termed *little leaguer's elbow*. Radiographically, there may be fragmentation of the medial epicondylar apophysis and medial displacement/avulsion of the ossification center. An avulsed medial epicondylar ossification center may become entrapped into the joint or cause ulnar nerve damage. On magnetic resonance imaging, high signal intensity may be seen on T2W images in the marrow of the medial epicondyle secondary to edema. There may be overgrowth of the medial apophysis as seen in this patient. Treatment is typically conservative with immobilization and rest, but occasionally internal reduction and fixation may be required.

Notes

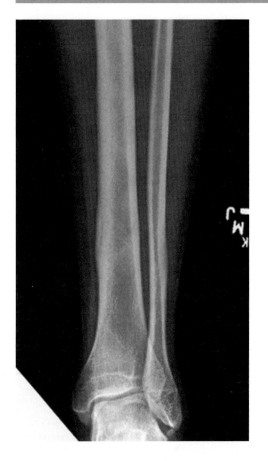
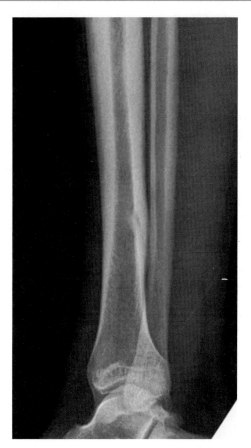
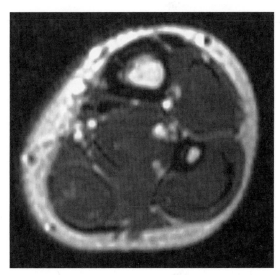

1. What is the diagnosis?

2. In the absence of lucency, what would be the differential diagnosis?

3. What do you expect to find on bone scintigraphy?

4. What is the typical appearance on computed tomography?

Longitudinal Tibial Stress Fracture

1. Longitudinal stress fracture of the tibia.

2. Cortical metastasis, osteoid osteoma, round cell tumor, osteomyelitis, prior fracture, and stress fracture.

3. A focal area of increased radionuclide uptake.

4. A linear lucency in the cortex associated with periosteal and endosteal callus.

References

Allen GJ: Longitudinal stress fractures of the tibia: Diagnosis with CT. *Radiology* 167:799–801, 1988.

Umans HR, Kaye JJ: Longitudinal stress fractures of the tibia: Diagnosis by magnetic resonance imaging. *Skeletal Radiol* 25:319–324, 1996.

Cross-Reference

Musculoskeletal Imaging: THE REQUISITES, 3rd ed, pp 12-14.

Comment

Exercise-induced stress reactions and stress fractures involving the tibia are common and may account for up to 75% of exertional leg pain and stress fractures. Detection is important to prevent complications and to lead to early recovery. The pathogenesis of stress fracture is not well understood but there is stimulation of bone remodeling, initially beginning with increased osteoclastic bone resorption. As the stimulus persists, an imbalance between bone resorption and bone replacement leads to weakening of the bone. Weight-bearing, muscle actions, and fatigue may all be contributing factors. Accelerated intracortical remodeling causes microscopic fractures, diminished density, and formation of resorption cavities that may coalesce and ultimately produce failure of the cortical or trabecular bone. This patient is atypical because the fracture is very evident radiographically. Often, radiographs are normal. A longitudinal stress fracture is depicted on computed tomography as a linear lucency in the cortex associated with periosteal and endosteal callus. On magnetic resonance imaging, this lesion appears as a linear abnormality oriented along the long axis of the tibial shaft. Edema surrounding the fracture or the fracture itself often begins at the level of the nutrient foramen. Endosteal and periosteal callus manifest as thickening of the cortex surrounding the stress fracture.

Notes

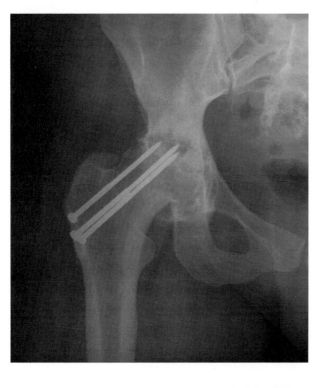

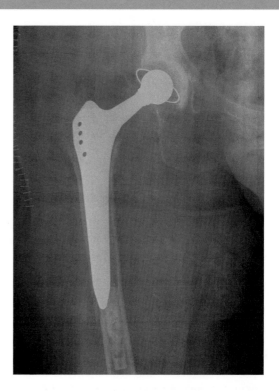

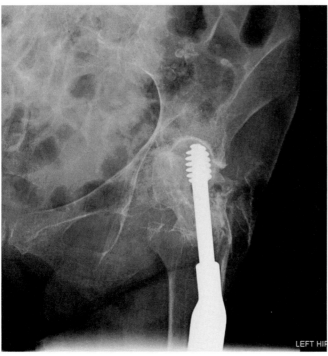

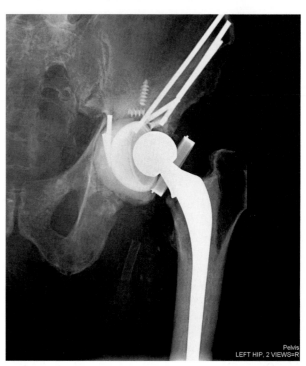

You are shown radiographs of four different patients with hip pain.

1. What is the main finding?

2. What is the main finding?

3. What is the main finding?

4. What is the main finding?

Hip Surgery Complications

1. Femoral head avascular necrosis resulting in penetration of Knowles pins.

2. Fracture of the femoral shaft involving lateral cortex at the tip of femoral implant from varus placement.

3. Dynamic hip screw migration and acetabular erosion from fracture collapse.

4. Rotation of acetabular cup from loosening.

Reference

Manaster B: Total hip arthroplasty: Radiographic evaluation. *Radiographics* 16:645–660, 1996.

Cross-Reference

Musculoskeletal Imaging: THE REQUISITES, 3rd ed, pp 199–200 and 360–365.

Comment

Every year thousands of patients have surgery in their hips. The two most common procedures are proximal femoral fracture fixation and various types of hip replacements. Fortunately, postoperative complications are not common, yet as many as 3% to 10% of complications can be sufficiently significant to require additional or repeat surgery. Infection, nerve injury, heterotopic ossification, and thromboembolism are notable complications. Hardware failure is an important finding, and this has many different manifestations.

Femoral neck fractures are often fixated after reduction with Knowles pins, set in triad for optimal stabilization. When patients develop osteonecrosis of the femoral head, the tips of the pins can penetrate through the cortex of the femoral head and erode the superior acetabulum. A similar situation occurs with a collapse of an intertrochanteric femur fracture fixated with a dynamic hip screw. The change in fracture position can cause the tip of the screw to migrate. Fracture of these pins and screws are also potential complications. In a total hip arthroplasty, loosening of the acetabular cup is depicted by a zone of lucency surrounding the implant. When the implant changes in position, the diagnosis is unequivocal. In the femur, subsidence, lucency in the cement or prosthesis, and scalloping of the bone are suggestive of loosening. Incorrect varus placement of a femoral implant may result in a fracture of the lateral femoral cortex.

Notes

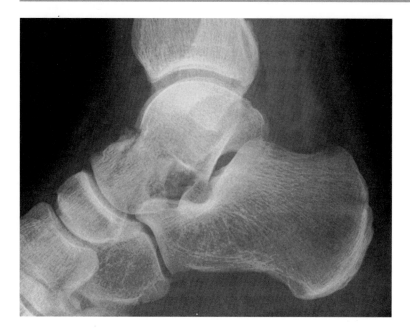 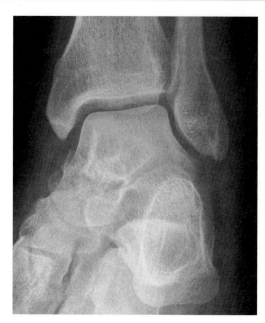

1. Describe the mechanism of injury.

2. What is the Hawkins sign and what does it mean?

3. In the Hawkins classification, what is the risk of developing avascular necrosis (AVN) for each classification?

4. What is a "snowboarder's fracture"?

Talar Neck Fracture

1. Abrupt dorsiflexion of the forefoot, probably from a motor vehicle collision or fall.

2. Subchondral lucency in the talar dome from disuse osteoporosis, which indicates an intact vascular supply.

3. AVN occurs in less than 5% of Type I fractures, 33% of Type II fractures, and two thirds of all of Type III fractures.

4. Avulsion fracture of the lateral talar process.

References

Canale ST, Kelley FB: Fractures of the neck and the talus. *J Bone Joint Surg* 60-A:143–156, 1978.

Vallier HA, Nork SE, Barei DP, et al: Talar neck fractures: Results and outcomes. *J Bone Joint Surg* 86-A; 1616–1624, 2004.

Cross-Reference

Musculoskeletal Imaging: THE REQUISITES, 3rd ed, pp 274–275.

Comment

Fractures of the talar neck are uncommon in adults and rare in children but this injury accounts for the second most frequently occurring type of fracture involving the talus. It is most often associated with motor vehicle accidents and falls, but occasionally a direct impaction to the dorsum of the foot may cause this fracture. When evaluating a talar neck fracture, recall the vascular supply to this bone. The main blood supply enters the talus through the tarsal tunnel as a branch of the posterior tibial artery. It supplies the inferior neck and most of the body. The dorsalis pedis artery and its branches enter the superior aspect of the neck and supply the dorsum of the neck and head regions. The peroneal artery supplies a portion of the lateral talus.

The Hawkins classification prognosticates the risk of developing avascular necrosis in patients who have fractures of the talus. Type I fractures are nondisplaced and bisect the subtalar joint between the middle and posterior facets. The vascular supply is generally preserved. Type II fractures are displaced with subluxation or dislocation of the subtalar joint, disrupting two (occasionally three) of the vascular supplies. Type III fractures are displaced with dislocation of the body from both the tibiotalar and subtalar joints, disrupting all three vascular supplies. Type IV fractures has an associated talonavicular subluxation or dislocation.

Eighty percent of talar neck fractures are Type II or III fractures. The incidence of Type I fractures is about 15% and Type IV fractures make up the remaining 5%.

Notes

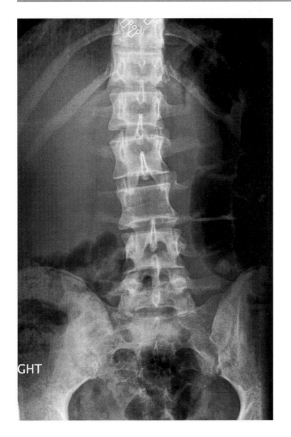 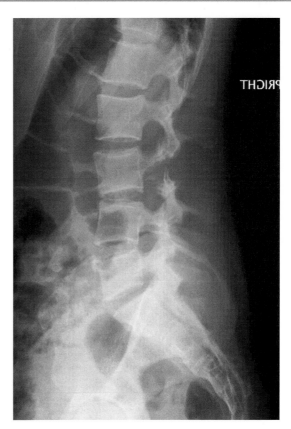

1. What is the diagnosis?

2. Is this considered a stable or unstable injury acutely? What is the prognosis?

3. Is this a common injury?

4. Which part of the spine is most likely to be affected?

CASE 75

Chance Fracture (L3)

1. Chance fracture of L3.

2. Acutely, this fracture is considered unstable. Pure osseous fractures have excellent healing potential and long-term stability is likely, but pure ligamentous injuries have a low healing potential and a high risk of residual instability.

3. No, but it is not uncommon either since it makes up about 10% of all major fractures of the spine.

4. The fractures occur between T12 and L4, with 50% occurring at L2, L3, and L4.

Reference

Ashman CJ, Yu JS, Chung CB: The Chance fracture: Anteroposterior radiographic signs. *Emegency Radiol* 4:320–325, 1997.

Cross-Reference

Musculoskeletal Imaging: THE REQUISITES, 3rd ed, pp 176–177.

Comment

The Chance fracture was initially described as the horizontal fracture that started in the spinous process and neural arch, extended into the vertebral body, and exited through the superior end plate anterior to the neural foramen. Since then, three additional patterns have been described. These range from a purely ligamentous injury to fractures that involve all three columns of the spine. Compression of the vertebral body is not a major finding. The mechanism of injury is related to the anterior position of the fulcrum of force during forced flexion of the torso. The restraint of a lap seatbelt or a fall onto the abdomen results in only tensile forces on the spine so that the primary injury is distraction.

A good lateral view generally is diagnostic, but often this cannot be obtained in a patient who has sustained multiple trauma. Computed tomography through the area of interest with sagittal reformatted images may be helpful, but the diagnosis can be achieved through careful inspection of an anteroposterior radiograph of the thoracolumbar spine. Pertinent observations include an increased interspinal distance (empty hole sign), splitting of the pedicle and/or transverse processes, fracture of the spinous process, fracture of the lamina, widening of the disc space or facet joints, and widening of the intercostal space.

Notes

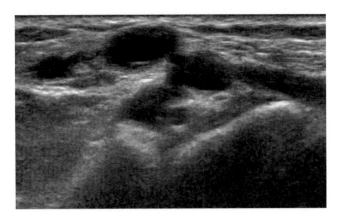
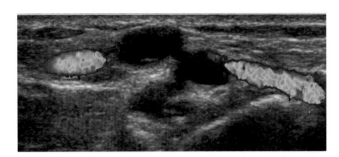

You are shown a longitudinal (right side is distal) sonogram without and with Doppler over the radial artery at the level of the distal radius.

1. What are the findings?

2. What is the most common mass presenting in the wrist?

3. Where can these lesions occur?

4. Which digit is most frequently affected and where does it occur?

Ganglion Cyst

1. There is an anechoic, multilobulated cyst.

2. About 50% to 70% of lesions in the hand and wrist are ganglion cysts.

3. Most arise from the joint capsule or tendon sheath, but they may also be intratendinous or intraosseous.

4. The middle finger, with 69% located in between the A1 and A2 pulleys.

References

Hoglund M, Tordai P, Muren C: Diagnosis of ganglions in the hand and wrist by sonography. *Acta Radiol* 35:35–39, 1994.

Nguyen V, Choi J, Davis KW: Imaging of wrist masses. *Curr Probl Diagn Radiol* 33:147–160, 2004.

Cross-Reference

Musculoskeletal Imaging: THE REQUISITES, 3rd ed, p 157.

Comment

The wrist is a complex joint with numerous articulations. Furthermore, the passing of tendons on the volar and dorsal surfaces and the presence of nerves and vessels contribute to an extensive differential diagnosis of conditions that present with a soft tissue mass. In the wrist, common lesions include ganglion cysts, giant cell tumors of the tendon sheath, hemangiomas, lipomas, and tumors of neural origin. Clinically, the diagnosis may not be discernable. Ganglion cysts are the most common disorder presenting as a mass in the hand and wrist, accounting for 50% to 70% of lesions. The majority of patients are women and most present with an enlarging asymptomatic mass in the second through fourth decades of life. Conservative management is typical but if the cyst causes pain, interference with activity, or nerve compression, then surgery is the treatment of choice, although 5% to 15% of these cysts recur. Aspiration alone has a recurrence rate greater than 50%.

Ganglion cysts contain free water and have a characteristic sonographic appearance of a well-circumscribed uniloculate or multiloculate anechoic cyst with posterior acoustic enhancement. When the lesion arises from the joint, you should attempt to identify the point of communication to the joint, since resected ganglia tend to recur if the neck of the ganglia is not removed.

Notes

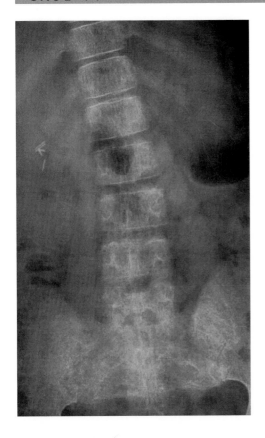

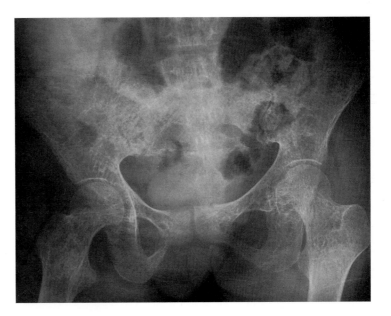

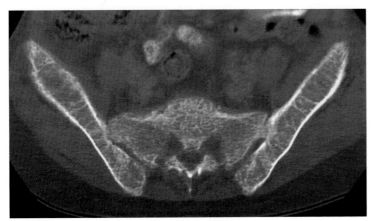

1. What diseases would you consider?

2. What does the "hair-on-end" appearance in the skull represent?

3. If the patient has right upper quadrant abdominal pain, what should be done?

4. What is a posterior mediastinal mass likely to represent?

Thalassemia Major

1. Thalassemia, thalassemia variants, sickle cell thalassemia, sickle cell anemia.

2. Marrow hyperplasia.

3. Ultrasound to look for gallstones.

4. Extramedullary hematopoiesis.

References

Tsitouridis J, Stamos S, Hassapopoulou E, et al: Extramedullary paraspinal hematopoiesis in thalassemia: CT and MRI evaluation. *Eur J Radiol* 30:33–38, 1999.

Tunaci M, Tunaci A, Engin G, et al: Imaging features of thalassemia. *Eur Radiol* 9:1804–1809, 1999.

Cross-Reference

Musculoskeletal Imaging: THE REQUISITES, 3rd ed, pp 566–569.

Comment

Thalassemia syndromes are a group of disorders of hemoglobin synthesis characterized by a decreased production of either the alpha or beta polypeptide chains of the hemoglobin molecules as a result of markedly decreased amounts of globin messenger ribonucleic acid. Beta-thalassemia major is the most common. Decreased or absent production of beta chains lead to decreased synthesis of total hemoglobin producing severe hypochromic anemia. Inclusion bodies in erythrocytes from excess alpha chains lead to hemolysis of the erythrocytes and ineffective hematopoiesis. This is associated with marrow hyperactivity, with excess production of fetal hemoglobin. Marrow hypertrophy and extramedullary hematopoiesis result in hepatosplenomegaly, skull and facial deformities, and pathologic fractures and growth retardation. The osseous structures also appear osteopenic with thin cortices and coarse trabeculation.

The radiographic appearance of intrathoracic extramedullary hematopoiesis is that of a paraspinal mass in the posterior mediastinum at the level of the middle to lower thorax. The process may be either unilateral or bilateral. These masses generally appear rounded or lobulated and do not contain calcifications. Patients with polycythemia, myelofibrosis, leukemia, Hodgkin's disease and other marrow replacement processes also occasionally demonstrate a need for extramedullary hematopoiesis. In thalassemia, the "hair-on-end" appearance of the skull from marrow expansion occurs with maxillary hypertrophy and forward displacement of the incisors producing a characteristic "rodent facies" appearance.

Notes

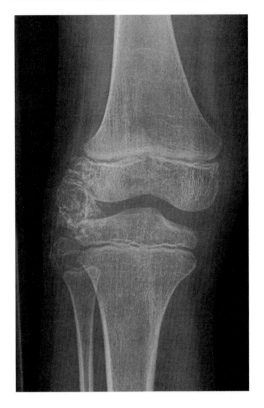
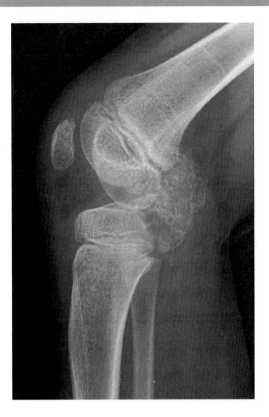

1. What is the most likely diagnosis?

2. What is the definition of hemimelia? Which side is more commonly involved in this condition?

3. There are three different types of this disease. What are they and which is most common?

4. Does it ever occur in the upper extremity?

Dysplasia Epiphysealis Hemimelica

1. Trevor-Fairbank disease.

2. Affects only one side of the bone. Medial side is twice as common as lateral side.

3. Localized form, classic form, and generalized form; classic form accounts for 67% of cases.

4. Yes, but it is rare.

Reference

Murphey MD, Choi JJ, Kransdorf MJ, et al: Imaging of osteochondroma: Variants and complications with radiologic-pathologic correlation. *Radiographics* 20:1407–1434, 2000.

Cross-Reference

Musculoskeletal Imaging: THE REQUISITES, 3rd ed, pp 450 and 453.

Comment

Dysplasia epiphysealis hemimelica (DEH), also known as Trevor-Fairbank disease, is an uncommon disorder manifested by osteochondromas arising from the epiphysis. The lower extremity is almost always involved (usually a single extremity). It is three times more common in boys. DEH is usually restricted to either the medial or lateral side of the limb (hemimelic). DEH is categorized into three different forms: a localized form (monostotic involvement), a classic form (more than one area of osseous involvement in a single extremity), and a generalized or severe form (disease involving an entire single extremity). The localized form affects the hind foot or ankle. The classic form shows characteristic hemimelic distribution and accounts for more than two thirds of cases, typically involving the knee and ankle. In the generalized form, the hip may appear dysplastic. Radiographic findings are characteristic. In infants and toddlers, the ossification center affected appears asymmetrically enlarged. Stippled calcification may be seen in the anomalous cartilage. As the child grows, the calcification becomes disorganized and is accompanied by irregular ossification. Subsequently, the ossifying epiphyseal osteochondroma becomes confluent with adjacent bone and eventually appears as a lobulated ossific mass, identical to any other exostosis, although marrow and cortical continuity with the underlying bone may not be as apparent. Magnetic resonance imaging is useful for identifying the extent of epiphyseal involvement, joint deformity, and effect on surrounding soft tissue.

Notes

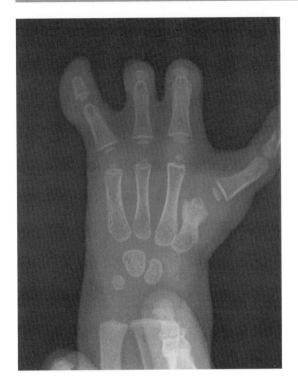 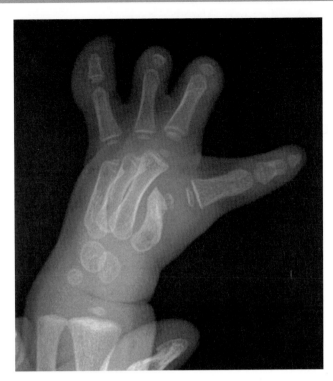

1. What is the most likely diagnosis?

2. What is the best method for diagnosis in utero?

3. Is there any treatment available?

4. Is there any association with the umbilical cord length?

CASE 79

Amniotic Band Constriction Syndrome

1. Amniotic band constriction syndrome.

2. Sequential fetal sonography.

3. Endoscopic release of the amniotic band in utero if there is threatened limb amputation.

4. There may be an association with a short umbilical cord.

References

Fisher RM, Cremin BJ: Limb defects in the amniotic band syndrome. *Pediatr Radiol* 26:24–29, 1976.

Pedersen TK, Thomsen SG: Spontaneous resolution of amniotic bands. *Ultrasound Obstet Gynecol* 18: 673–674, 2001.

Cross-Reference

Musculoskeletal Imaging: THE REQUISITES, 3rd ed, pp 647–649.

Comment

Amniotic band constriction syndrome is a sporadic condition that comprises a group of congenital anomalies characterized by amputations, constriction bands, pseudosyndactylism, and multiple craniofacial, visceral, and body wall defects. It occurs in approximately 1 in 1200 to 1 in 15,000 live births. Some of the cases present with congenital anomalies that are incompatible with life, but some only show isolated limb constrictions such as this patient. There are two mechanisms proposed for this condition: (1) as the amniotic ring constricts around a limb, the blood flow distal to the obstruction is compromised, leading to the demise of the limb and autoamputation, and (2) early amnion rupture leads to development of fibrous bands that entrap the fetal body.

Sequential fetal sonography affords the ability to observe in utero the process of limb strangulation. Prenatal diagnosis with three-dimensional sonography with multiplanar imaging and surface rendering has been shown to depict the relationship between the amniotic band and the fetal limb accurately. Doppler studies document vascular integrity. Although endoscopic fetal therapy with lysis of the constriction ring in utero is an option, intervention is not always warranted since spontaneous resolution can occur.

Notes

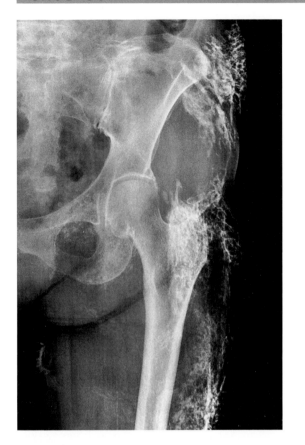
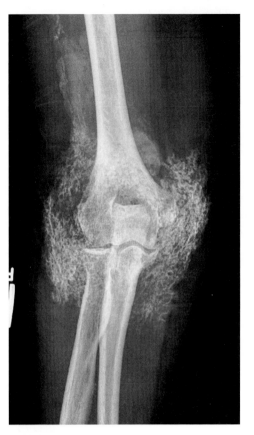

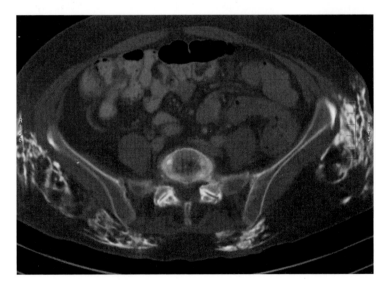

1. What is the diagnosis?

2. What is the disease process?

3. Is there an association with neoplastic processes?

4. What percentage of patients have lung manifestations? What do they get?

Dermatomyositis

1. Dermatomyositis.

2. An inflammatory myopathy with deposition of complement in the skeletal muscle and subcutaneous tissue.

3. Yes, dermatomyositis may be associated with malignant neoplasms, including genitourinary, gynecologic, esophageal, and lung cancer, as well as melanoma.

4. About 67%; interstitial lung disease.

References

Garcia J: MRI in inflammatory myopathies. *Skeletal Radiol* 29:424–438, 2000.

Hanlon R, King S: Overview of the radiology of connective tissue disorders in children. *Eur J Radiol* 33: 74–84, 2000.

Cross-Reference

Musculoskeletal Imaging: THE REQUISITES, 3rd ed, pp 331–334.

Comment

The inflammatory myopathies, characterized by an inflammatory infiltrate of the skeletal muscle, are the largest group of acquired and potentially treatable myopathies. They comprise a group of autoimmune diseases of unknown cause that produce inflammation and muscle degeneration. Based on clinical, histopathological, immunological, and demographic features, they are differentiated into three distinct subsets: dermatomyositis, polymyositis, and inclusion-body myositis. Dermatomyositis is a microangiopathy affecting the skin and muscle. Activation and deposition of complement causes lysis of endomysial capillaries and muscle ischemia. Patients usually present between the third and fifth decades of life although a juvenile form is well known, and females are more frequently affected. Patients present with muscle weakness and tenderness, which leads to atrophy and contracture. Muscle edema occurs early in the disease process, followed by calcification and atrophy. Magnetic resonance imaging has been useful in evaluating the disease, depicting high signal intensity on T2W images suggesting edema early in the disease, and fatty infiltration in the muscle late in the disease. Radiographically, the most common manifestation is nonspecific subcutaneous calcification. "Sheetlike" calcifications along fascial or muscle planes of the proximal large muscles are less common but is pathognomonic for the disease. Periarticular calcifications may occur but are uncommon.

Notes

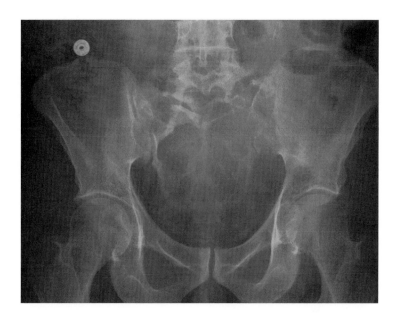

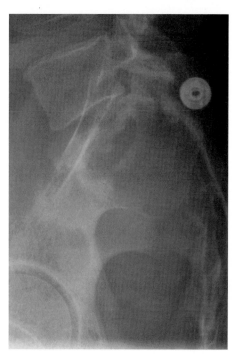

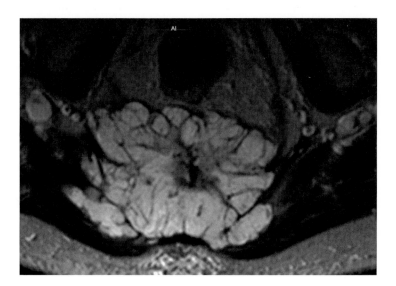

1. What is the most likely diagnosis in this 70-year-old man?

2. Explain the characteristic location of involvement.

3. What is the characteristic cell of this tumor?

4. A patient in remission has been followed for 5 years. Is the patient considered cured?

Chordoma

1. Sacral chordoma. If you had only the radiographs, plasmacytoma and primary sarcoma are also considerations.

2. Ectopic rests of notochordal tissue are found in the sacrococcygeal region and the base of the skull, and also in the nuclei pulposi of the intervertebral discs.

3. The physaliphorous cell with cytoplasm distended from mucus droplets.

4. No, a chordoma can recur at any time, even as much as 20 years later.

Reference

Sung MS, Lee GK, Kang HS, et al: Sacrococcygeal chordoma: MR imaging in 30 patients. *Skeletal Radiol* 34:87–94, 2005.

Cross-Reference

Musculoskeletal Imaging: THE REQUISITES, 3rd ed, pp 526–527.

Comment

A chordoma is a tumor arising from ectopic rests of primitive notochordal tissue and is most common in the two ends of the spine. It is slow growing but progressively invasive. The most common symptom is pain but it develops insidiously over months to years. The five-year survival is 50% to 60% but recurrences can occur much later than five years. Over one-half of tumors occur in the sacrococcygeal region, 35% affect the spheno-occipital region, and the remaining 15% are found in the spine. The peak incidence of sacrococcygeal tumors is in the sixth and seventh decades of life. In other areas of the spine, the peak incidence is in the fourth or fifth decades. When it presents in a child, it is limited to the spheno-occipital region or the cervical spine. It is twice as common in men as in women. The characteristic magnetic resonance imaging appearance is a polylobulated mass with occasional cysts, with a firm pseudocapsule that surrounds the tumor except where it has destroyed bone and septations. In the sacrum, it may be covered by the periosteum. The radiographic finding is bone destruction with a soft tissue mass that may be very sizable. In the sacrum, the average size is 10 cm and usually involves the midline. It may show dystrophic calcification. The classic appearance of multiple lucencies in the sacrum resembling a honeycomb is not a common finding.

Notes

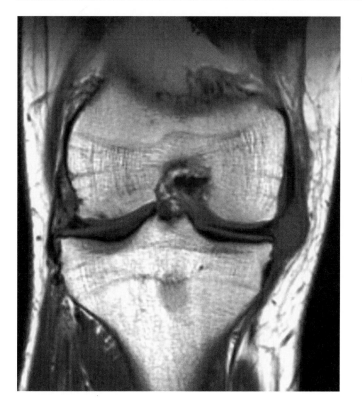 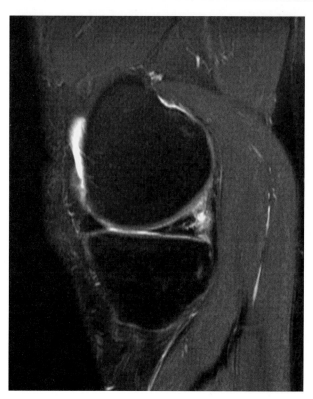

1. What is the diagnosis?

2. What is the classic clinical description of this entity?

3. What is the appropriate treatment? What if you were to aspirate the fluid?

4. Which side is more common, medial or lateral?

Atlas Posterior Arch Fracture

1. Fracture of the posterior arch of C1.

2. Yes.

3. Ninety percent are bilateral.

4. Pull of the rectus capitis muscle that attaches to the posterior ring of C1.

Reference

Rao SK, Wasyliw C, Nunez DB, Jr: Spectrum of imaging findings in hyperextension injuries of the neck. *Radiographics* 25:1239–1254, 2005.

Cross-Reference

Musculoskeletal Imaging: THE REQUISITES, 3rd ed, pp 166–169.

Comment

The most common fracture of the atlas (C1 vertebra) involves the posterior arch. It is the result of a hyperextension injury, causing the posterior arch of C1 to be compressed between the basiocciput and posterior arch of the axis (C2 vertebra). These injuries can produce either a unilateral or a bilateral arch disruption. Note that in this patient, the dorsal fragment is angulated cranially owing to the traction of the rectus capitis muscle and this frequently occurs with bilateral posterior ring fractures. These fractures when isolated to the posterior ring are considered stable and are not associated with prevertebral soft tissue swelling. Radiographically, the diagnosis is apparent with careful inspection of the spine. Computed tomography should be performed to determine if other parts of the atlas are fractured. The differential diagnosis is a congenital cleft, which has well-defined and sclerotic margins in contradistinction to a fracture, which appears sharp and noncorticated.

Notes

Meniscal Tear with Meniscal Cyst

1. Meniscal cyst.

2. Masslike swelling at the joint line that fluctuates in size with either a change in knee position or with manipulation.

3. Repair or debride the meniscal tear either arthroscopically or with open excision. The cyst would recur.

4. Medial by a ratio of 2 to 1.

References

Campbell SE, Sanders TG, Morrison WB: MR imaging of meniscal cysts: Incidence, location, and clinical significance. *AJR Am J Roentgenol* 177:409–413, 2001.

De Maeseneer M, Shahabpour M, Vanderdood K, et al: MR imaging of meniscal cysts: Evaluation of location and extension using a three-layer approach. *Eur J Radiol* 39:117–124, 2001.

Cross-Reference

Musculoskeletal Imaging: THE REQUISITES, 3rd ed, p 232.

Comment

The clinical symptoms of a meniscal cyst vary although joint line pain associated with a palpable mass is a classic presentation. The incidence of meniscal cysts has been reported to be between 1% and 2% in knees that undergo a diagnostic study, but as high as 8% in patients undergoing surgery. A meniscal cyst is caused by decompression of synovial fluid through a meniscal tear. Stretching of the knee capsule and parameniscal soft tissues by the cystic mass is thought to be the cause of the pain. Most patients are in their third or fourth decades of life when first evaluated, and men are more frequently affected than women. These cysts are common after a meniscectomy, trauma, or significant degeneration of a meniscus. When a tear is horizontally oriented, it is more likely to communicate with a cyst. Remember that three fourths of these cysts are palpable. One important clue to the diagnosis is that the size of the meniscal cyst may increase and decrease with different knee positions. Long-standing cysts may be large, contain extruded meniscal debris, and cause erosive changes in the adjacent tibial cortex.

Notes

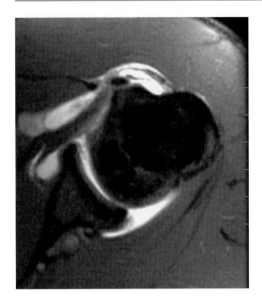
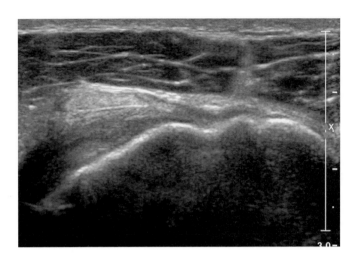

You are shown an axial gradient-recalled-echo magnetic resonance image and a transverse (right side is lateral) sonogram of the shoulder.

1. What is the diagnosis? Why does it happen?

2. Where does the biceps brachii muscle attach in the shoulder?

3. List the restraints of the tendon of the long head of the biceps in the shoulder.

4. What is a Buford complex?

Medial Dislocation of the Biceps Tendon

1. Extra-articular dislocation of the biceps tendon. A defect in the transverse ligament that bridges the bicipital groove allows displacement of the tendon anterior to the subscapularis tendon adjacent to the lesser tuberosity.

2. The short head—tip of the coracoid process adjacent to the coracobrachialis muscle. The long head—superior rim of the glenoid at the bicipital tubercle and the glenoid labrum.

3. The corocohumeral ligament, superior glenohumeral ligament, and transverse humeral ligament, with contributions from the subscapularis tendon.

4. Congenital absence of the anterosuperior labrum with a cordlike middle glenohumeral ligament.

References

Cervilla V, Schweitzer ME, Ho C, et al: Medial dislocation of the biceps brachii tendon: Appearance at MR imaging. *Radiology* 180:523–526, 1991.

Martinoli C, Bianchi S, Prato N, et al: US of the shoulder: Non–rotator cuff disorders. *Radiographics* 23:381–401, 2003.

Cross-Reference

Musculoskeletal Imaging: THE REQUISITES, 3rd ed, p 96.

Comment

Degenerative changes of the rotator cuff tendons may sometimes cause a dislocation of the tendon of the long head of the biceps brachii muscle. Impingement can be an important factor by causing disruption of the coracohumeral ligament, one of the intrarticular restraints of the biceps tendon, and the anterior fibers of the supraspinatus tendon. This allows the biceps tendon to dislocate out of the bicipital groove. Clinically, patients complain of shoulder pain or a snapping sensation in the shoulder during flexion and rotation of the elbow. Dislocation of the biceps tendon is shown best on axial magnetic resonance or transverse sonographic images. A normal tendon sits within the bicipital groove as either an ovoid or semilunar low-signal intensity or hyperechoic structure. In this case, the tendon has displaced medially, coming to rest anterior to the lesser tuberosity. The bicipital groove is empty ("empty groove" sign). When evaluating a potential tendon dislocation, it is critical to take note of the integrity of the transverse humeral ligament and subscapularis tendon to correctly classify the biceps tendon dislocation. This can be difficult since the tendon may come to rest in a number of locations from the lesser tuberosity to the anterior glenoid. Occasionally, a dislocated tendon mimics an anterior labral tear or a Buford complex on magnetic resonance imaging.

Notes

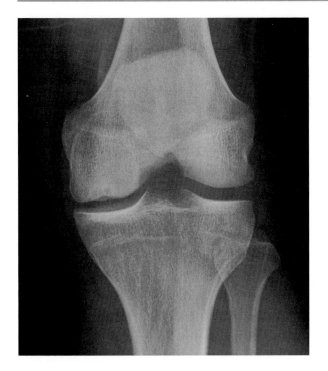

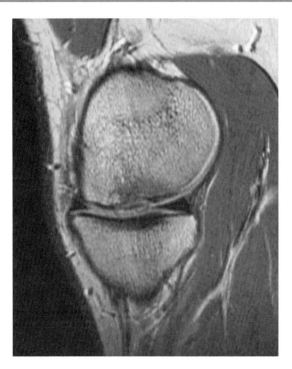

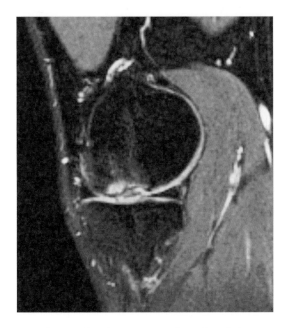

1. What is the diagnosis? What else did you consider?

2. What are associated risk factors for this condition?

3. What is the underlying pathology?

4. In the acute phase of the disease, what imaging modality would you choose to make the diagnosis, magnetic resonance imaging or bone scan?

Spontaneous Osteonecrosis of the Knee

1. Spontaneous osteonecrosis of the knee.
   Osteochondritis dessicans, post-traumatic
   osteochondral defect, and neuroarthropathy.

2. Obesity, trauma, corticosteroid administration, and
   meniscal tears.

3. An insufficiency fracture.

4. Magnetic resonance imaging is preferred over bone
   scintigraphy owing to superior spatial resolution
   and increased specificity.

References

Bjorkengren AG, AlRowaih A, Lindstrand A, et al: Spontaneous osteonecrosis of the knee: Value of MR imaging in determining prognosis. *AJR Am J Roentgenol*
154:331–336, 1990.

Valenti N, Jr, Leyes M, Schweitzer D: Spontaneous
osteonecrosis of the knee: Treatment and evolution.
Knee Surg Sports Traumatol Arthrosc 6:12–15, 1998.

Cross-Reference

Musculoskeletal Imaging: THE REQUISITES, 3rd ed,
pp 244–246.

Comment

Spontaneous osteonecrosis of the knee (SONK) is a
distinct clinical entity that occurs predominantly over
the load-bearing surface of the medial femoral condyle.
It actually is an insufficiency fracture and not true
osteonecrosis. Most patients are elderly, the majority
presenting over the age of 50 years, and this condition
has its highest incidence in the sixth and seventh
decades of life. The hallmark of this disease is a sudden onset of pain and an association with the development of a meniscal tear has been suggested. In some
patients, the disease evolves quickly, resulting in collapse of the articular surface and development of secondary osteoarthritis. Initial radiographs obtained
during the acute phase of the disease are often normal.
However, soon after the acute phase, flattening of the
weight-bearing surface of the medial femoral condyle
develops and a narrow zone of increased density
reflecting trabecular compression surrounds the devitalized area. Over time, a radiolucent crescent in the
subchondral bone becomes evident (a clue that should
always be sought). As the lesion progresses, joint space
narrowing, subchondral eburnation, and the development of periostitis and osteophytosis may eventually
obscure some or all of the features of osteonecrosis.

Magnetic resonance imaging is advocated in patients
of this age to avert the complications of a "missed"
diagnosis.

Notes

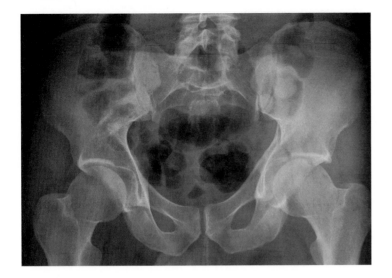

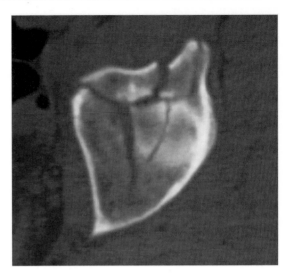

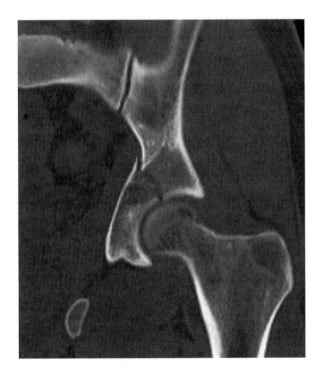

1. What is the diagnosis? Is this a common injury?

2. Why is fracture orientation on computed tomography (CT) important?

3. What are the radiographic landmarks of the hip?

4. What fracture typically accompanies a posterior dislocation?

Acetabular Fractures

1. Transverse acetabular fracture. Yes, acetabular fractures constitute 25% of all pelvic fractures.

2. Because it helps to identify the type of fracture. A column fracture is oriented in the coronal plane of the pelvis while a transverse fracture is oriented in the sagittal plane.

3. The iliopectineal and ilioischial lines identify the columns and the anterior and posterior rim lines identify the acetabular margins.

4. Posterior wall fractures and femoral head fractures.

Reference

Yu JS: Hip and femur trauma: Imaging of trauma to the extremities. *Semin Musculoskeletal Radiol* 4:205–220, 2000.

Cross-Reference

Musculoskeletal Imaging: THE REQUISITES, 3rd ed, pp 189–193.

Comment

Fractures of the acetabulum occur as a result of high-energy trauma and are frequently complex because of comminution. The displacement of multiple fragments may result in incongruity of the articular surface and ultimate development of post-traumatic osteoarthritis. The Judet-Letournel classification has been widely recognized as a useful surgical classification. Fractures of the acetabulum are divided into five simple fracture types and five associated fracture types representing a combination of different simple fracture types. The simple fracture types are posterior acetabular wall, posterior column, anterior acetabular wall, anterior column, and transverse acetabular fractures. The five associated fracture types are transverse and posterior acetabular wall, T-shaped, anterior column and posterior hemitransverse, posterior column and posterior acetabular wall, and both column fractures.

CT is advocated for evaluating acetabular fractures. The advantage of CT over conventional radiography is unimpeded visualization of complex fractures, allowing more accurate assessment of the size, relationship, and degree of displacement of fracture fragments, incongruity at fracture lines, and disruption of the acetabular column. Column and transverse fractures have characteristic imaging patterns on CT. Anterior and posterior column fractures are oriented in a medial to lateral orientation (coronal plane). These fractures extend into the obturator foramen. Transverse fractures bisect the innominate bone and are oriented in the anterior to posterior direction (sagittal plane).

Notes

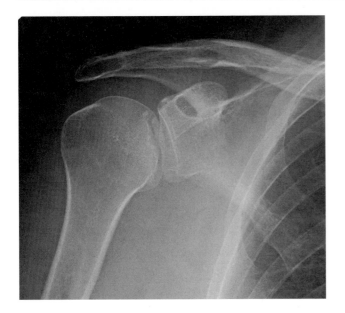 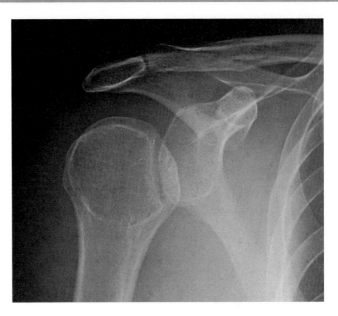

1. What is your diagnosis?

2. How does this injury occur?

3. If this injury remains untreated, what eventually happens to the joint?

4. What are two common humeral fractures associated with this injury, and how frequently do they occur?

C A S E   8 6

Posterior Shoulder Dislocation

1. Posterior shoulder dislocation.

2. Indirect trauma, such as electrocution or seizure, but occasionally as a result of direct impaction against the anterior shoulder or a fall on an outstretched hand.

3. Development of pseudoarthrosis and glenohumeral instability.

4. Lesser tuberosity fracture (25%) and humeral head (10%).

References

Cisternino SJ, Rogers LF, Stufflebam BC, Kruglik GD: The trough line: A radiographic sign of posterior shoulder dislocation. *AJR Am J Roentgenol* 130:951–954, 1978.

Schwartz E, Warren RF, O'Brien SJ, Fronek J: Posterior shoulder instability. *Orthop Clin North Am* 18:409–419, 1987.

Cross-Reference

Musculoskeletal Imaging: THE REQUISITES, 3rd ed, pp 105–106.

Comment

A posterior dislocation of the glenohumeral joint is one of the most commonly misdiagnosed injuries in trauma patients. About 50% of these injuries are missed on initial radiographic evaluation. Several factors contribute to the errors in diagnosis. An adequate study may be impossible to perform because the shoulder is locked in internal rotation. Clinically, important findings that are indicative of a dislocation may be masked by a concomitant hematoma, muscle spasm, or associated fractures. A lesser tuberosity fracture of the proximal humerus should raise your suspicion for a potential posterior glenohumeral dislocation. There are three types of posterior shoulder dislocations; however, the subacromial type is by far the most common. Posterior subglenoid and subspinous dislocations are rare. Important radiographic observations include the trough sign as in this patient (a vertical compression fracture of the anterior humeral head), rim sign (widening of the joint beyond 6 mm), absent half moon sign (loss of humeral head/glenoid rim overlap), Velpeau's sign (superior subluxation of humeral head), and disruption of the scapulohumeral arch. Computed tomography should be performed when a posterior dislocation is suspected to search for a reverse Bankart lesion, a tear of the posterior labrum, and stripping of the posterior periosteum.

Notes

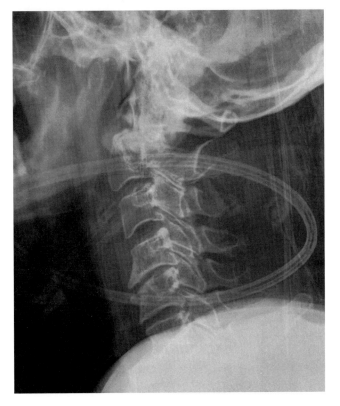 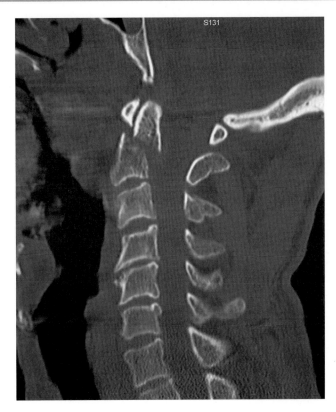

1. What is the diagnosis and is it stable?
2. What percentage of spine injuries involves this area?
3. What are some variations of these injuries?
4. What is the implication of these different types?

Fractures of the Odontoid

1. Oblique odontoid base fracture; unstable because it frequently leads to nonunion and generally requires a C1-C2 fusion.

2. About 10%.

3. The fracture line can be horizontal, slope forward, or slope backward.

4. If the fracture is horizontal, the odontoid fragment can displace either anteriorly or posteriorly; if the fracture slopes forward, the odontoid fragment displaces anteriorly; and if it slopes posteriorly, the odontoid fragment displaces posteriorly.

References

Anderson LD, D'Alonzo RT: Fractures of the odontoid process of the axis. *J Bone Joint Surg* 56-A:1663–1674, 1978.

Maak TG, Grauer JN: The contemporary treatment of odontoid injuries. *Spine* 31(suppl 11): S53–S60, 2006.

Cross-Reference

Musculoskeletal Imaging: THE REQUISITES, 3rd ed, pp 167–171.

Comment

An odontoid fracture remains one of the most difficult fractures to identify in the cervical spine. Fractures of the odontoid process are usually the result of head trauma transmitted to the C1-C2 area. Pain is common but neurological injuries are not. If the dens is displaced, its direction is dictated by the force that is transmitted. The most common classification is the Anderson and D'Alonzo classification, which describes three odontoid fracture types. In type 1, the fracture involves the tip of the odontoid process and most likely represents an avulsion by the alar ligaments. In type 2, the most common type, a fracture occurs at the base of the odontoid process or below the level of the superior articular facet of C2. In type 3, a fracture involves the body of C2. The availability of computed tomography has allowed expeditious delineation of the extent of injury including assessment of the insertion of the anterior longitudinal ligament. More recently, magnetic resonance imaging has been more widely used because it enables evaluation of the attachments of the alar and transverse ligaments, which also can be indicators of an unstable situation when avulsed. Opinions vary as to the optimal treatment of a type 2 fracture and include long-term external immobilization with a collar or halo and surgical stabilization with a C1-C2 fusion.

Notes

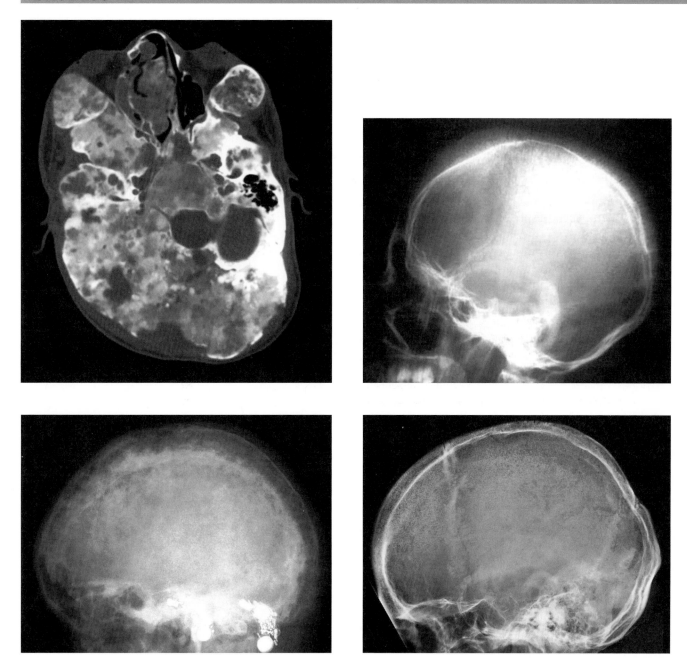

1. You are shown four different skulls. What is the diagnosis or main observation?

2. What is the diagnosis or main observation?

3. What is the diagnosis or main observation?

4. What is the diagnosis or main observation?

Skull Abnormalities

1. Fibrous dysplasia.

2. Diffuse "hair-on-end" appearance.

3. Paget's disease, chronic phase.

4. "Salt-and-pepper" skull appearance of hyper-parathyroidism.

Reference

Tehranzadeh J, Fung Y, Donohue M, et al: Computed tomography of Paget disease of the skull versus fibrous dysplasia. *Skeletal Radiol* 27:664–672, 1998.

Cross-Reference

Musculoskeletal Imaging: THE REQUISITES, 3rd ed, pp 374–375, 413, 462–463.

Comment

There are many diseases that have characteristic manifestations in the skull. Changes in the skull can affect the diploic space, outer table, inner table, skull base, frontal bones, cranial vault morphology, and density of the bones, among other findings. This case is designed to help you familiarize yourself with four common skull manifestations. Although some are typical of certain processes (Paget's disease and fibrous dysplasia), others only allow you to develop a differential diagnosis. Fibrous dysplasia is characterized by a "ground-glass" appearance, asymmetry, and involvement of the paranasal sinuses and facial bones. Latent Paget's disease is symmetric and has a "cotton-wool" appearance accompanied by typical cortical thickening. A hair-on-end appearance indicates a need for additional hematopoiesis. The differential diagnosis includes thalasemia, sickle cell disease, polycythemia, and hereditary spherocytosis and sometimes myelofibrosis, leukemia, Hodgkin's disease, and other marrow replacement processes. The salt-and-pepper skull is characteristic of hyperparathyroidism although multiple myeloma and diffuse metastasis can occasionally have a similar appearance.

Notes

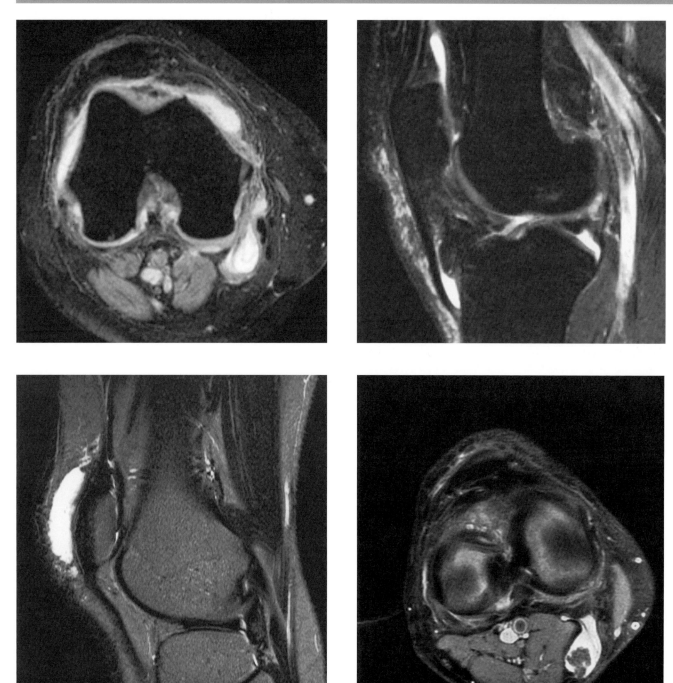

1. You are shown images from four different patients. What is the lesion and what symptoms does it elicit?

2. What is the lesion and what symptoms does it elicit?

3. What is the lesion and what symptoms does it elicit?

4. What is the lesion and what symptoms does it elicit?

Cystic Knee Lesions

1. Pes anserine bursitis; pain, tenderness, and firm swelling over the pes anserinus.

2. Deep infrapatellar bursitis; anterior knee pain aggravated by palpation over distal patellar tendon.

3. Prepatellar bursitis; pain and swelling over patella.

4. Baker's cyst; painless mass unless ruptured, when symptoms are similar to acute deep venous thrombosis.

Reference

McCarthy CL, McNally EG: The MRI appearance of cystic lesions around the knee. *Skeletal Radiol* 33:187–209, 2004.

Cross-Reference

Musculoskeletal Imaging: THE REQUISITES, 3rd ed, pp 243–245.

Comment

There are many knee lesions that appear cystic on magnetic resonance imaging. Many present with pain or as a palpable mass. Bursal distention is a common finding in the knee. Commonly visualized bursae include those around the patella as well as the pes anserine, tibial collateral ligament, semimembranosus-tibial collateral ligament, iliotibial, and fibular collateral ligament-biceps femoris tendon regions. The most common lesion is a baker's cyst, which is a popliteal cyst that communicates with the joint through a weakened posteromedial capsule between the medial head of the gastrocnemius and the semimembranosus tendon. Distension is usually related to an intra-articular abnormality of the knee that increases the intra-articular pressure. The pes anserine bursa lies deep to the pes anserinus and superficial to the tibial insertion of the medial collateral ligament. Distension is common in overweight elderly females with arthritis or from overuse in runners. The prepatellar bursa is situated anterior to the patella and proximal patellar tendon. Most cases are related to direct trauma. The deep infrapatellar bursa is located between the posterior margin of the distal patellar tendon and the anterior aspect of the tibia, beneath Hoffa's fat pad. Bursitis is usually the result of overuse of the knee, particularly in runners and jumpers.

Notes

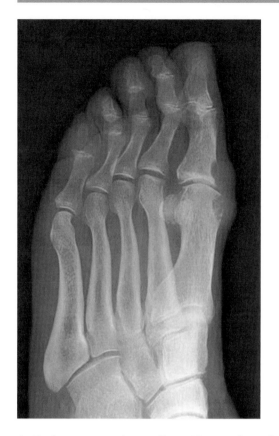
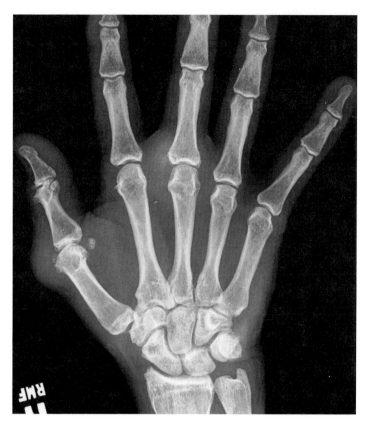

1. Is there a genetic predisposition to the primary form of this disease?
2. What is a typical time interval from the onset of symptoms to radiographically detectable changes in the joints?
3. Explain the radiographic finding in the fifth toe.
4. On magnetic resonance imaging, what finding is *most* characteristic of this disease?

Gout

1. Yes, autosomal dominant with weak penetrance in females (90% of patients affected are male).

2. Many years (average 7 to 12 years).

3. Lysis of bone secondary to an intraosseous tophus.

4. The tophus may have low signal intensity on both T1W and T2W images.

Reference

Yu JS, Chung C, Recht M, et al: MR imaging of tophaceous gout. *AJR Am J Roentgenol* 168:523–527, 1997.

Cross-Reference

Musculoskeletal Imaging: THE REQUISITES, 3rd ed, pp 335–339.

Comment

Gout is a condition caused by the deposition of urate monohydrate crystals in tissues. Gout can be divided into an idiopathic form and those that are secondary to other disorders. The idiopathic form is characterized by an overproduction of uric acid due to abnormal renal excretion of urate, caused by a deficiency of the enzyme phosphorylribosyltransferase. There are numerous causes of secondary gout. In some diseases, the increased production of uric acid is caused by an excessive breakdown of nucleoproteins (polycythemia vera, myelofibrosis, leukemia, multiple myeloma, anemias, psoriasis, and glycogen storage disease), whereas in others it is on the basis of renal failure.

The radiographic findings in the foot are characteristic of this disease. Soft tissue masses adjacent to erosions in the first metatarsal head and proximal phalanx have sclerotic rims and typical "overhanging" edges. Calcifications within the tophi are not uncommon. In the hand, the tophi are more prominent in the thumb and third metacarpophalangeal joints but the joint spaces are not severely narrowed. On MRI, gout can sometimes mimic a neoplastic process, because it can provoke a significant periosteal reaction and bone marrow edema. Destruction of the bone and the presence of juxta-articular masses (which do enhance) can appear ominous to the wearied observer. The key to interpreting gout on magnetic resonance imaging is to identify a lesion that is low in signal intensity on both T1W and T2W images. There are not many "bad things" that have low signal intensity on T2W images. Once you have performed this task, then you can resume your search for features that are typical of gout.

Notes

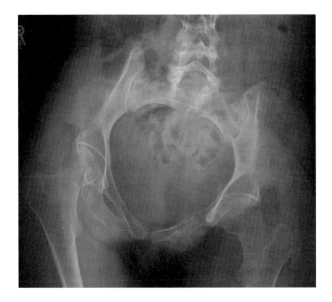 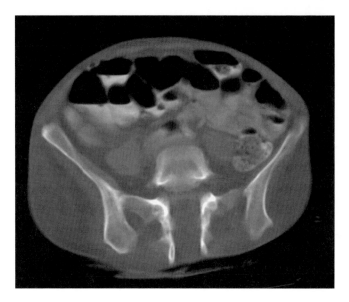

1. What is the diagnosis? What observations did you make?

2. What etiologic factors have been reported?

3. What is the severest expression of the syndrome in the pelvis?

4. Is this associated with "mermaid" syndrome?

CASE 91

Caudal Regression Syndrome

1. Caudal regression syndrome. Partial sacral agenesis and spina bifida.

2. Maternal diabetes mellitus, genetic predisposition, and vascular hypoperfusion.

3. Complete agenesis of the sacrum and lumbar spine.

4. Although caudal regression syndrome has occurred in patients with sirenomelia, the two entities are most likely unrelated.

References

Adra A, Corder D, Mejides A, et al: Caudal regression syndrome: Etiopathogenesis, prenatal diagnosis, and perinatal management. *Obstet Gynecol Surg* 49:508–516, 1994.

Estin D, Cohen AR: Caudal agenesis and associated caudal spinal cord malformations. *Neurosurg Clin N Am* 6:377–391, 1995.

Cross-Reference

Musculoskeletal Imaging: THE REQUISITES, 3rd ed, pp 595–596.

Comment

The caudal regression syndrome is a spectrum of caudal axial skeletal and associated neurologic and soft tissue defects caused by an insult to the developing caudal mesoderm and ectoderm during the first trimester. Defects include partial to complete sacral agenesis, spina bifida, spinal stenosis, an angular and wedge-shaped conus medullaris, tethering of the cord, and a presacral meningocele. In the absence of the sacrum, the ilia articulate with the lumbar spine, drawing these bones to the midline so that the pelvis appears narrowed. Scoliosis is common and seen in over 50% of cases. Clinically, findings depend on the severity of disease expression and include leg weakness, bowel and bladder incontinence, anorectal atresia, renal aplasia, and pulmonary hypoplasia. Patients with sirenomelia, congenital fusion of the lower extremities, have presented with caudal regression syndrome but this is likely incidental and not part of the syndrome.

Notes

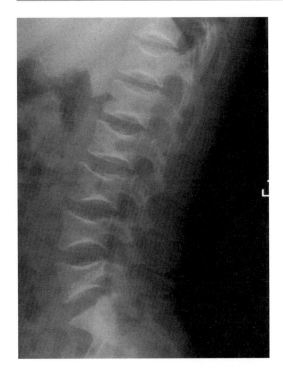
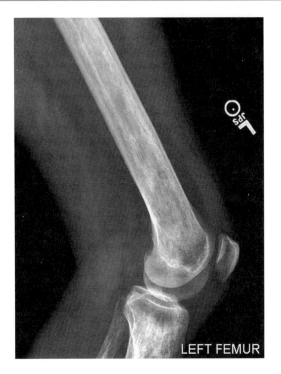
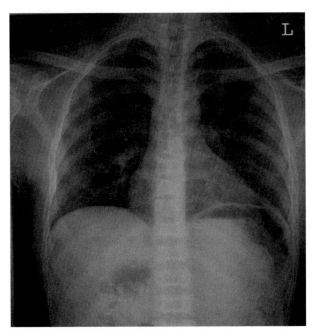

1. What is the diagnosis?
2. What is the most important determinant of disease severity?
3. What finding did you observe in the femur? What caused this?
4. Describe hand-foot syndrome. Whom does it affect?

Sickle Cell Disease

1. Sickle cell disease.

2. Oxygen tension.

3. Bone-in-bone appearance. Medullary infarction.

4. Acute dactylitis from ischemia. Black infants 6 to 18 months of age (uncommon after 6 years of age).

Reference

Crowley JJ, Sarnaik S: Imaging of sickle cell disease. *Pediatr Radiol* 29:646–661, 1999.

Cross-Reference

Musculoskeletal Imaging: THE REQUISITES, 3rd ed, pp 567–568.

Comment

Sickle cell disease occurs primarily in blacks and in persons of Mediterranean descent. It is an inherited disorder that is characterized by reversible sickling of the red blood cells. People who carry two genes for sickle hemoglobin (HbSS) have sickle cell anemia. People who have only one gene for sickle hemoglobin have sickle cell variants. Only a few of these variants have important clinical expressions. When HbS is found in combination with HbC or thalassemia, the process is referred to as sickle cell disease. Several factors influence the severity of the disease. Oxygen tension is the most important factor in patients with sickle cell disease because sickling begins when the oxygen tension drops below 40 mm Hg. Other important considerations include the pH, blood viscosity, mechanical fragility of the RBCs, and the percentage of HbS. Clinically, patients present with anemia caused by rapid destruction of the abnormal erythrocytes. The increased blood viscosity causes thrombosis and infarction in end vessels, which may present as dactylitis in infants.

Radiographically, there is coarsening of the osseous trabeculation and diminished bone density. The vertebral bodies demonstrate characteristic biconcave contours ("fish vertebrae") or central depressions that are the result of diminished bone growth induced by sludging of red blood cells. The bone-in-bone appearances in the long bones are created by infarctions. Hip and shoulder pain may indicate the presence of avascular necrosis. Did you notice the right shoulder in the chest radiograph?

Notes

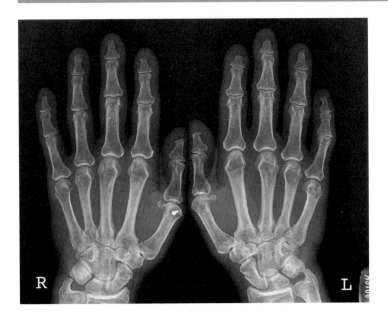 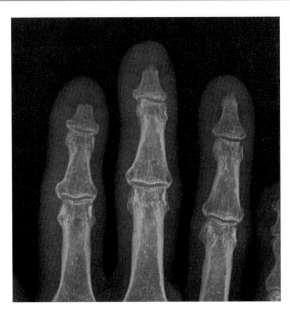

1. List the differential diagnosis for the different patterns.

2. What neoplasm is associated with exposure to polyvinyl chloride?

3. What neuropathic disorder does this finding and calcification of digital nerves characterize?

4. In a skeletally immature person, what part of the distal phalanx is most vulnerable to thermal injuries?

Acro-osteolysis

1. Diffuse pattern: collagen vascular disease and vasculitis, Raynaud's disease, neuropathic disease, thermal injuries, hyperparathyroidism, trauma, epidermolysis bullosa, abnormal stresses, psoriasis, frostbite, sarcoid, hypertrophic osteoarthropathy, pyknodysostosis. Bandlike resorption: polyvinyl chloride exposure and Hadju-Cheney disease.

2. Angiosarcoma of the liver.

3. Leprosy (Hansen's disease).

4. The growth plate.

References

Destouet JM, Murphy WA: Acquired acro-osteolysis and acronecrosis. *Arthritis Rheum* 26:1150–1154, 1983.

Kemp SS, Dalinka MK, Schumaker HR: Acro-osteolysis: Etiologic and radiological considerations. *JAMA* 255:2058–2061, 1986.

Cross-Reference

Musculoskeletal Imaging: THE REQUISITES, 3rd ed, pp 330–333.

Comment

Destruction/resorption of the distal phalanges of the hand describes acro-osteolysis, and this process is associated with numerous etiologies. In many situations, it is impossible to determine the precise cause of the bone lysis when one is asked to rely exclusively on radiographs of the hands. It is important to observe findings elsewhere in the skeleton and to make use of relevant clinical history to render a more specific diagnosis. The pattern of bone lysis is helpful in narrowing the diagnostic considerations, however. There are two patterns of acro-osteolysis in adults. One pattern preferentially involves the tufts of the terminal phalanges, while the other pattern creates a band of osteolysis in the midportion of these bones. The differential diagnosis for bandlike resorption is narrower than for the diffuse pattern of lysis. Bandlike resorption should bring to mind polyvinyl chloride toxicity and Hajdu-Cheney disease and occasionally hyperparathyroidism, collagen vascular diseases, and abnormal stresses. In the latter three situations, more classic resorption of the tuft of the distal phalanges typically coexists.

Notes

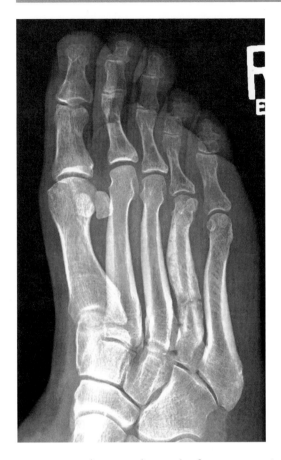 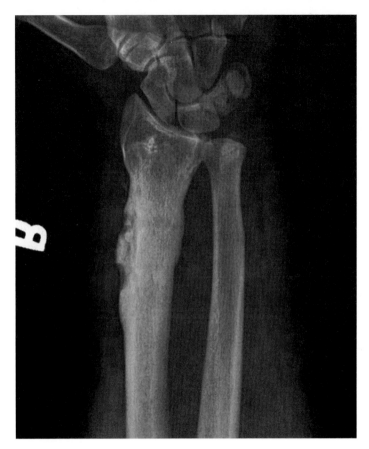

1. You are shown radiographs from two patients. What do they have in common?

2. What is peculiar about the chronic phase of the disease?

3. What would be an appropriate imaging technique to further evaluate this patient?

4. What is important to remember about chronic draining sinus tracts?

CASE 94

Chronic Osteomyelitis with Proliferative Periostitis

1. Chronic osteomyelitis with a pathologic fracture.

2. Chronic osteomyelitis may remain clinically inactive for years then reactivate.

3. A combination of single-photon emission computed tomography/computed tomography and tagged leukocyte scintigraphy is more specific because the pathologic fracture would obscure pertinent findings in the bone marrow on magnetic resonance imaging.

4. Squamous cell carcinoma can develop in them.

References

Bunyaviroch T, Aggarwal A, Oates ME: Optimized scintigraphic evaluation of infection and inflammation: Role of singe-photon emission computed tomography/computed tomography fusion imaging. *Semin Nucl Med* 36:295–311, 2006.

Tehranzadeh J, Wong E, Wang F, Sadighpour M: Imaging of osteomyelitis in the mature skeleton. *Radiol Clin North Am* 39:223–250, 2001.

Cross-Reference

Musculoskeletal Imaging: THE REQUISITES, 3rd ed, pp 550–554.

Comment

This is a straightforward case once you detect the cortical lysis in the fourth metatarsal and distal radius as well as adjacent soft tissue swelling. When a bone infection progresses to a chronic infection, it can be associated with significant periosteal bone formation, giving rise to a markedly thickened cortex of variable density. Often, the bony trabecular pattern alters also with an increased number and size of spongy trabeculae, which further add to the density of the bone. Cysts in the sclerotic areas are common particularly in the diaphysis. The appearance mimics fibrous dysplasia, Paget's disease, and occasionally a neoplastic process. Although the bone appears denser, it is structurally weakened by the infection and vulnerable to the formation of a pathologic fracture, especially if there is increased stress on the bone. Chronic osteomyelitis can sometimes be associated with a chronically draining sinus tract. If this occurs for a period of years, the development of squamous cell carcinoma is an important consideration to keep in mind.

Notes

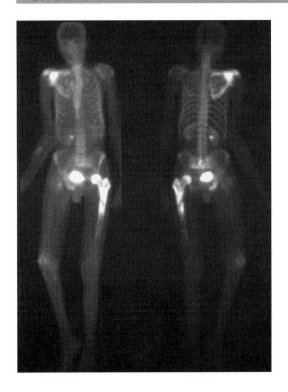

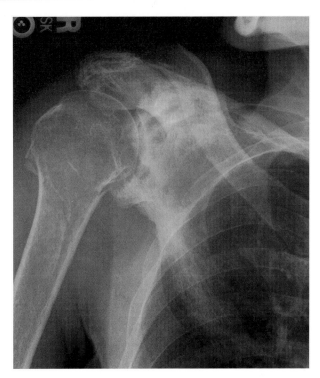

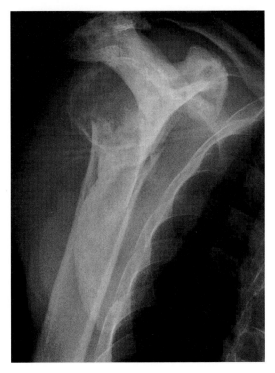

1. What caused the changes in this patient's scapula? What complication do you see?

2. What does a "mosaic pattern" refer to in this disease?

3. Does osteoporosis circumscripta involve the outer table, inner table, or both?

4. If this patient has a sudden rise in the serum alkaline phosphatase level, what does it indicate?

Paget's Disease

1. Paget's disease. A fracture of the infraglenoid region.

2. A patternless arrangement of coarsened and enlarged osseous trabeculae.

3. It generally involves only the outer table of the skull.

4. Sarcomatous degeneration.

References

Griffiths HJ: Radiology of Paget's disease. *Curr Opin Radiol* 4:124–128, 1992.

Mirra JM, Brien EW, Tehranzadeh J: Paget's disease of bone: Review with emphasis on radiologic features, Part II. *Skeletal Radiol* 24:173–184, 1995.

Cross-Reference

Musculoskeletal Imaging: THE REQUISITES, 3rd ed, pp 397–403.

Comment

This case would be challenging without the aid of a corresponding bone scan. Paget's disease is characterized by destruction (lytic phase) of bone followed by attempts at repair (reparative phase). The cause of this disease is unknown. It is most common in middle-aged people, affecting twice as many men as women. The lytic phase of the disease may predominate early in the disease process, but more frequently, there is a combination of destruction and repair. The osteosclerotic phase is characterized by osteoblastic activity. In the quiescent phase, bone resorption and cellular activity is absent. Histologically, lesions are characterized by fibrosis and marked vascularity. The haversian canals are abnormally enlarged, resulting in poor distinction between cortical and medullary bone. When Paget's disease is widely disseminated, the serum alkaline phosphatase level may be elevated. An acute elevation, however, heralds malignant transformation.

About 10% to 35% of patients present with monostotic disease. In the long bones, it begins at the ends of the bones and moves toward the diaphysis. The leading edge represents the osteolytic phase and has been described as having a "blade of grass" appearance. A mixed and sclerotic phase follows resulting in a pattern of disorganization with bone expansion, thickening of the cortex, and trabecular coarsening. The bones are soft and prone to fracture, as in this patient. In the spine, involvement may be monostotic or polyostotic. The thickened cortex produces a classic "picture frame" appearance. Coarsening of the vertical trabeculation, along with the cortical changes, contributes to an increased density of the vertebral body. The lumbar spine and sacrum are the most common sites of involvement in the vertebral column.

Notes

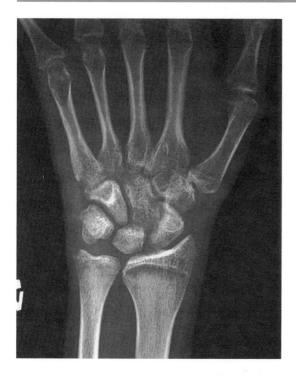

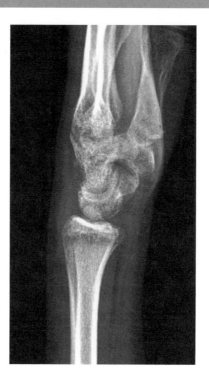

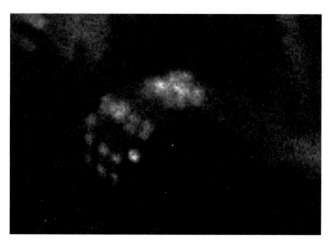

1. What are the radiographic findings and what is the main diagnostic consideration?

2. List the neoplasms that may be associated with this condition.

3. What are the characteristic clinical features of this disorder?

4. What do you see on magnetic resonance imaging?

Reflex Sympathetic Dystrophy

1. Diffuse periarticular osteopenia and soft tissue swelling; reflex sympathetic dystrophy.

2. Malignant tumors of the brain, lung, ovary, breast, pancreas, and bladder.

3. Stiffness, pain, tenderness, and weakness associated with swelling, hyperesthesia, and vasomotor changes.

4. About 50% of patients depict marrow edema during the warm phase, but none do in the cold phase of reflex sympathetic dystrophy.

References

Crozier F, Champsaur P, Pham T, et al: Magnetic resonance imaging in reflex sympathetic dystrophy syndrome of the foot. *Joint Bone Spine* 70:503–508, 2003.

Doury P: Algodystrophy. Reflex sympathetic dystrophy syndrome. *Clin Rheumatol* 7:173–180, 1988.

Cross-Reference

Musculoskeletal Imaging: THE REQUISITES, 3rd ed, pp 394–395.

Comment

Reflex sympathetic dystrophy (RSD), also known as algodystrophy, is a painful condition most commonly caused by trauma. Myocardial infarction, hemiplegia, cerebrovascular accident, disc herniation, surgery, infection, vasculitis, and neoplasms may also elicit this disorder. Although the pathogenesis of RSD is not clear, the most widely accepted theory is that an injury or lesion produces painful impulses that are sent to the spinal cord through afferent pathways establishing a series of reflexes. These reflexes stimulate efferent pathways that travel to the peripheral nerves, producing the findings associated with this condition. There is data that supports the suggestion that RSD is related to overactivity of the sympathetic nervous system. One fourth to one half of cases are bilateral although it tends to affect one side more severely than the other.

There are two phases to the disease: a warm phase associated with pain, stiffness, and vasomotor symptoms, followed by a cold phase, characterized by fibrosis, leading to disabling trophic symptoms. The radiographic findings of this condition are characteristic. Soft tissue swelling and regional osteoporosis are prominent features of the warm phase. Resorption of cancellous or trabecular bone in the metaphyseal region leads to peri-articular osteoporosis. Although this finding may also occur in synovial inflammatory arthropathies, the absence of joint space loss and erosions are notable observations. Bone scintigraphy demonstrates increased radionuclide uptake in an articular distribution caused by increased vascularity of the synovial membrane and bones.

Notes

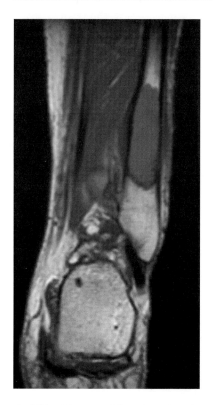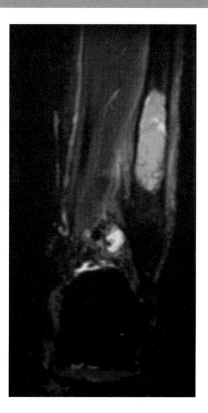

1. This 21-year-old patient has increasing pain and fever. What entities should you consider?

2. What features indicate that this is an aggressive lesion?

3. What are the two least common radiographic presentations of Ewing's sarcoma?

4. Can Ewing's sarcoma be confused with infection clinically?

Ewing's Sarcoma

1. Osteomyelitis, eosinophilic granuloma, Ewing's sarcoma, and intraosseous osteosarcoma.

2. Endosteal scalloping, cortical breakthrough, periostitis, and a soft tissue mass.

3. "Normal" radiographs from diffuse involvement (rare) and a well-marginated lesion (less than 4%).

4. Yes, since fever, leukocytosis, and elevated erythrocyte sedimentation rate may be typical presenting symptoms and signs.

References

Enneking WF: Staging of musculoskeletal neoplasms. *Skeletal Radiol* 13:183–194, 1985.

Ma LD, Frassica FJ, Scott WW, et al: Differentiation of benign and malignant musculoskeletal tumors: Potential pitfalls with MR imaging. *Radiographics* 15:349–366, 1995.

Cross-Reference

Musculoskeletal Imaging: THE REQUISITES, 3rd ed, pp 489–491.

Comment

Ewing's sarcoma is a common malignant tumor of bone. It accounts for about 10% of all primary bone tumors. Nearly 95% of patients are between the ages of 4 and 25 years at presentation, with a peak age between 10 and 15 years. Males are twice as likely to be affected. Pain is the presenting symptom in one half of patients, initially characterized as intermittent but increasing in severity over time. Frequently, patients may present with nonspecific symptoms such as fever, increased erythrocyte sedimentation rate, and leukocytosis, which suggests an infection, or with weight loss and anemia. There may be a significant delay in rendering a diagnosis due to the indolent nature of this tumor early in the disease. As a result, by the time the tumor is discovered, 15% to 30% of patients have evidence of metastases. The pelvis and long bones are involved in 75% of cases, but the spine (usually sacrum) may be involved in 6% of patients.

The magnetic resonance imaging findings demonstrated by this patient are uncommon and represent one of the least common presentations of this tumor, a well-marginated lesion. More typical findings of Ewing's sarcoma are poor margination, permeative or moth-eaten osteolysis, cortical erosion, exuberant periostitis, and a soft tissue mass. Osteosclerosis (mimicking osteosarcoma) and sequestration (mimicking osteomyelitis) can be confusing observations. Radiographs tend to underestimate the size of tumors.

Notes

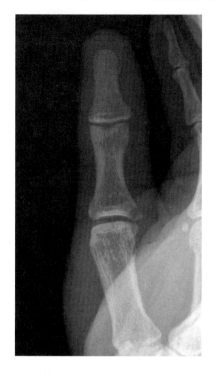 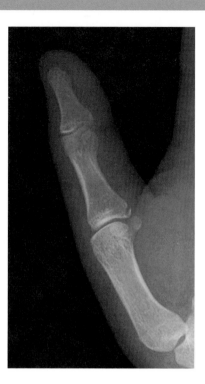

1. What do you call this injury? Define it.

2. How is this injury produced?

3. What is the treatment of choice in this patient? Why is this appropriate?

4. What is a Stener lesion?

Gamekeeper's Thumb

1. Gamekeeper's or skier's thumb. Avulsion of the base of the proximal phalanx of the thumb at the attachment of the ulnar collateral ligament (UCL).

2. Sudden valgus stress with hyperextension, which either disrupts the UCL or causes an avulsion of its osseous insertion.

3. Conservative therapy with immobilization. The UCL is a capsular ligament and nonsurgical management is adequate for healing, as with medial collateral ligament injuries of the knee.

4. The torn end of a ruptured UCL becomes displaced superficially to the adductor pollicis aponeurosis.

Reference

Spaeth HJ, Abrams RA, Bock GW, et al: Gamekeeper thumb: Differentiation of nondisplaced and displaced tears of the ulnar collateral ligament with MR imaging. *Radiology* 188:553–556, 1993.

Cross-Reference

Musculoskeletal Imaging: THE REQUISITES, 3rd ed, pp 159–161.

Comment

An injury to the ulnar collateral ligament (UCL) of the metacarpophalangeal joint of the thumb is termed gamekeeper's or skier's thumb. It accounts for approximately 6% of all skiing injuries but is also a frequent injury in athletic activities such as football, wrestling, baseball, and hockey. In the past, the diagnosis was based on clinical examination and stress radiography. More recently, magnetic resonance imaging has been advocated for evaluation of UCL injuries. When the UCL ruptures, the torn end may become displaced superficially to the adductor pollicis aponeurosis. This complex, called the Stener lesion, may interfere with healing because the interposed aponeurosis prevents apposition of the ligament to the bone. In this situation, surgery has been advocated as the treatment of choice because instability may persist if the injury is left untreated. When the UCL avulses from the base of the proximal phalanx of the thumb, the relative position of the bone fragment may allow differentiation between a nondisplaced tear and a Stener lesion. If radiographic evaluation fails to demonstrate an osseous avulsion, then further evaluation with MRI is recommended to ensure that the ligament is not displaced. Stress radiography is no longer recommended because a nondisplaced tear may convert to a Stener lesion with this maneuver, thus requiring surgical repair.

Notes

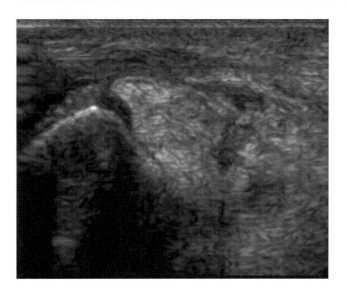 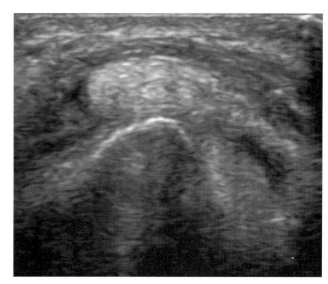

1. You are shown transverse sonograms of the peroneal tendons in neutral position and then with the ankle everted and dorsiflexed. The right side of the images is posterior. What is the diagnosis?

2. Why do you think this occurred in this patient? How does it appear?

3. Is this a common abnormality? How is it treated?

4. What is the best method for diagnosing this disorder?

Peroneus Longus Tendon Dislocation

1. Dislocation of the peroneus longus tendon.

2. There is a tear of the superior peroneal retinaculum anteriorly. Hypoechoic defect of the retinaculum anteriorly.

3. It is relatively uncommon, seen in only 0.3% to 0.5% of ankle trauma. Surgery.

4. Dynamic sonography or kinematic magnetic resonance imaging are the preferred techniques for diagnosis.

References

Fessel DP, van Holsbeeck MT: Ultrasound of the foot and ankle. *Semin Musculoskelet Radiol* 2:271–282, 1998.

Neustadter J, Raikin SM, Nazarian LN: Dynamic sonographic evaluation of peroneal tendon subluxation. *AJR Am J Roentgenol* 183:985–988, 2004.

Cross-Reference

Musculoskeletal Imaging: THE REQUISITES, 3rd ed, pp 252 and 267.

Comment

The peroneus longus and peroneus brevis tendons function as evertors of the foot and dynamic stabilizers of the lateral ankle. Plantar flexion of the ankle and pronation and abduction of the foot are additional functions. The peroneus brevis tendon descends anteromedial to the peroneus longus tendon at the level of the common peroneal sheath, which begins 4 cm proximal to the lateral malleolus. This sheath passes through a fibro-osseous tunnel that is stabilized posterolaterally by the superior peroneal retinaculum; medially by the posterior talofibular ligament, calcaneofibular ligament, and posteroinferior tibiofibular ligament; and anteriorly by the fibular groove. Peroneal tendon subluxation/dislocation is an uncommon sequela of ankle trauma and can involve one or both tendons. Most cases are related to tears of the superior peroneal retinaculum although a flattened fibular groove can also predispose to this condition. The mechanism of injury in acute subluxation is a sudden passive dorsiflexion and eversion of the ankle, which is followed by a reflexive contraction of the peroneal muscles. In chronic subluxation, the development of a lax and incompetent superior peroneal retinaculum may cause a snapping sensation and lateral pain. Dynamic sonography is the best method for diagnosis, because many patients present with transient subluxation. Imaging in the provocative position shows movement of one or both hyperechoic tendons anteriorly, over the fibula. The superior peroneal retinaculum can be evaluated and hypoechoic or anechoic defects are diagnostic of tears.

Notes

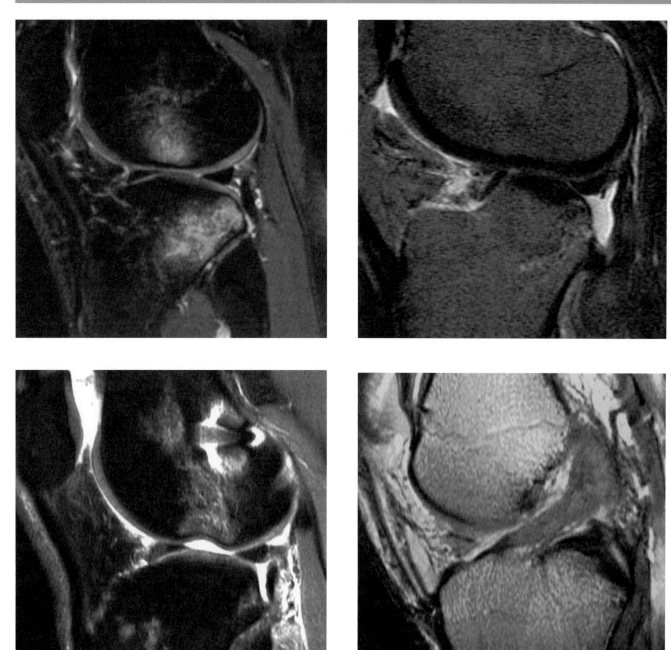

Match the sign with its name; then give its definition.

1. What is this sign called?

2. What is this sign called?

3. What is this sign called?

4. What is this sign called?

Indirect Signs of ACL Tear

1. Rotary contusion pattern. Edema in the lateral notch and posterolateral tibia.

2. Exposed lateral meniscus sign. Posterior displacement of the lateral meniscus exceeding 3.5 mm.

3. Deep notch sign. A lateral condylopatellar sulcus deeper than 1.5 mm. (Did you notice the exposed meniscus sign also?)

4. Anterior cruciate ligament (ACL) angle sign. An angle with Blumenstaat's line exceeding 15 degrees.

References

Gentili A, Seeger LL, Yao L, Do HM: Anterior cruciate ligament tear: Indirect signs at MR imaging. *Radiology* 193:835–840, 1994.

McCauley TR, Moses M, Kier R, et al: MR diagnosis of tears of anterior cruciate ligament of the knee: Importance of ancillary findings. *AJR Am J Roentgenol* 162:115–119, 1994.

Cross-Reference

Musculoskeletal Imaging: THE REQUISITES, 3rd ed, pp 233–237.

Comment

In the setting of acute trauma to the knee, bone marrow edema visualized on MR images in the lateral femoral condyle and posterolateral tibia is nearly pathognomonic of a complete ACL tear. This contusion pattern occurs when the femur externally rotates on a fixed tibia, allowing impaction of the articular surface of the lateral femoral condyle against the posterolateral aspect of the tibia when the ACL ruptures. This frequently produces an impaction fracture of the lateral femoral condyle at the lateral condylopatellar sulcus region. When the lateral condylopatellar sulcus depth exceeds 1.5 mm, it is called a deep lateral notch sign. The buckled posterior cruciate ligament sign is produced when there is anterior translation of the tibia and is positive when the angle is less than 107 degrees. A positive ACL angle sign is defined as an angle subtended by the anteromedial ACL bundle and Blumenstaat's line exceeding 15 degrees. When the posterior edge of the lateral meniscus hangs over the posterior edge of the tibia by more than 3.5 mm, it is referred to as a positive exposed or displaced lateral meniscus sign. There are several other abnormalities that, when visualized, should prompt close inspection of the ACL; these include a chip fracture of the posterolateral cortex of the proximal tibia created by shearing forces during subluxation of the femur, an avulsion of the anterior tibia at the attachment of the ACL, and an avulsion of the lateral tibial cortex (Segond fracture).

Notes

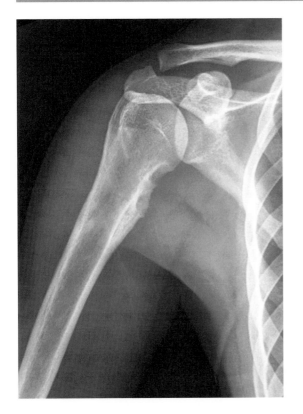

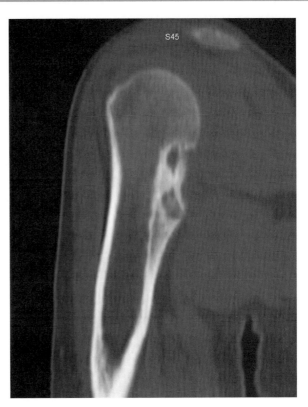

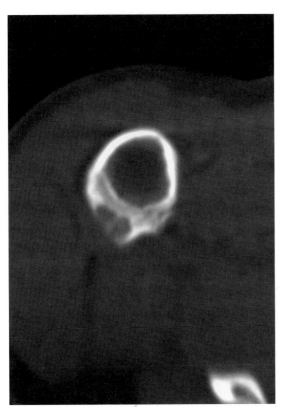

1. What do you observe and what lesions would you consider?

2. List some observations that do not support a diagnosis of osteosarcoma.

3. What is the single most important feature that suggests benignity?

4. Are these lesions more common in flat bones or tubular bones?

Periosteal (Juxtacortical) Chondroma

1. Saucerization of the bone; periosteal chondroma, periosteal chondrosarcoma, parosteal osteosarcoma, periosteal desmoid, benign osteoblastoma, neurofibroma, and subperiosteal hemangioma.

2. The absence of radiating osseous spicules that extend into the soft tissues excludes periosteal osteosarcoma; smoothness of the cortical saucerization and absence of pedunculated mass excludes parosteal osteosarcoma.

3. Size. Periosteal chondrosarcomas usually are larger than benign chondromas.

4. They occur exclusively in tubular bones.

References

Robinson P, White LM, Sundaram M, et al: Periosteal chondroid tumors: Radiologic evaluation with pathologic correlation. *AJR Am J Roentgenol* 177:1183–1188, 2001.

Woertler K, Blasius S, Brinkschmidt C, et al: Periosteal chondroma: MR characteristics. *J Comput Assist Tomogr* 25:425–430, 2001.

Cross-Reference

Musculoskeletal Imaging: THE REQUISITES, 3rd ed, pp 450–452 and 454.

Comment

A periosteal chondroma is a benign neoplasm that occurs in the surface of tubular bones, characteristically in the metaphysis. The lesion is slow growing and ranges from 1 cm to 7 cm at presentation (average is less than 3 cm). Most patients are in their third and fourth decades of life. Radiographically, the classic appearance is a single cartilaginous mass in the metaphyseal periosteum causing a well-defined depression or "saucerization" of the adjacent cortex. Calcifications occur in about 50% of cases. On magnetic resonance imaging, the lesions are typically polylobulated and show a low signal intensity rim. Peritumoral edema is typically absent but if observed, you should be concerned that the lesion may be a periosteal low-grade chondrosarcoma. On T1W images, lesions depict hypo- to isointense signal intensity to muscle and hyperintensity to fat on T2W images. Areas of calcification show low signal intensity on all pulse sequences. Administration of contrast depicts peripheral enhancement. Histologically, the lesion comprises lobules of hyaline cartilage with frequent areas of hypercellularity, binucleate chondrocytes, and focal mild cytologic atypia. Peripheral fibrovascular bundles surrounding the lobules are responsible for peripheral enhancement.

Notes

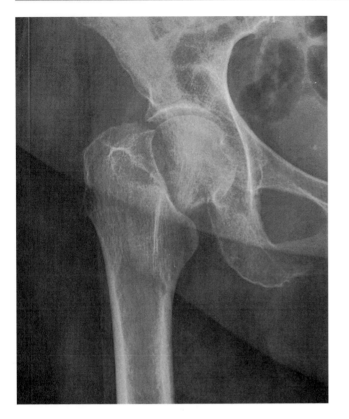 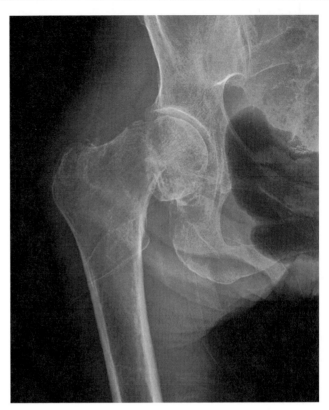

1. These two images were taken 3 days apart. What has happened?

2. How would you classify this injury?

3. What vessels supply the femoral head?

4. Does this patient have a high risk for developing avascular necrosis of the femoral head? Why?

Subcapital Femur Fracture

1. The subcapital femur fracture has become displaced.

2. Garden type III.

3. Medial and lateral epiphyseal arteries and the artery of the ligamentum teres.

4. Yes. Subcapital fractures are at highest risk and the more angulated the fracture, the more likely it is that avascular necrosis will develop.

Reference

Yu JS: Hip and femur trauma: Imaging of trauma to the extremities. *Semin Musculoskeletal Radiol* 4:205–220, 2000.

Cross-Reference

Musculoskeletal Imaging: THE REQUISITES, 3rd ed, pp 196–198.

Comment

Subcapital fractures occur just distal to the articular margin of the femoral head. Fractures that occur through the neck are referred to as transcervical fractures and those that occur at the junction of the neck and the shaft are referred to as basicervical. Two important potential complications of subcapital fractures include nonunion and avascular necrosis of the femoral head. The more proximal the fracture line, the greater the incidence of both complications. The femoral head is supplied by three terminal arterial sources. The main arterial supply of the adult femoral head originates from the medial and lateral femoral circumflex arteries, which may arise from either the femoral artery or the deep femoral artery. At the base of the femoral neck, terminal branches of the medial circumflex artery (medial epiphyseal artery) and lateral circumflex artery (lateral epiphyseal artery) converge to form a vascular ring that supplies numerous ascending cervical arterial vessels. The artery of the ligamentum teres also contributes blood supply to the femoral head epiphyseal region. The leading factors contributing to the development of avascular necrosis of the femoral head are disruption of the epiphyseal arteries or the vessels that supply these terminal vessels, and an unstable reduction of a fracture. Angulated and displaced neck fractures tether these end-arteries, disrupting the blood supply. The most common classification for intracapsular hip fractures is the *Garden classification* (four stages): I, incomplete or impacted fracture; II, complete fracture without displacement; III, complete fracture with varus angulation; and IV, complete fracture with total displacement.

Notes

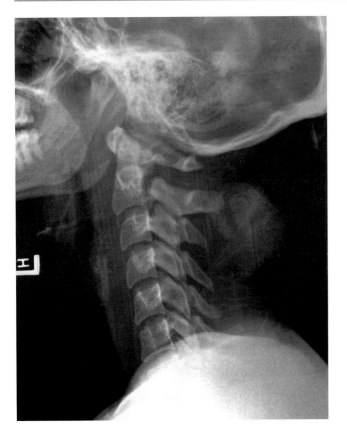
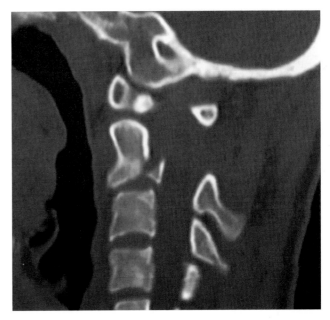

1. What is the diagnosis?

2. What is the Effendi classification?

3. What does anterior displacement of C2 on C3 indicate? Is it unstable?

4. Reportedly, what percentage of people present with neurologic deficits?

Hangman's Fracture

1. Hangman's fracture.

2. Classification of hangman's fractures based on the relationship of C2 on C3.

3. Damage to the C2 disk and anterior longitudinal ligament. Yes.

4. Ten percent.

Reference

Effendi B, Roy D, Cornish B, et al: Fractures of the ring of the axis. *J Bone Joint Surg* 63-B:319–327, 1981.

Cross-Reference

Musculoskeletal Imaging: THE REQUISITES, 3rd ed, pp 170–171.

Comment

Bilateral fractures of the neural arch of C2 are called a *hangman's fracture*. It is usually caused by a hyperextension injury, although flexion-compression and flexion-distraction injuries occasionally may cause this fracture. The vast majority of these fractures are caused by motor vehicle accidents. Because there is no encroachment of the spinal canal, neurologic deficits are uncommon in this injury and generally are not permanent. Hangman's fractures have been classified by Effendi et al. into three types, based on the relationship of C2 on C3. In type 1 fractures, there is no forward displacement of C2 on C3 and the fractures involve only the posterior elements. In type 2 fractures, there is anterior displacement of C2 on C3 exceeding 3 mm or with a 15-degree angulation. In type 3 fractures, there is anterior displacement of both anterior and posterior fragments. Generally, both type 2 and 3 require halo immobilization. Other fractures of the cervical spine also are common in patients with a hangman's fracture. Fractures of the C1 arch occur in 15% of cases, fractures of the body of C2 (as in this patient) occur in another 15% of cases, and 10% of patients also have a fracture in the thoracic spine.

Notes

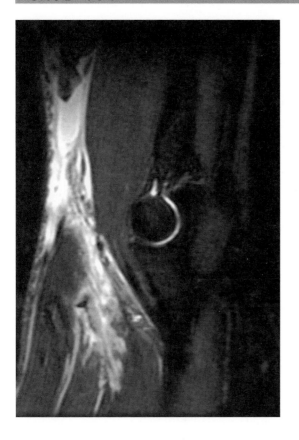
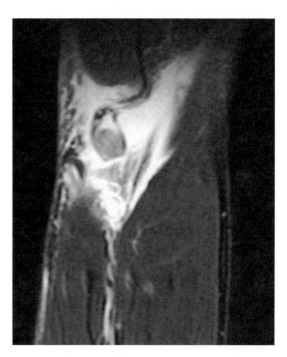
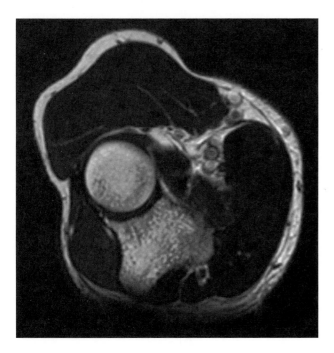
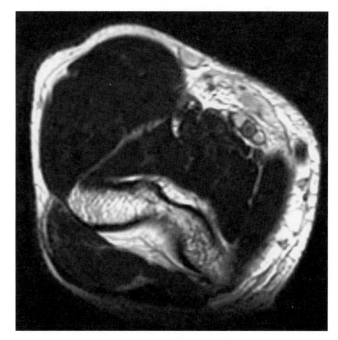

1. What is the injury?

2. How is this injury sustained?

3. Is this a common location for this injury?

4. What information should you report?

Biceps Tendon Avulsion

1. Avulsion of the biceps tendon from the bicipital tuberosity of the proximal radius.

2. Forced hyperextension of a flexed elbow or forced flexion against resistance.

3. Yes, most occur at the radial insertion.

4. Location of rupture, degree of retraction, integrity of biceps aponeurosis, and presence of hematoma.

Reference

Jorgensen U, Hinge K, Rye B: Rupture of the distal biceps brachii tendon. *J Trauma* 26:1061–1062, 1986.

Cross-Reference

Musculoskeletal Imaging: THE REQUISITES, 3rd ed, pp 129–130.

Comment

The biceps brachii muscle originates from two locations on the scapula, the supraglenoid tubercle and the tip of the coracoid process, and inserts on the bicipital tuberosity of the proximal radius. Its primary action is flexion of the elbow joint but it also contributes to supination of the forearm. Magnetic resonance imaging is the preferred method for evaluating ruptures of the biceps tendon. When it occurs, patients complain of a tearing sensation and pain in the antecubital space, most frequently when lifting a heavy object. On examination, there is ecchymosis of the anterior arm about the elbow, tenderness in the antecubital fossa, and proximal retraction with flexion of the elbow. Weakening of elbow flexion and supination are notable findings.

On magnetic resonance imaging, the abnormality may be observed in the coronal, sagittal, and transaxial planes. On sagittal images, there is often a gap between the avulsed tendon and bicipital tuberosity. On T2W images, edema in and around the tendon may be noted and the gap may be filled with fluid. On transaxial images, absence of the distal tendon just proximal to the bicipital tuberosity and interstitial edema in the soft tissues confirm the diagnosis. More proximally, there may be intense edema around a thickened tendon between the brachioradialis and brachialis muscles, as well as distally, anterior to the supinator muscle. Treatment is primary reattachment of the biceps tendon to the tuberosity within the first few days of the injury.

Notes

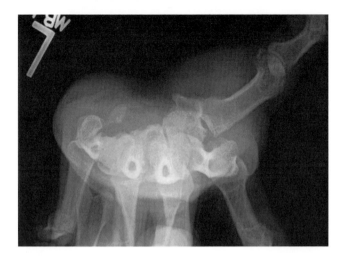

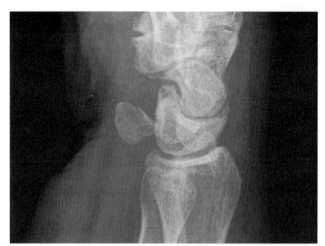

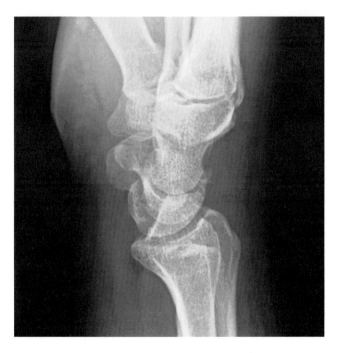

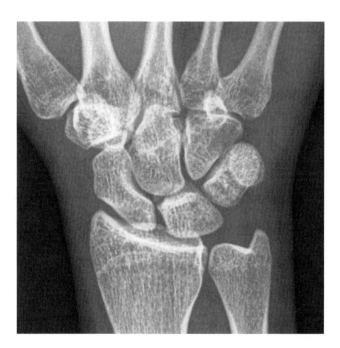

You are shown radiographs from four different patients.

1. What is the diagnosis?

2. What is the diagnosis?

3. What is the diagnosis?

4. What is the diagnosis?

C A S E   1 0 5

Subtle Wrist Fractures/Injuries

1. Displaced hamate hook fracture.

2. Dislocated pisiform.

3. Triquetral chip fracture.

4. Lunate fracture.

References

Goldfarb CA, Yin Y, Gilula LA, et al: Wrist fractures: What the clinician wants to know. *Radiology* 219:11–28, 2001.

Vigler M, Aviles A, Lee SK: Carpal fractures excluding the scaphoid. *Hand Clin* 22:501–516, 2006.

Cross-Reference

Musculoskeletal Imaging: THE REQUISITES, 3rd ed, pp 143–150.

Comment

Fractures of the carpus frequently involve multiple bones or a single bone in association with significant ligamentous injury. Many of these injuries are difficult to identify radiographically unless films are closely scrutinized. A dedicated approach to every film (particularly frontal and lateral views) should include identification of soft tissue swelling, carpal alignment, joint integrity, and cortical defects with particular attention to the zones of vulnerability. Secondary soft tissue signs such as the scaphoid and pronator quadratus fat stripes, and peristyloid soft tissue distension are useful when positive in increasing the index of suspicion.

Triquetral fractures are the second most common bone injury in the carpus after the scaphoid. Most are dorsal avulsion injuries at the ulnotriquetral ligament insertion or chip fractures from direct impaction against the dorsal lip of the radius and are best seen in the lateral view. Fractures of the body may be vertical or transverse and are best seen on oblique views. Lunate fractures are usually from a fall on an outstretched hand with compression. They are extremely difficult to identify on radiographs and generally require cross-sectional imaging modalities for confirmation. Hamate hook fractures occur from direct trauma or an avulsion. This is a common injury in racquet sports. Pisiform injuries are usually from a direct blow resulting in a linear or comminuted fracture or rupture of the flexor carpi ulnaris tendon.

Notes

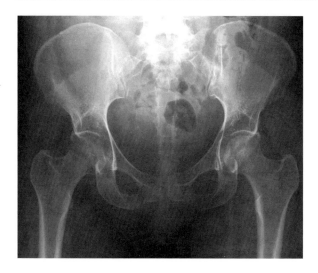
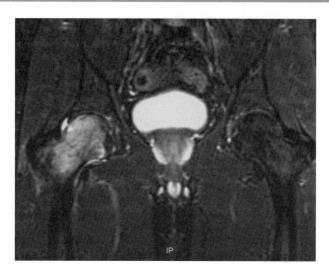

1. What is the differential diagnosis?

2. This 40-year-old man had sudden onset of right hip pain without trauma. What is the most likely disorder?

3. What should you recommend?

4. If an arcuate low signal intensity abnormality paralleling the superior cortex of the femoral head develops over time, what is the most likely condition? Will it resolve?

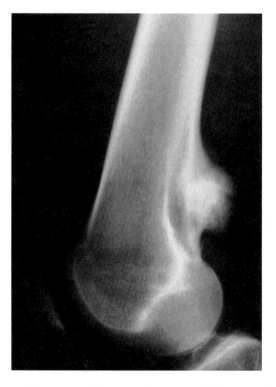
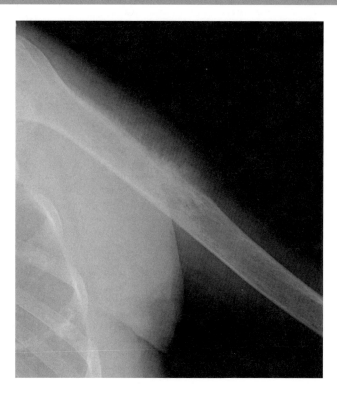

1. These two films are from two different patients. What is their commonality?

2. What is the differential diagnosis for the first patient?

3. Which is more aggressive?

4. What is the prognosis of each lesion?

Transient Osteoporosis of the Hip

1. Transient osteoporosis of the hip, regional migratory osteoporosis, osteonecrosis, bone contusion, infiltrative neoplasm, and transient bone edema syndrome.

2. Transient osteoporosis of the hip.

3. Sequential magnetic resonance imaging studies.

4. An insufficiency fracture of the femoral head. If it is thicker than 4 mm or longer than 12 mm, it will not resolve spontaneously.

Reference

Beltran J, Opsha O: MR imaging of the hip: Osseous lesions. *Magn Reson Imaging Clin N Am* 13:665–676, 2005.

Cross-Reference

Musculoskeletal Imaging: THE REQUISITES, 3rd ed, pp 354, 393–394.

Comment

Transient osteoporosis of the hip is a painful hip condition that affects most frequently middle-aged men and pregnant women. It is characterized by a sudden onset of severe hip pain in the absence of trauma and in people with no risk factors for avascular necrosis. It is a self-limiting process that usually reverses within several months of onset with conservative therapy but may last as long as 9 or 10 months. Radiographically, the affected hip appears diminished in bone density compared with the asymptomatic hip. This is particularly conspicuous in the femoral head and in the region of the tensile and compressive trabeculation of the neck. Magnetic resonance imaging depicts low signal intensity on T1W images and high signal intensity on fluid sensitive images within the marrow of the femoral head and neck, indicating the presence of edema. Administration of gadolinium solution shows diffuse enhancement of the abnormal marrow. A joint effusion is common. In some patients, transient osteoporosis of the hip may be a manifestation of regional migratory osteoporosis, which affects multiple consecutive joints.

Notes

Surface Osteogenic Sarcomas

1. Both patients have a surface osteosarcoma. The first patient has parosteal osteosarcoma and the second has periosteal osteosarcoma.

2. Myositis ossificans, parosteal osteosarcoma, juxtacortical chondroma and chondrosarcoma, and osteochondroma.

3. Periosteal osteosarcoma.

4. Both have better prognosis than conventional osteogenic sarcoma until there is marrow invasion, at which time the prognosis becomes the same as for conventional osteosarcoma.

References

Murphey MD, Robbin MR, McRae GA, et al: The many faces of osteosarcoma. *Radiographics* 17:1205–1231, 1997.

Yu JS, Weis LD: MR imaging of parosteal osteosarcoma in two skeletally immature patients. *Clin Imaging* 21:63–68, 1997.

Cross-Reference

Musculoskeletal Imaging: THE REQUISITES, 3rd ed, pp 435–439.

Comment

A parosteal osteogenic sarcoma (POS) is a slow-growing malignant tumor of bone arising from the periosseous tissues adjacent to the cortex. It accounts for 1.7% of all bone tumors and 4% of osteosarcomas. The most common location is about the knee (70% of cases), with a predilection for the posterior surface of the distal femur. Generally, medical attention is sought after a long duration of symptoms, which include localized or painful swelling, development of a mass, joint dysfunction, or joint pain. POS has a relatively good prognosis if it is detected before significant extension into the medullary cavity. POS is frequently detected in the third and fourth decades of life, although 10% to 25% of lesions occur in patients who are under 19 years of age. POS presents as an osteoblastic, exophitic mass arising from the surface of the bone. As it enlarges, the tumor has a tendency to encircle the bone resulting in a thin radiolucent zone that separates the tumor from the underlying bone. The cortex usually does not become invaded until late in the course of the disease.

Periosteal osteosarcoma is rare and presents in the second or third decade of life. The appearance is that of a scalloped lesion in the diaphysis of the femur or tibia, with a circumferential soft tissue mass that produces spicules of bone that give a sunburst pattern of periostitis. A Codman's triangle is not unusual.

Notes

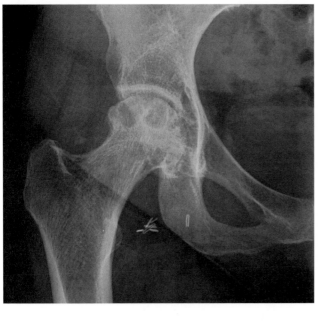
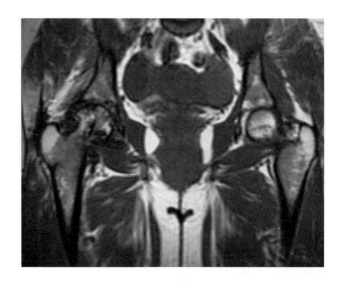
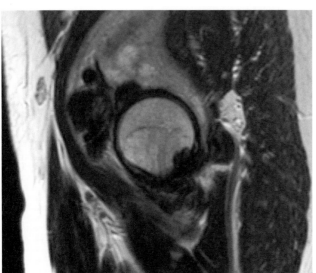
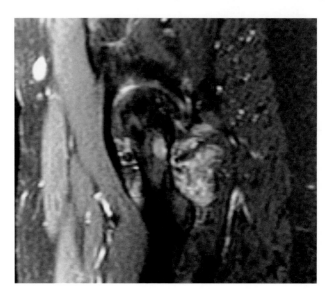

1. What is your differential diagnosis based on the hip radiograph? Do the magnetic resonance images help narrow the differential diagnosis?

2. What is a characteristic symptom of this disorder?

3. Histologically, what is peculiar about this process?

4. Would you advocate radiation therapy for treatment?

Pigmented Villonodular Synovitis

1. Pigmented villonodular synovitis (PVNS), synovial chondromatosis, amyloidosis, and, occasionally, hemophilia, gout, and synovial sarcoma. Yes, hemosiderin implicates PVNS.

2. Recurrent serosanguinous joint effusions.

3. Mitotic figures may be seen in proliferating fibroblasts, macrophages, and synovial cells.

4. Radiation therapy is generally reserved for older patients and recurrences, although long-term results are equivalent to surgery.

References

Bancroft LW, Peterson JJ, Kransdorf MJ: MR imaging of tumors and tumor-like lesions of the hip. *Magn Reson Imaging Clin N Am* 13:757–774, 2005.

Dorwart RH, Genant HK, Johnston WH, Morris JM: Pigmented villonodular synovitis of synovial joints: Clinical, pathologic, and radiologic features. *AJR Am J Roentgenol* 143:877–885, 1984.

Cross-Reference

Musculoskeletal Imaging: THE REQUISITES, 3rd ed, pp 503–507.

Comment

PVNS is a diffuse synovial proliferative disorder that affects the joints, bursae, and tendon sheaths. It is a monoarticular process of unknown etiology and 50% of patients affected are younger than 40 years of age. Nearly 80% of PVNS cases occur in the knee joint. Symptoms are generally long in duration, characterized by recurrent joint effusions, decreased range of motion, and joint locking. Grossly, the lesion appears brown owing to the extensive hemosiderin deposition. Radiographically, periarticular soft tissue swelling may be evident with an associated joint effusion. As the disease progresses, synovial hypertrophy and erosions become more evident as well as subchondral cysts. Intra-articular calcification is absent. Periarticular osteopenia is a late finding, as is joint space narrowing. Juxta-articular erosions are typical, particularly in the hip, elbow, and wrist joints. On magnetic resonance imaging, low signal intensity mass(es) on all pulse sequences owing to hemosiderin in the synovium is/are notable, especially on gradient-recalled images. This process becomes more diffuse as the disease progresses to involve the entire joint. The differential diagnosis on magnetic resonance imaging includes gout, amyloid, and synovitis of infection early in the disease. Treatment is with surgical resection of the synovium through an open arthrotomy if diffuse, or arthroscopically if the disease is more focal.

Notes

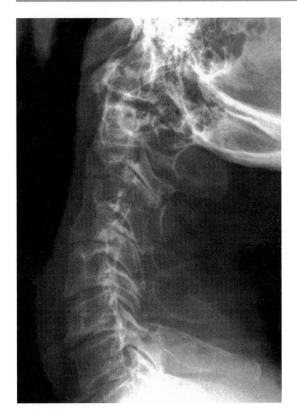

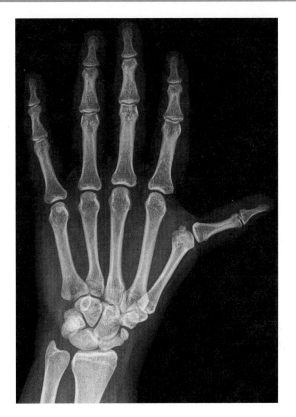

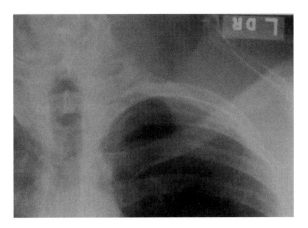

1. What is the diagnosis?

2. What does the shoulder radiograph show?

3. In the spine, what is the risk for neurologic sequelae?

4. What do you see in the hand?

Klippel-Feil Syndrome

1. Klippel-Feil syndrome.

2. Sprengel's deformity.

3. Low. Neurologic sequelae are more commonly seen with hypermobility of the upper cervical from fusion of the lower segments. In this patient, degenerative disc disease is the most likely complication.

4. Hypoplasia of the first metacarpal bone and navicular.

References

Pizzutillo PD, Woods M, Nicholson L, MacEwen GD: Risk factors in Klippel-Feil syndrome. *Spine* 19:2110–2116, 1994.

Tracy MR, Dormans JP, Kusumi K: Klippel-Feil syndrome: Clinical features and current understanding of etiology. *Clin Orthop Relat Res* 424:183–190, 2004.

Cross-Reference

Musculoskeletal Imaging: THE REQUISITES, 3rd ed, pp 594–595.

Comment

Klippel-Feil syndrome is a congenital disorder characterized by failure of cervical segmentation at multiple levels. Patients have a short neck with a low hairline, and limited cervical motion. Scoliosis, spina bifida, and rib anomalies can also occur. It is associated with numerous abnormalities affecting the renal (unilateral renal ectopia, agenesis, horseshoe), nervous (Chiari malformation, meningocele), and vascular (persistent trigeminal artery, aneurysms) systems and deafness from abnormalities of the inner, middle, and outer ear (Mondini's malformation, aplasia). Additionally, one third of patients have a Sprengel's deformity, which is caused by tethering of the scapula to the cervical spine by a fibrous band or an anomalous bone (omovertebral bone). As a result, the scapula has an elevated position and the shoulder is limited in motion. In the thumb, anomalies such as hypoplasia, abnormal segmentation (triphalangeal thumb), and polydactyly are also manifestations that are common.

Notes

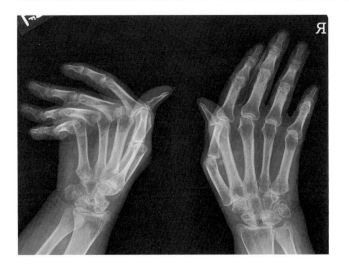
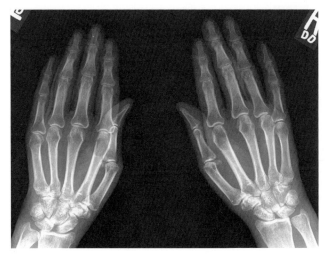

1. Both films were done on the same day. What is the diagnosis? What else could you consider?

2. What percentage of patients with this disease have arthralgia or arthritis? What is characteristic about the arthritis?

3. What are other target organs of this disease?

4. Is the risk of osteonecrosis in patients treated after corticosteroid therapy similar to other arthropathies?

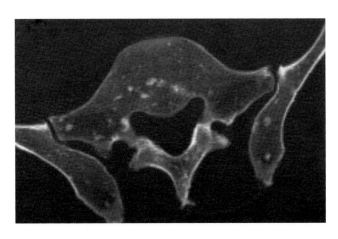
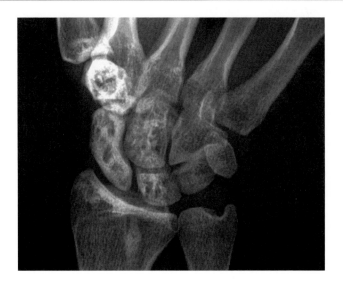

1. Is there a differential diagnosis?

2. What is a common cutaneous lesion associated with this disorder and how frequently is this seen?

3. What other disorders have an association with this condition?

4. What does each lesion represent histologically?

Systemic Lupus Erythematosus

1. Arthropathy of systemic lupus erythematosus. Jaccoud's arthropathy and rheumatoid arthritis.

2. Nearly 95%. Nonerosive but inflammatory.

3. Renal, thorax (pleura, pericardium), and neurologic and hematologic organs.

4. No, it is much higher (four- to fivefold increase).

References

Cronin ME: Musculoskeletal manifestations of systemic lupus erythematosus. *Rheum Dis Clin North Am* 14: 99–116, 1988.

Leskinen RH, Skrifvars BV, Laasonen LS, Edgren KJ: Bone lesions in systemic lupus erythematosus. *Radiology* 153:349–352, 1984.

Cross-Reference

Musculoskeletal Imaging: THE REQUISITES, 3rd ed, pp 328–329.

Comment

Systemic lupus erythematosus (SLE) is a collagen vascular disorder that is common in females. Females are 5 to 10 times more likely to be affected by SLE, and it is more common in blacks than in whites. Nearly 95% of patients manifest joint pain and the proximal interphalangeal, metacarpophalangeal, wrist, and knee joints are most frequently involved. In some patients, the clinical presentation is similar to rheumatoid arthritis, with the notable difference of frequent remissions and exacerbations without residual deformation of the joint and the discrepancy between severe symptoms that is associated with few radiographic abnormalities.

Radiographically, the arthropathy of SLE is classified as a nonerosive inflammatory arthropathy. Soft tissue swelling and periarticular osteopenia are typical. Deformities of the digits without erosions such as swan neck or boutonniere deformities, hyperextension of the interphalangeal joints of the thumbs, ulnar deviation, and joint subluxation are common. Ligament laxity contributes to these deformities, which can be reduced on a typical posteroanterior radiographic position of the hands seen on the second image of this patient. In the distal phalanx, there may be tuft resorption or localized areas of sclerosis (acral sclerosis). Soft tissue calcifications occur in 7% of cases.

Notes

Osteopoikilosis

1. Osteopoikilosis, epiphyseal dysplasia, melorheostosis, osteoblastic metastasis, and, rarely, sclerotic form of multiple myeloma and sarcoidosis.

2. Dermatofibrosis lenticularis disseminata; 25% of cases.

3. Scleroderma, cleft palate, dwarfism, syndactyly, endocrine disorders, melorheostosis, and dystocia.

4. A focus of lamellar bone containing haversian systems.

Reference

Lagier R, Mbakop A, Bigler A: Osteopoikilosis: A radiological and pathological study. *Skeletal Radiol* 11: 161–168, 1984.

Cross-Reference

Musculoskeletal Imaging: THE REQUISITES, 3rd ed, pp 629–630.

Comment

Osteopoikilosis is a rare bone dysplasia characterized by the presence of numerous round or oval foci of compact bone within the spongiosa. The etiology is unknown although a familial occurrence has been reported, believed to be transmitted as an autosomal dominant. This disorder may become evident at any age and has no sexual predilection. Clinically, the manifestations are usually mild or absent. The radiographic findings in this case are characteristic of osteopoikilosis. Small, numerous well-defined areas of sclerosis measuring a few millimeters to several centimeters in size are the principal finding. These lesions tend to cluster in a periarticular distribution with a predilection for the epiphysis and metaphysis of a bone. Lesions also commonly involve the carpus, tarsus, pelvis, and scapula. Involvement of the skull, clavicle, ribs, mandible, sternum, and vertebral bodies are unusual. Bone scintigraphy usually shows no radionuclide uptake except on rare occasions. The differential diagnosis is limited when you consider the symmetric distribution, clustering about the joints, and uniformity of the size of lesions, which are distinctive features not present in other disorders. In this patient's wrist, there is likely an overlap with melorheostosis because there is cortical thickening of the second metacarpal bone.

Notes

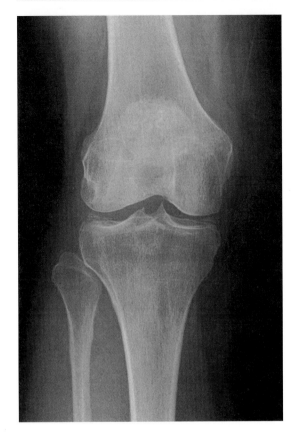 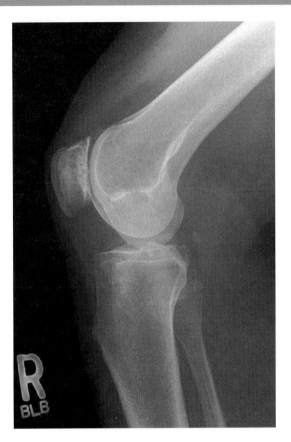

1. What is the best diagnosis?

2. What specific finding led you to come to this conclusion?

3. Where is this arthritis most commonly detected?

4. Describe "rapidly progressive osteoarthritis."

CPPD (Pyrophosphate) Arthropathy

1. Calcium pyrophosphate dihydrate (CPPD) deposition arthropathy.

2. Disproportionate involvement of the patellofemoral joint and meniscal chondrocalcinosis.

3. Knee, wrist, and second and third MCP joints.

4. Condition (usually in the hip) characterized by rapid development of degenerative changes depicted by extensive subchondral bone collapse and fragmentation, eburnation, joint space loss, and joint disorganization that often mimics neuroarthropathy. It is a misnomer because it represents a form of pyrophosphate arthropathy, not osteoarthritis.

Reference

Rubenstein J, Pritzke KPH: Crystal-associated arthropathies. *AJR Am J Roentgenol* 152:685–695, 1989.

Cross-Reference

Musculoskeletal Imaging: THE REQUISITES, 3rd ed, pp 339–342.

Comment

There are two important observations in this patient: chondrocalcinosis and disproportionate involvement of the patellofemoral joint. Note that the medial and lateral compartments are not narrowed. Calcium pyrophosphate dihydrate (CPPD) crystals can accumulate both in and around joints and affect the articular cartilage, synovium, capsule, tendons, and ligaments. When it occurs in fibrocartilaginous tissues, such as the menisci of the knee, triangular fibrocartilage of the wrist, labrum of the hip, and annular ligaments of the spine, the calcifications tend to appear thick, shaggy, and irregular but often conform to the shape of the structure that they occupy. This is in contradistinction to hydroxyapatite crystal deposition, which tends to be dense and chunky, and is often described as "cloudlike." Synovial deposition of CPPD crystals may appear irregular, whereas capsular calcifications are either linear or irregular. In the articular hyaline cartilage, calcifications appear thin, and parallel the contour of the bony articular surface. Tendinous and ligamentous calcifications also have a characteristic appearance of thin, linear radiodense strands that often extend for a considerable distance from the bone.

Acute goutlike presentations are referred to as *pseudogout*, manifested by joint inflammation, pain, and redness. Although early disease shows erosive change, more advanced disease appears primarily productive with sclerosis, osteochondral fragments, and osteophytes resembling osteoarthritis. The distinctive finding is the location of the abnormalities and the presence of large subchondral cysts, such as in the patellofemoral joint in the knee.

Notes

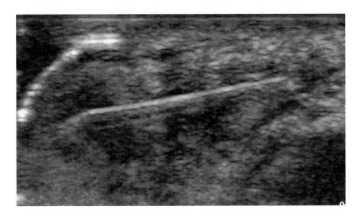 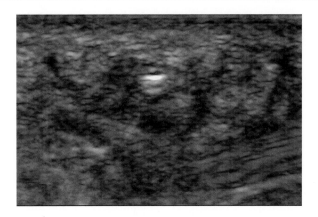

You are shown longitudinal and transverse sonograms of the foot in a patient with pain.

1. What are the findings?

2. What is the diagnosis?

3. What sonographic manifestation is seen deep to the linear abnormality?

4. What should be done next?

Foreign Body—Wood Splinter

1. A linear, echogenic structure with acoustic shadowing within heterogenously hypoechoic soft tissues.

2. Foreign body with abscess formation.

3. Posterior reverberation artifact deep to the wood splinter.

4. Incision and drainage, and removal of the foreign body.

References

Horton LK, Jacobson JA, Powell A, et al: Sonography and radiography of soft-tissue foreign bodies. *AJR Am J Roentgenol* 175:1155–1159, 2001.

Peterson JJ, Bancroft LW, Kransdorf MJ: Wooden foreign bodies: Imaging appearance. *AJR Am J Roentgenol* 178:557–562, 2002.

Cross-Reference

Musculoskeletal Imaging: THE REQUISITES, 3rd ed, pp 47–48.

Comment

Wood particles are ubiquitous, and despite advances in numerous imaging techniques, the ability to visualize retained wooden foreign bodies in the soft tissues remains a difficult task. In the absence of a history of penetrating injury, the diagnosis may be delayed months to years. When there is a high index of suspicion of a retained foreign body, localization of the body is challenging. Even if patients have extracted the wood splinter at the time of injury, frequently, fragmented particles remain. The most common presentation is a painful swollen soft tissue mass or pseudotumor. Wood is porous and organic, and serves as an ideal nidus for infection, and retained particles can lead to cellulitis, abscess formation, or a fistula. Sonography is the best modality for detecting retained wooden foreign bodies and has been shown to be both sensitive and specific. There is a marked difference in the impedance of wood and soft tissues so that the leading edge of the wood appears hyperechoic, resulting in marked acoustic shadowing. Magnetic resonance imaging and computed tomography, though commonly used in the initial evaluation of possible foreign bodies, have been shown to be significantly less effective than sonography in identifying retained wooden particles. On MR imaging, wood appears low in signal intensity and is usually surrounded by nonspecific granulation tissue of variable intensity. On CT, wood usually shows a linear area of increased attenuation.

Notes

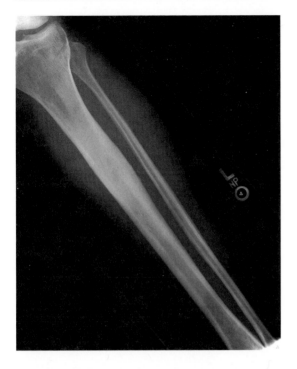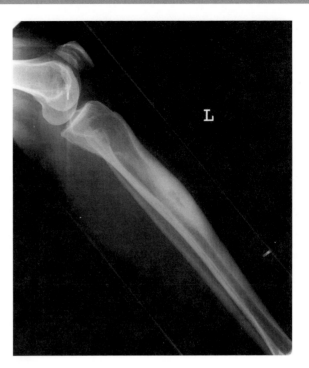

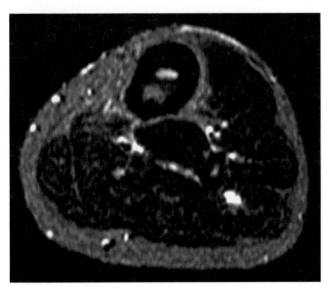

1. List the entities that you would consider.

2. What is sclerosing osteitis of Garre?

3. What percentage of patients with this abnormality develop a sequestrum? Is it more common in adults or children?

4. If this lesion is identified in a child, what should you look for?

Brodie's Abscess

1. Brodie's abscess, fibrous dysplasia, adamantinoma, and ossifying fibroma. On initial radiographic inspection, you may consider stress fracture and osteoid osteoma but the MR findings exclude them.

2. Uncommon manifestation of a low-grade infection, which causes a sclerotic reaction without bone destruction or sequestration.

3. About 20%. Children.

4. Communication to the growth plate by a tortuous sinus tract.

Reference

Lopes TD, Reinus WR, Wilson AJ: Quantitative analysis of the plain radiographic appearance of Brodie's abscess. *Invest Radiol* 32:51–58, 1997.

Cross-Reference

Musculoskeletal Imaging: THE REQUISITES, 3rd ed, pp 527–528 and 550–556.

Comment

When a bone infection becomes a chronic condition, it may produce a spectrum of radiographic appearances. A Brodie's abscess is a painful lesion characterized by a well-defined geographic, radiolucent focus surrounded by diffuse sclerosis. Two thirds of these lesions occur in the metaphysis of a bone, while the remaining one third of lesions occurs in the diaphysis. Rarely, it can involve the epiphysis. While most lesions present as an intramedullary lytic lesion with well-defined and broad sclerotic margins along the long axis of the bone, occasionally it is cortically based with associated periosteal reactive changes. A Brodie's abscess represents a cavity in the bone lined by inflammatory granulation tissue and is filled with purulent or mucoid fluid. It is hypothesized that the bone abscess develops when the organism has a reduced virulence or the host demonstrates increased resistance to the infection. Clinically, patients with Brodie's abscess may not have associated fever or elevated erythrocyte sedimentation rate.

Notes

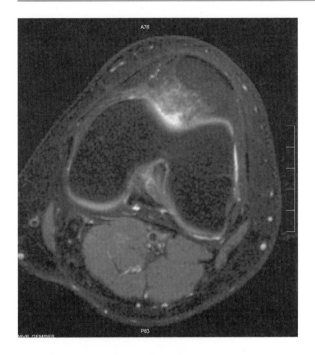

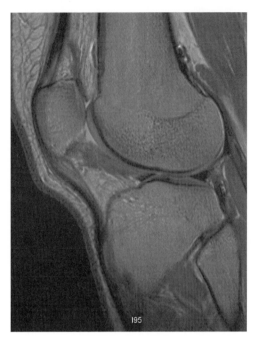

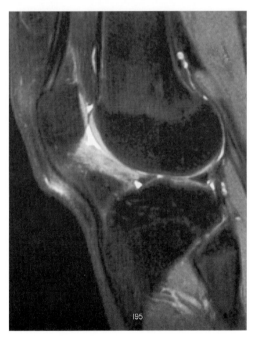

1. List the differential diagnosis.

2. How would you expect this patient to present?

3. In chronic cases, what tissues/substances affect the magnetic resonance imaging appearance?

4. What is peculiar about Hoffa's fat pad that enables neoplastic conditions of synovium to remain isolated within the fat pad?

Hoffa's Syndrome

1. Hoffa's syndrome/disease, intracapsular chondroma, focal nodular synovitis, and contusion.

2. Pain in the anterior aspect of the knee, exacerbated by extension.

3. Fibrin and hemosiderin deposition.

4. It contains residual synovial tissue.

References

Jacobson JA, Lenchik L, Ruhoy MK, et al: MR imaging of the infrapatellar fat pad of Hoffa. *Radiographics* 17:675–691, 1997.

Saddik D, McNally EG, Richardson M: MRI of Hoffa's fat pad. *Skeletal Radiol* 33:433–444, 2004.

Cross-Reference

Musculoskeletal Imaging: THE REQUISITES, 3rd ed, pp 247–248.

Comment

The infrapatellar fat pad of Hoffa is a triangular fat compartment in the anterior aspect of the knee. Hoffa's disease is a painful condition caused by a single, acute traumatic episode or repetitive trauma to the anterior knee producing hemorrhage and necrosis in the fat pad. The inflamed fat pad becomes hypertrophied, further predisposing it to traumatic impingement between the femur and tibia. Hoffa's syndrome is a similar entity to Hoffa's disease but occurs in the absence of known trauma. It is generally accepted that joint space narrowing secondary to degenerative joint disease such as osteoarthritis contributes to the development of the syndrome when there is synovial trapping. Clinically, patients complain of long-standing pain in the anterior compartment of the knee. Swelling may be evident on both sides of the patellar tendon. Forced extension exacerbates the pain due to increased pressure on the fat pad. Infrapatellar bursitis may accompany the disease process.

The diagnosis is conspicuous on magnetic resonance imaging. Patients with Hoffa's disease demonstrate areas of intense edema within the infrapatellar fat pad during the acute phase of the disease. Bowing of the patellar tendon from mass effect may be evident. When the condition is chronic or subacute, fibrin and hemosiderin deposition affect the signal intensity in the fat, producing regions of low signal intensity on T1W and T2W images.

Notes

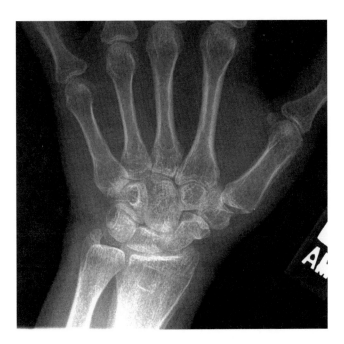
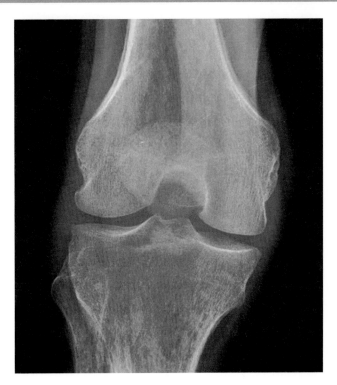

1. What is the diagnosis?

2. Is this a painful condition?

3. What would you expect to see on a bone scan? Is a bone scan more sensitive than radiographs?

4. Is there an association with acro-osteolysis?

CASE 116

Secondary Hypertrophic Osteoarthropathy

1. Secondary hypertrophic osteoarthropathy, probably from lung cancer.

2. Yes. In fact, pain differentiates hypertrophic osteoarthropathy from thyroid acropachy, which is painless.

3. "Parallel track" sign (tracer uptake along the cortical margins of the metaphysis and diaphysis of the tubular bones of the extremities). Yes.

4. There can be focal areas of tuftal resorption that mimic acro-osteolysis.

References

Pineda C, Fonseca C, Martinez-Lavin M: The spectrum of soft tissue and skeletal abnormalities of hypertrophic osteoarthropathy. *J Rheumatol* 17:626–632, 1990.

Pineda CJ, Martinez-Lavin M, Goobar JE, et al: Periostitis in hypertrophic osteoarthropathy: Relationship to disease duration. *AJR Am J Roentgenol* 148:773–778, 1987.

Cross-Reference

Musculoskeletal Imaging: THE REQUISITES, 3rd ed, pp 358–359.

Comment

Secondary hypertrophic pulmonary osteoarthropathy (HOA) is a chronic proliferative bone disorder characterized by painful periostitis of long tubular bones, clubbing of the finger and toes, and synovitis. The periostitis causes a relatively acute, deep-seated pain in the extremities, often described as a severe burning, and the adjacent skin may be swollen and warm. In contradistinction to primary HOA (pachydermoperiostosis), a form that is often hereditary but occasionally idiopathic, secondary HOA is associated with an underlying neoplastic, infectious, or inflammatory process, which accounts for 95% of all cases. About 10% to 25% of patients with bronchogenic carcinoma develop HOA, as do as many as 50% of patients with pleural mesothelioma.

Radiographically, periosteal new bone may be evident in the diaphysis of the tibia and fibula, radius and ulna, femur, humerus, metacarpals and metatarsals, and phalanges. It is a bilateral process. As the disease progresses, the metaphyseal regions of these bones become involved. The differential diagnosis includes primary HOA, thyroid acropachy, and venous stasis. In thyroid acropachy, the periostitis is asymptomatic and occurs principally in the small bones of the hands and feet. It does not involve the long tubular bones.

Other clinical findings such as exophthalmos and pretibial myxedema generally are present as well. Periosteal reaction in venous stasis tends to occur in the lower extremities.

Notes

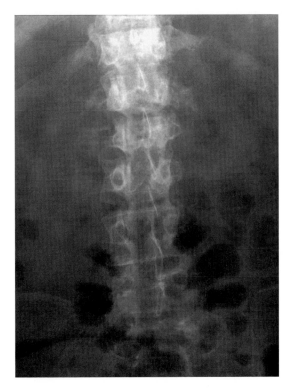 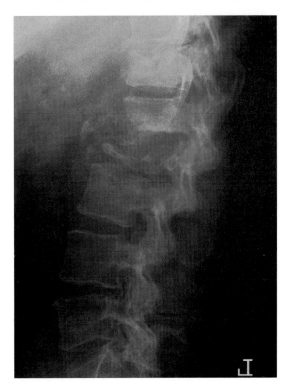

1. What is your diagnosis and what findings support your diagnosis?

2. What is the expected course of this disease?

3. List three mechanisms by which the spine may become infected.

4. How do you explain the involvement at multiple levels?

Tuberculous Spondylitis (Pott's Disease)

1. Tuberculous spondylitis (Pott's disease); L1-2 discitis associated with a calcified psoas abscess and skip lesion with discitis involving T11-12.

2. Slow progression with initial preservation of the disc. Eventually, an angular (gibbus) deformity develops as the disc is destroyed.

3. Hematogenous source, direct implantation by way of the venous system (Batson's plexus), or direct extension from an adjacent infection.

4. Infection spreads under the longitudinal ligaments.

References

Almeida A: Tuberculosis of the spine and spinal cord. *Eur J Radiology* 55:193–201, 2006.
Shanley DJ: Tuberculosis of the spine: Imaging features. *AJR Am J Roentgenol* 164:659–664, 1995.

Cross-Reference

Musculoskeletal Imaging: THE REQUISITES, 3rd ed, pp 558–560.

Comment

This patient presented with characteristic findings of a tuberculous spondylitis. Clinically, patients present with back pain, although localized tenderness and stiffness and a neurologic deficit also are common initial complaints. The disease progresses slowly and affects the thoracolumbar region most frequently. The infection can erode the articular cortex and then penetrate into the disc, where the infection is then free to spread to the adjacent vertebral body. Remember that tuberculous spondylitis has several notable differences to bacterial infections, since the posterior elements, disc, epidural space, and paraspinous soft tissues also can become primarily infected in addition to the vertebral body. The loss of cortical distinction in the anterior or posterior aspect of the vertebral body correlates with extension of the infection beneath the longitudinal ligaments, and this process is often expressed in the form of periostitis. The development of an acute, angular kyphosis (gibbus deformity) is strongly suggestive of tuberculosis. Tuberculosis may also directly infect the paraspinal soft tissues creating large abscesses, particularly in the psoas muscles, resulting in large calcified abscesses. The infection can extend via the longitudinal ligaments, paraspinal soft tissues, and muscles, producing skip lesions far removed from the initial source of infection. Another typical feature of tuberculosis is a "burrowing" abscess. These tubular tracts can also course for a long distance and perforate the internal organs of the peritoneal cavity or communicate to the skin through a sinus.

Notes

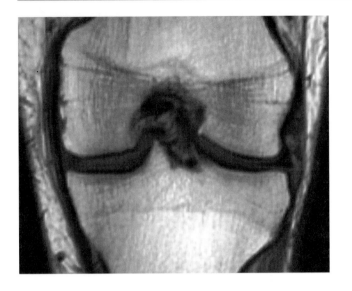
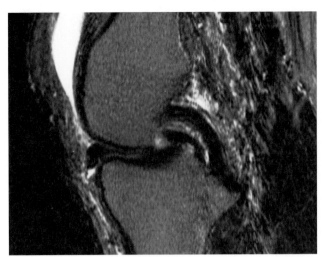
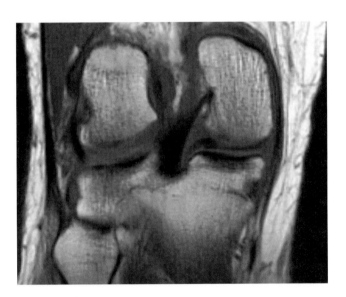
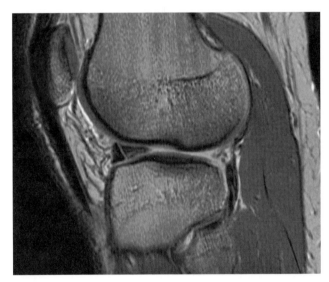

1. You are shown two pairs of images. Both patients have the same diagnosis but different findings. What are the findings?

2. Is this injury considered a relative emergency? Why?

3. What other conditions should you consider when you see an "absent meniscus" sign?

4. What is the sensitivity of this injury on magnetic resonance imaging?

CASE 118

Meniscal Buckethandle Tear

1. The first patient has a buckethandle tear of the medial meniscus with a "double PCL" (posterior cruciate ligament) sign. The second has a buckethandle tear of the lateral meniscus with a displaced posterior horn or "flipped fragment" sign.

2. Yes. Patients should be treated expeditiously because these tears may cause joint locking.

3. Prior meniscectomy, large meniscal tear, congenital hypoplasia or aplasia, and severe degeneration.

4. Sixty percent.

Reference

Magee TH, Hinson GW: MRI of meniscal bucket-handle tears. *Skeletal Radiol* 27:495–499, 1998.

Cross-Reference

Musculoskeletal Imaging: THE REQUISITES, 3rd ed, pp 225–230.

Comment

Buckethandle tears of the knee have been reported to occur in 9% to 24% of patients with a meniscal tear. It is the most common cause of a displaced meniscal injury and is considered a vertical-longitudinal tear that involves three portions of the meniscus. It often involves the entire length of the meniscus, although isolated involvement of the anterior or posterior horn can occur. A meniscal fragment can be displaced into the intercondylar notch or the anterior compartment.

Magnetic resonance imaging is the best noninvasive technique for detecting buckethandle tears. A key to making the diagnosis on the coronal images is to inspect the intercondylar region closely for abnormal structures and the menisci for a cleft that divides the peripheral fragment (bucket) from the displaced fragment (handle). Several important signs that are indicative of a buckethandle tear have been identified on the sagittal images. The "double PCL" sign indicates that a displaced intercondylar fragment lies inferior to the PCL, paralleling the orientation of this ligament. This finding has been reported only with medial meniscal tears. The "flipped meniscus" sign refers to a buckethandle tear that has a tear at two points. When the peripheral posterior horn fragment displaces anteriorly, it becomes juxtaposed to the anterior horn, giving the appearance that the meniscal horn has a "piggyback" companion. This finding is frequently accompanied with an "absent meniscus" sign.

Notes

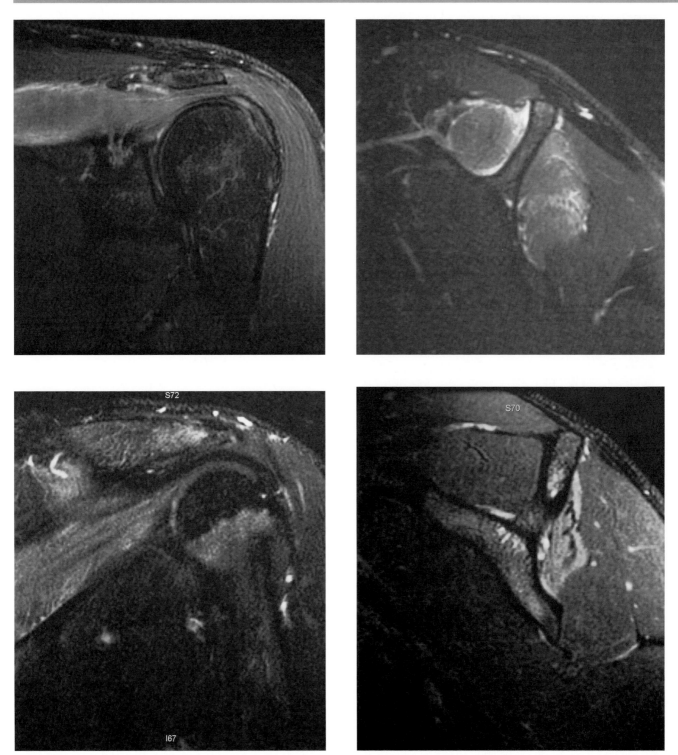

1. The first set of images is from one patient and the second set is from another. What is the main difference?

2. When assessing scapular fractures, what is a critical observation to include in your report?

3. What is the most common cause of this condition?

4. What is quadrilateral space syndrome? What does it affect in the shoulder?

Suprascapular Notch Syndrome

1. The level of suprascapular nerve impingement (the second patient's lesion is below the spinoglenoid notch).

2. Extension of a fracture line to the suprascapular notch. They can present with nerve palsy.

3. Perilabral cyst from a superior labral tear.

4. Axillary nerve compression. The teres minor and the posterior deltoid muscles.

Reference

Fritz RC, Helms CA, Steinbach LS, Genant HK: Suprascapular nerve entrapment: Evaluation with MR imaging. *Radiology* 182:437–444, 1992.

Cross-Reference

Musculoskeletal Imaging: THE REQUISITES, 3rd ed, pp 46, 97–98.

Comment

The suprascapular nerve is a mixed motor and sensory nerve that contains pain fibers to the shoulder and provides the motor supply to the supraspinatus and infraspinatus muscles of the rotator cuff. When entrapped or injured, it is referred to as suprascapular notch syndrome. Some common causes of this syndrome include a suprascapular notch ganglion, perilabral cyst, and tumors. If the nerve is injured or entrapped, the location of insult determines which muscles are affected. A lesion below the spinoglenoid notch affects only the infraspinatus muscle innervation, whereas a lesion within the suprascapular notch affects innervation to both the supraspinatus and infraspinatus muscles. The typical appearance of subacute muscle denervation is high signal intensity on T2W images in the affected muscle. The altered signal intensity in the muscle reflects an increase in the extracellular water space, which increases the T1 and T2 relaxation times. The total water content of the muscle is only minimally increased, a finding attributed to simultaneous shrinking of the myoplasm. These changes may be detected as early as two weeks from the time of injury or entrapment, and the outcome is dependent on the promptness of treatment. If the nerve entrapment is not treated, there usually is progression to irreversible fatty change and atrophy of the muscle. On T1W images, this is reflected by an increase in high signal intensity tissue in between the muscle fibers, producing a striated appearance in the muscle.

Notes

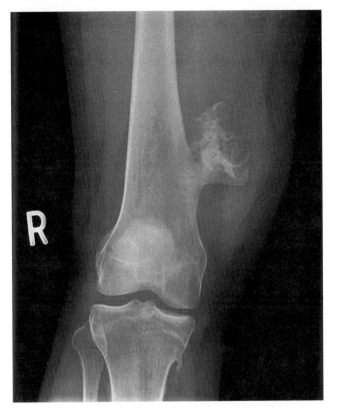

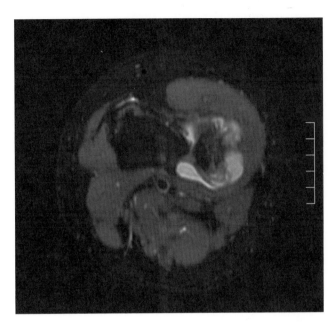

1. Where are the majority of these lesions found?

2. What is the appropriate diagnosis?

3. What are some clinical signs that indicate aggressive behavior?

4. What observations did you make on the magnetic resonance image?

Osteochondroma—Malignant Degeneration

1. Ninety-five percent are located in the extremities and over one third occur in the region of the knee.

2. Pedunculated osteochondroma of the femur with malignant degeneration.

3. Pain and growth.

4. Irregular cartilage cap, focal thickening exceeding 1 cm, destruction of underlying bone, and bursal formation.

Reference

Woetler K, Lindner N, Gosheger G, et al: Osteochondroma: MR imaging of tumor-related complications. *Eur Radiol* 10:832–840, 2000.

Cross-Reference

Musculoskeletal Imaging: THE REQUISITES, 3rd ed, pp 445–451.

Comment

An osteochondroma is the most common benign bone-forming tumor. It is the result of displaced growth plate cartilage that produces new bone, creating an osseous excrescence growing laterally from the metaphyseal region of the bone. The typical features of an osteochondroma are continuity of the periosteum, cortex, and bone marrow, and coverage by a cartilaginous cap that continues to grow until skeletal maturation. There are two characteristic appearances, pedunculated and sessile. About 95% occur in the extremities and over one third congregate around the knee. Pedunculated lesions grow away from the adjacent joint. The imaging appearance of an osteochondroma is pathognomonic, particularly when pedunculated. Occasionally, it may have similar features to a parosteal osteosarcoma or myositis ossificans but careful inspection easily differentiates these lesions from an exostosis. The presence of an overlying bursa is common and this can become inflamed.

Malignant degeneration is uncommon, occurring in less than 1% of solitary lesions. What you must look for includes destruction or lysis of bone, deformation of the matrix in the cartilaginous cap, thickening or irregularity of the cap, and growth of the cap with or without new matrix calcification. When a patient presents with new onset pain, a magnetic resonance imaging study is particularly useful in demonstrating these aggressive features.

Notes

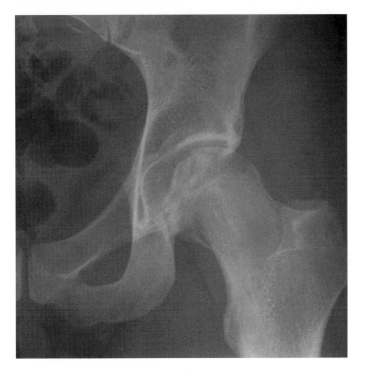
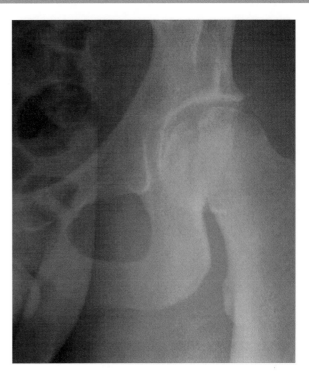

1. What is the diagnosis?

2. How are these injuries classified?

3. What is the most common mechanism of injury?

4. What should be the next step? Why?

Femoral Head Fracture

1. Femoral head fracture.

2. By fracture location with respect to fovea capitis, and presence of a fracture of the femoral neck or acetabulum.

3. Hip dislocation, both anterior and posterior.

4. Computed tomography to evaluate for displacement. To characterize the size, location, and degree of involvement of the weight-bearing surface; to identify any intra-articular fragments; and to determine if displacement exceeds 2 mm.

References

Richardson P, Young JWR, Porter D: CT detection of cortical fracture of the femoral head associated with posterior hip dislocation. *AJR Am J Roentgenol* 155: 93–94, 1990.

Tehranzadeh J, Vanarthos W, Pais MJ: Osteochondral impaction of the femoral head with associated hip dislocation: CT study in 35 patients. *AJR Am J Roentgenol* 155:1049–1052, 1990.

Cross-Reference

Musculoskeletal Imaging: THE REQUISITES, 3rd ed, pp 194–196.

Comment

Femoral head fractures occur most commonly in association with hip dislocations. The incidence of femoral head fractures is about 7% in patients with posterior dislocation and ranges from 10% to 68% in patients with anterior dislocation. Fractures may be either the result of a shearing injury or direct impaction. The Pipkin classification has been popularized and divides femoral head fractures into one of four types. In type 1 fractures, a hip dislocation results in a fracture of the femoral head below the fovea capitis femoris. In type 2 fractures, a hip dislocation results in a fracture of the femoral head above the fovea capitis femoris. In type 3 fractures, a type 1 or 2 fracture is associated with a femoral neck fracture. In type 4 fractures, a type 1 or 2 fracture is associated with a fracture of the acetabular rim. A more comprehensive classification has been suggested by others because Pipkin's classification does not differentiate anterior from posterior dislocation or categorize acetabular fractures. In general, femoral head fractures are associated with a poor outcome in about one third of patients. Complications include heterotopic ossification, avascular necrosis, recurrent dislocation, and infection.

Notes

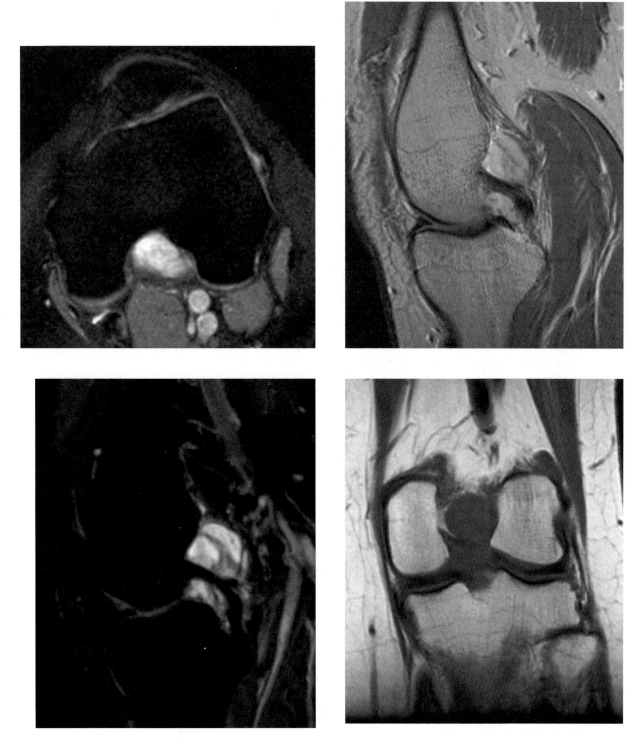

1. What are some conditions that can cause this appearance?

2. Can these lesions cause osseous erosion?

3. What is the most common presentation of a patient with this lesion?

4. How are these lesions treated?

CASE 122

Posterior Cruciate Ganglion Cyst

1. Cruciate ganglion cyst, meniscal cyst, synovial cyst.

2. Yes.

3. Pain and limitation of the range of motion.

4. Arthroscopic resection. Occasionally cysts may regress with conservative treatment.

References

Kim RS, Kim KT, Lee JY, Lee KY: Ganglion cysts of the posterior cruciate ligament. *Arthroscopy* 19:E36–E40, 2003.

Recht MP, Applegate G, Kaplan P, et al: The MR appearance of cruciate ganglion cysts: A report of 16 cases. *Skeletal Radiol* 23:597–600, 1994.

Cross-Reference

Musculoskeletal Imaging: THE REQUISITES, 3rd ed, pp 244–246.

Comment

Extra-articular cysts arising about the knee joint are common and likely represent popliteal cysts, meniscal cysts, and ganglion cysts. Intra-articular cysts, however, are uncommon and most likely represent either meniscal cysts or ganglion cysts. A cruciate ganglion cyst is an unusual entity that presents as a well-defined, multilocular lesion arising from either the posterior or anterior cruciate ligament. On T1W images, these cysts vary from hypo- to slightly hyperintense with respect to the signal intensity of muscle. On T2W images, the majority of cysts demonstrate homogeneously high signal intensity, although hemorrhage may alter the signal characteristics of a particular lesion. The differential diagnosis is limited. Trapped joint effusion can be eliminated owing to the multilocular nature of the majority of posterior cruciate ligament lesions and the fusiform appearance of anterior cruciate ligament lesions. Occasionally, a large intra-articular meniscal cyst arising from the posterior horn of either meniscus can mimic this ganglion cyst but the presence of a large meniscal tear should be evident.

Notes

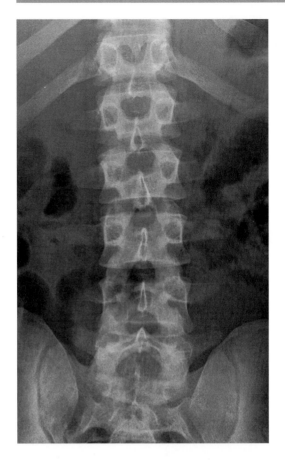 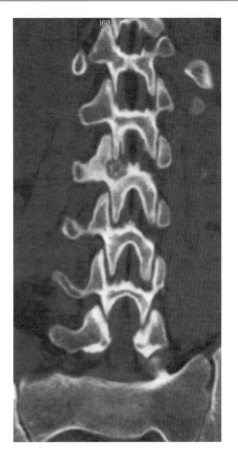

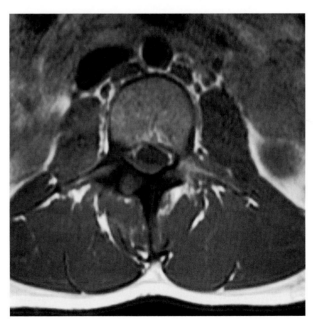

1. What findings did you observe in the spine?

2. Describe a "double density" sign on a bone scan.

3. What is the characteristic appearance of this lesion when it involves a carpal or tarsal bone?

4. Where is its typical location in the long bones?

Osteoid Osteoma

1. Dense L2 lamina with a round intermediate intensity soft tissue nidus and thickening of the cortex of the L2 spinous process.

2. A small focal area of intense radionuclide uptake superimposed upon a larger region of less intense activity typical of an osteoid osteoma.

3. Round, well-circumscribed calcified lesion surrounded by a lucent rim with no reactive sclerosis.

4. In the periosteum or outer cortex.

References

Flemming DJ, Murphey MD, Carmichael BB, Bernard SA: Primary tumors of the spine. *Semin Musculoskeletal Radiol* 4:299–320, 2000.

Shankman S, Desai P, Beltran J: Subperiosteal osteoid osteoma: Radiographic and pathologic manifestations. *Skeletal Radiol* 26:457–462, 1997.

Cross-Reference

Musculoskeletal Imaging: THE REQUISITES, 3rd ed, pp 420–424.

Comment

Osteoid osteoma is a tumor that affects young people; 90% of cases occur in people under the age of 25 years. There is a predilection for males by a 3:1 ratio. Pain, which tends to be worse at night and ameliorated by small doses of aspirin, is the hallmark of this benign lesion. Initially, the pain is mild and transient but then becomes severe and persistent. Soft tissue swelling and tenderness may accompany the pain when severe. The nidus of an osteoid osteoma, the essential lesion of this tumor, is usually small, measuring less than one centimeter in diameter. This nidus may eventually calcify but is initially devoid of calcium. Reactive sclerosis, such as cortical thickening and periostitis, is a dominant secondary feature of this lesion. The degree of reactive bone is influenced by the location of the nidus. An intracapsular osteoid osteoma, for example, elicits less reactive sclerosis than a subperiosteal lesion in the shaft of the femur.

In the long bone and spine, computed tomography is essential in demonstrating the location of the radiolucent nidus, which is often obscured by reactive bone on radiographs. The superficial location is helpful in differentiating an osteoid osteoma from a longitudinal stress fracture in the long bones. Reactive sclerosis may be more difficult to identify when the osteoid osteoma involves the spine. Look for a scoliotic curvature, which identifies the side of the lesion (concavity of the curve) but take notice that there is no rotatory component, a typical finding in patients with idiopathic scoliosis. Notable observations include a dense pedicle, lamina, transverse process, or spinous process.

Notes

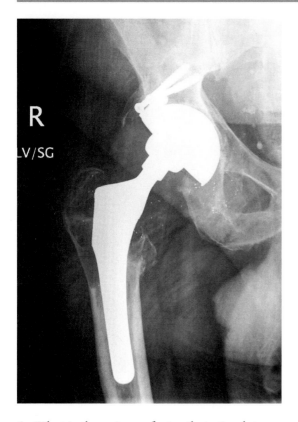

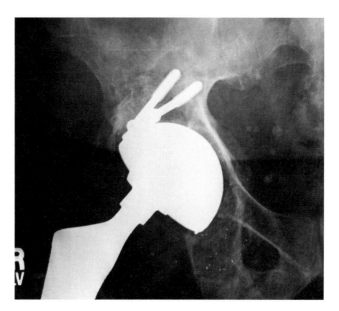

1. What is the primary factor that stimulates new bone formation around a total joint prosthesis?

2. List some factors that can lead to bone resorption.

3. What is the hypothesized effect of cytokines in this condition?

4. What radiographic findings are most helpful in identifying an infected prosthesis?

Particle-Related Inflammatory Disease

1. Mechanical load.

2. Infection, particle disease, insufficient mechanical load, and implant motion.

3. Probably acts directly on osteoclasts or its precursors.

4. Ill-defined periprosthetic resorption, acute periosteal reaction, and multiple sites of subacute periosteal reaction.

References

Bauer TW, Schils J: The pathology of total joint arthroplasty. II. Mechanisms of implant failure. *Skeletal Radiol* 28:483–497, 1999.

Manaster B: Total hip arthroplasty: Radiographic evaluation. *Radiographics* 16:645–660, 1996.

Cross-Reference

Musculoskeletal Imaging: THE REQUISITES, 3rd ed, pp 365–366.

Comment

Periprosthetic lucencies about hip arthroplasties are an important radiologic observation. It is the most common radiographic sign of loosening or particle-related inflammatory disease. Progressive widening of an area of lucency around the implants and/or cement fractures are strong indicators of loosening. There are other important causes of radiolucencies about the components of a hip replacement. One of these causes is particle-related inflammatory disease (aggressive granulomatosis), a condition characterized by rapid and progressive resorption of bone. It can be unifocal or multifocal. This patient had lysis of bone around the acetabular screws, the acetabular implant medially, and around the proximal aspect of the femoral implant. Lysis of bone in the greater and lesser trochanteric area is very pronounced. The condition occurs when small metal, methylmethacrylate, or polyethylene fragments induce a foreign body reaction. Macrophages become activated after exposure to a foreign material. The release of cytokines, such as tumor necrosis factor, further contributes to bone loss around the prosthetic device, ultimately causing its failure through loosening, and development of stress fractures. Foreign-body-type giant cells also participate in this condition, as do osteoclasts. The differential diagnosis includes infection. The diagnosis is fairly straightforward when you identify displaced surface beads from the prosthesis around the joint (as in this patient). Aspiration of the hip joint is required for most diagnoses.

Notes

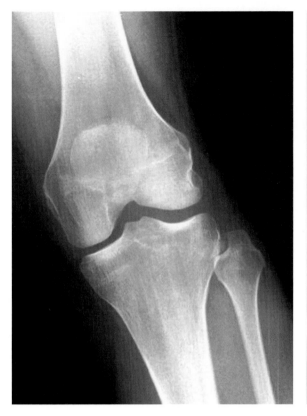 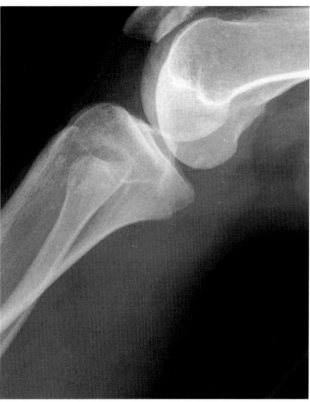

1. What is the diagnosis?

2. What are the types and which is most common?

3. What occupation is particularly at risk for this injury?

4. Is there an idiopathic type?

Dislocated Proximal Tibiofibular Syndesmosis

1. Dislocation of the proximal tibiofibular syndesmosis.

2. Anterolateral, posteromedial, and superior dislocations; anterolateral.

3. Parachutists.

4. Yes, some young people can have recurrent subluxation before adolescence. It responds to conservative management and does not recur with skeletal maturity.

References

Keogh P, Masterson E, Murphy B, et al: The role of radiography and computed tomography in the diagnosis of acute dislocation of the proximal tibiofibular joint. *Br J Radiol* 66:108–111, 1993.

Voglino JA, Denton JR: Acute traumatic proximal tibiofibular joint dislocation confirmed by computed tomography. *Orthopedics* 22:255–258, 1999.

Cross-Reference

Musculoskeletal Imaging: THE REQUISITES, 3rd ed, pp 209–212.

Comment

Dislocations of the proximal tibiofibular syndesmosis are an unusual but important diagnosis. The final position of the fibular head dictates the type of dislocation, and these can occur in the anterolateral, posteromedial, and superior directions. The tibiofibular joint is maintained by the articular capsule, anterior and posterior tibiofibular ligaments, lateral collateral ligament, and biceps tendon. Most injuries are the result of falls or a twisting injury of the knee. Radiographically, the typical appearance is anterior displacement of the fibular head, as seen in this patient on the lateral view (if you extrapolate a line on the dorsal cortex of the fibula, it should intercept the dorsal surface of the lateral femoral condyle). The head of the fibula usually lies adjacent to the posterolateral tibia with a little overlap of the cortical surfaces on the frontal view, but notice that there is no overlap in this patient. Posterior dislocations are rare but important since the peroneal nerve is frequently injured as well. Computed tomography is the preferred imaging modality for diagnosis of subluxation of this joint and for further characterizing a dislocation if surgery is required.

Notes

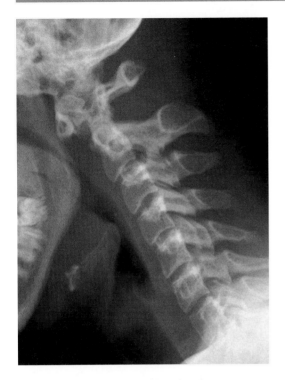

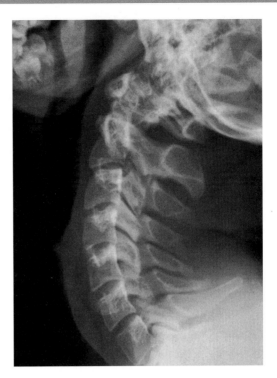

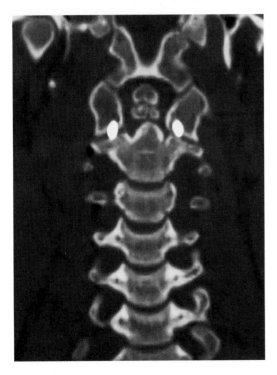

1. What is the diagnosis?

2. What determines atlantoaxial instability when this anomaly is observed?

3. Can this abnormality occur after trauma?

4. What do you observe on the flexion and extension radiographs?

Os Odontoideum

1. An os odontoideum.

2. The juxtaposition of the transverse ligament of C1 to the ossicle.

3. Some cases actually represent a nonunion of a type 2 odontoid fracture.

4. The ossicle is fixed to the atlas and moves with C1.

Reference

Matsui H, Imada K, Tsuji H: Radiographic classification of os odontoideum and its clinical significance. *Spine* 22:1706–1709, 1997.

Cross-Reference

Musculoskeletal Imaging: THE REQUISITES, 3rd ed, pp 166–167.

Comment

An os odontoideum is a small bone that exists above a hypoplastic odontoid process. It has a characteristic appearance: a small, round or oval, well-corticated ossicle located above the tip of the odontoid process or more cephalad near the basion of the skull. When evaluating this anomaly, one clue is to search for coexisting abnormalities of the atlas including hypoplasia of the posterior neural arch and hypertrophy of the anterior arch. Most experts agree that an os odontoideum represents a congenital anomaly (overgrowth of the os terminale secondary to hypoplasia of the odontoid) although some cases do represent a post-traumatic condition. The importance of an os odontoideum is its association with atlantoaxial instability. Stability is dependent on the level of the cleft between it and the odontoid process, and on the degree of development of the dens. If the transverse ligament is juxtaposed to the ossicle, then the odontoid process is unable to form a stable relationship with the atlas, a configuration that is conducive to atlantoaxial instability. In severe cases of instability, the caliber of the spinal canal can be significantly compromised. Assessment of stability is performed with flexion and extension lateral radiographs. It is important to quantify the degree of motion of the ossicle and changes in the caliber of the spinal canal. Currently, computed tomography or magnetic resonance imaging is advocated for further evaluation of the integrity of the transverse ligament.

Notes

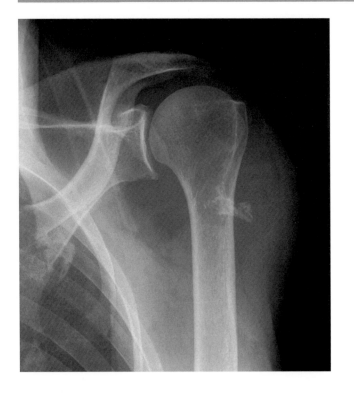 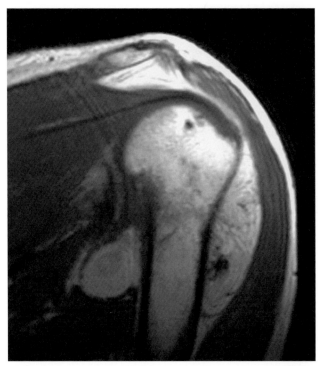

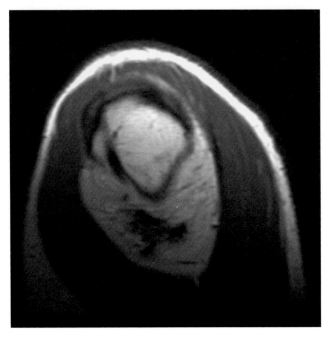 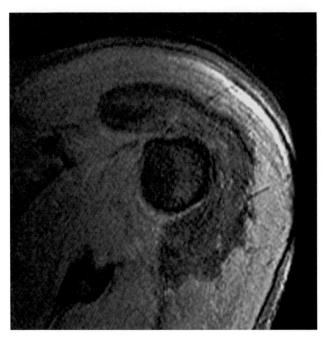

1. What is the diagnosis?

2. Is it common?

3. What is unusual about this lesion?

4. What is the typical patient profile?

Parosteal Lipoma

1. Parosteal lipoma.

2. Lipomas are common but this type of lipoma constitutes only 0.3% of all lipomas.

3. Its intimate relation with the periosteum.

4. Although one half of patients are older than 40 years of age, anyone can get it, so there is no characteristic profile.

Reference

Yu JS, Weis L, Becker W: MR imaging of parosteal lipoma. *Clin Imaging* 24:15–18, 2000.

Cross-Reference

Musculoskeletal Imaging: THE REQUISITES, 3rd ed, pp 475–477 and 481.

Comment

A parosteal lipoma is a rare lesion presenting as an enlarging, nontender mass in a middle-aged person. One half of patients affected are between the ages of 40 and 70 years, although it has been reported in children. The most common locations involved are the femur, radius, and humerus. Pathologically, a parosteal lipoma is a multilobulated, broad-based mass circumscribed by a thin, fibrous capsule. Microscopically, it is composed of normal adipose cells. The radiographic features of a parosteal lipoma are distinctive. A well-circumscribed radiolucent mass intimately abuts the adjacent cortex. Osseous changes at the site of attachment are variable and likely reactive. The underlying cortex may become thinned or saucerized from pressure erosion or fusiformly thickened from focal hyperostosis. On magnetic resonance imaging, a parosteal lipoma has signal intensity that is identical to that of subcutaneous fat on T1W images but it is sometimes lower in signal intensity on T2W images. Low signal intensity septa may be variably present and can enhance with contrast. The appearance at the site of attachment has been variable, but areas of persistently low intensity on all pulse sequences probably represent cortical bone at the attachment site. If the pedicle is small, the entire excrescence appears low in signal intensity, but if the area of ossification is larger, then only the periphery of the pedicle is of low intensity.

Notes

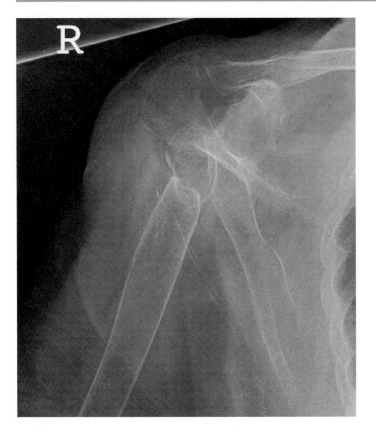
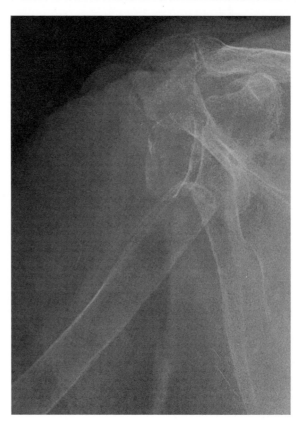

1. What is your differential diagnosis?
2. What disorder is most likely to cause the changes depicted in this patient?
3. List the characteristic radiographic features of the hypertrophic form of this condition.
4. What should be done if you detect periarticular soft tissue calcific/ossific densities?

Neuroarthropathy (Atrophic Type)

1. Atrophic neuroarthropathy. If only one joint, you may consider massive osteolysis of Gorham, post-traumatic osteolysis, metastasis, tumor, and infection.

2. Syringomyelia.

3. Recall the five "D"s: increased density, joint distension, intra-articular and periarticular debris, joint disorganization, and dislocation.

4. Magnetic resonance imaging to exclude a chondrosarcoma.

Reference

Yu JS: Diabetic foot and neuroarthropathy: Magnetic resonance imaging features. *Topics Magn Reson Im* 9:295–310, 1998.

Cross-Reference

Musculoskeletal Imaging: THE REQUISITES, 3rd ed, pp 311–314.

Comment

Neuropathic osteoarthropathy, or neuroarthropathy, is a complex complication of neuropathic disease. The pathogenesis of neuropathic disorders remains debatable, but many experts consider repetitive trauma and altered sympathetic control of blood flow to be significant factors. Loss of the protective sensations of pain and proprioception leads to chronic destabilization of the joint. The resultant changes in the articular cartilage cause fibrillation and degeneration, and eventual erosion of the cortical surfaces. Neuroarthropathy has three presentations: hypertrophic, atrophic, and mixed. In atrophic neuroarthropathy, there is resorption of the bone producing a well-demarcated transition between the lysed and remaining bone. Several important observations in this patient are notable. There is no evidence of a fracture or accompanying bone repair, the bone density at the margin of lysis is normal, and there is no indication of surgery. This presentation of neuroarthropathy is much more common in the upper extremity and is usually associated with syringomyelia or peripheral nerve injury. It is nearly always of the atrophic type. In the lower extremity, the hip and the knee are common locations of neuroarthropathy, which is more likely to be caused by either tabes dorsalis or syringomyelia. In the hip, soft tissue swelling caused by an effusion and capsular hypertrophy, and intra-articular debris, are important clues to the diagnosis. In the foot, it is nearly always hypertrophic and caused by diabetes mellitus or alcoholism.

Notes

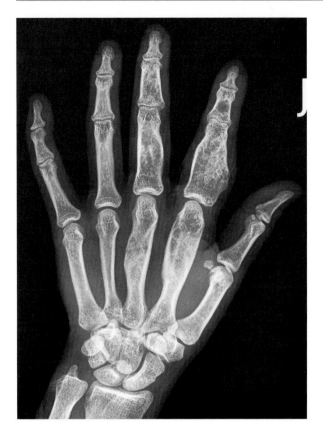 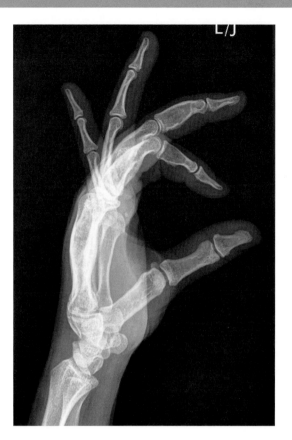

1. What is the most likely diagnosis?

2. Histologically, what is the essential lesion and is it similar to individual cases?

3. Is this usually a bilateral or unilateral process?

4. Is this an aggressive condition with widespread dissemination?

Ollier's Disease

1. Ollier's disease.

2. The lesions are typical enchondromas composed of lobules of cartilaginous cells, but there is often increased cellularity and focal atypia.

3. It has a tendency to involve only one side of the body.

4. No, it a slowly progressive disease although it may lead to severe deformity of the fingers and extremities.

Reference

Brien EW, Mirra JM, Kerr R: Benign and malignant cartilage tumors of bone and joint: Their anatomic and theoretical basis with an emphasis on radiology, pathology and clinical biology. I. The intramedullary cartilage tumors. *Skeletal Radiol* 26:325–353, 1997.

Cross-Reference

Musculoskeletal Imaging: THE REQUISITES, 3rd ed, pp 444–446.

Comment

Enchondromatosis, or Ollier's disease, is a condition that is characterized by the presence of numerous enchondromas, particularly in the hands, such as in this patient. It is a nonhereditary abnormality with a predilection for one side of the body. The source of the disease is abnormal cartilage growth, arising from either the growth plate or from metaplastic cartilage from the periosteum. Radiographically, the osseous lesions may be located in the medullary cavity of the metacarpals, phalanges, or the long bones. In the hand, multiple enchondromas produce thinning, expansion, and occasionally disappearance of the cortex, with focal calcifications within the lesions. In the long bones, the intraosseous lesion may be extensive in the diaphysis and metaphysis of the bone. In skeletally immature patients, involvement of the epiphysis may cause growth disturbances.

The consideration of malignant transformation should be raised when there is progressive destruction and breakthrough of the cortex with infiltration of the adjacent soft tissues beyond the cortical limits on sequential radiographs. Reportedly, this can occur in 30% of cases. The risk of malignancy increases the longer the patient has the disease, and most often the transformation is into a chondrosarcoma.

Notes

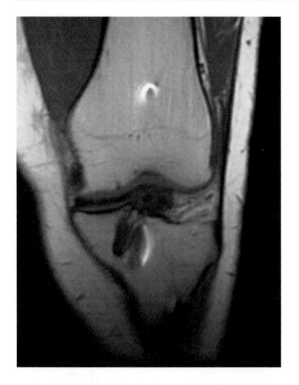

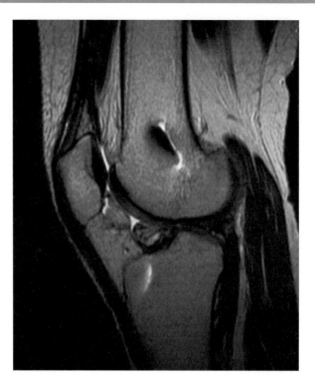

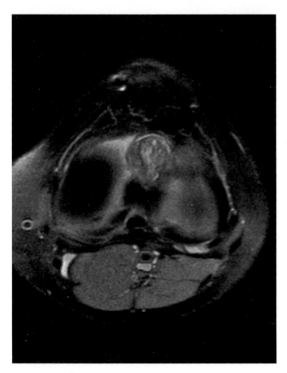

1. What is the diagnosis?

2. What is its arthroscopic appearance?

3. How do these patients present?

4. How does roof impingement occur and does it become apparent with full flexion or extension?

Localized Anterior Arthrofibrosis (Cyclops Lesion)

1. Localized anterior arthrofibrosis or a cyclops lesion.

2. Headlike nodule with reddish-blue discoloration resembling the eye of the cyclops.

3. Knee locking or restricted full extension.

4. The tibial tunnel is placed too far anterior on the tibia causing effacement and constriction of an anterior cruciate ligament (ACL) graft during the last 5 to 10 degrees of knee extension.

References

Huang GS, Lee CH, Chan WP, et al: Acute anterior cruciate ligament stump entrapment in anterior cruciate ligament tears: MR imaging appearance. *Radiology* 225:537–540, 2002.

Recht MP, Piraino DW, Applegate G, et al: Complications after anterior cruciate ligament reconstruction: Radiographic and MR findings. *AJR* 167:705–710, 1996.

Cross-Reference

Musculoskeletal Imaging: THE REQUISITES, 3rd ed, pp 237–238.

Comment

This patient had an ACL repair. The key observation in this patient is a nodular mass in the anterior joint recess adjacent to the ACL graft. On the coronal T1W image, it demonstrates heterogeneously isointense signal intensity to muscle. On the sagittal T2W image, it shows heterogeneous signal intensity as well. The axial gradient-echo image shows the overall size of the lesion. Localized anterior arthrofibrosis, otherwise known as a cyclops lesion because of its appearance on arthroscopy, represents a focal reactive fibrous nodule that is often attached to the ACL graft. It is an important cause of diminished range of motion and occasionally joint locking in postoperative patients. The increased frequency of ACL reconstructions has increased the need to be informed about the imaging features of this procedure, in both normal and pathologic situations, and potential postoperative complications. The majority of cyclops lesions are either the result of debris raised by drilling the tibial tunnel or an injury to the exposed fibers of the ACL graft by roof impingement. However, it can also occur in an acute rupture of the ACL when the fibers fold anteriorly on themselves.

Notes

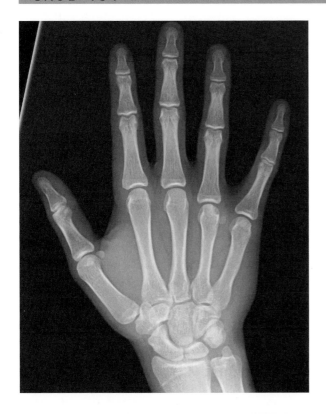

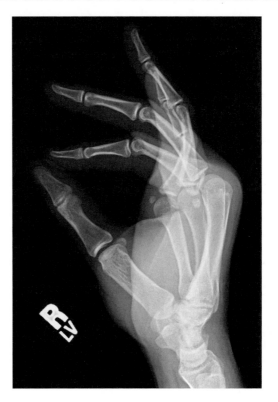

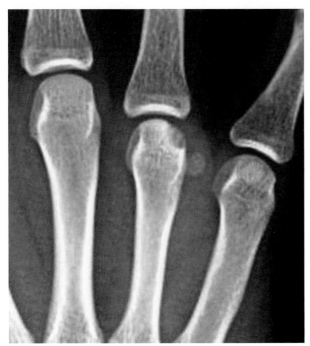

1. What is the diagnosis?

2. Is this a benign lesion?

3. What should be done?

4. Is recommending another imaging study an appropriate course of action?

Fight Bite

1. Impaction fracture of the head of the fourth metacarpal bone (fight bite) with cellulitis.

2. No, it represents a potentially serious injury that is infected with oral flora and may progress to septic arthritis, infectious tenosynovitis, and compartment syndrome.

3. This patient needs a surgical consultation, and likely an exploration of the metacarpophalangeal joint region.

4. Yes, magnetic resonance imaging can depict the full extent of infection and direct the surgeon's preoperative plan.

References

Chadaev AP, Juktin VI, Butkevich AT, Emkuzhev VM: Treatment of infected clench-fist human bite wounds in the area of metacarpophalangeal joints. *J Hand Surg* 21-A:299–303, 1996.

Perron AD, Miller MD, Brady WJ: Orthopedic pitfalls in the ED: Fight bite. *Am J Emerg Med* 20:114–117, 2002.

Cross-Reference

Musculoskeletal Imaging: THE REQUISITES, 3rd ed, pp 159–160.

Comment

A *fight bite* refers to an injury that occurs when a clenched fist strikes an open mouth, and this is considered one of the worst injuries associated with a human bite. The impaction fracture produces a wedge deformity on the metacarpal head, which occurs when it impacts against the tooth of an opponent. These injuries are often treated as minor injuries without recognition that the joint capsule, extensor tendon, or deep fascial spaces may have been violated and inoculated with oral bacteria. Significant morbidity can occur if the diagnosis is delayed or the initial management is inadequate. Injuries to the cartilage, joint capsule, and bone may be severe if the infection is allowed to progress. Generally, patients do not present after the initial altercation but present to medical attention after 1 or 2 weeks with a markedly swollen hand. Magnetic resonance imaging is optimal for depicting the full extent of infection and septic arthritis. Surgical debridement and exploration of the deep structures is the treatment of choice. If the capsule is not violated, irrigation is often sufficient, but as more tissues are involved, a more extensive debridement is required.

Notes

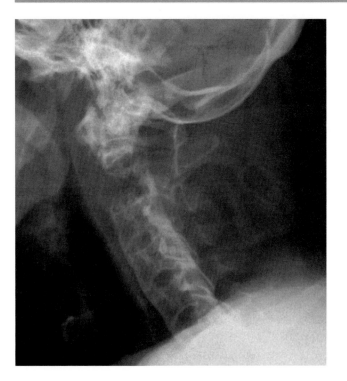
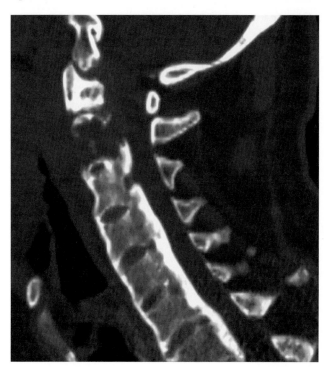

1. How would this patient present?

2. When do you expect cord signs (disturbances in motor and sensory function in the lower extremity) to be exhibited?

3. Can this disorder occur elsewhere in the spine? How may it present?

4. What other disorder commonly coexists in the spine?

Ossification of the Posterior Longitudinal Ligament

1. With neurologic symptoms or pain in the neck, shoulder, and upper extremity.

2. When the thickness of the ligament exceeds 60% of the sagittal diameter of the cervical spinal canal.

3. Yes, it occasionally may affect the thoracic (T4 to T7) and lumbar spine (L1 to L2). Urinary and rectal incontinence.

4. Diffuse idiopathic skeletal hyperostosis in 30% to 50% of patients.

References

Heller JG, Johnston RB, III, Goodrich A: Ossification of the posterior longitudinal ligament: A report of nine cases in non-oriental patients. *Skeletal Radiol* 23:601–606, 1994.

Ono K, Yonenobu K, Miyamoto S, Okada K: Pathology of ossification of the posterior longitudinal ligament and ligamentum flavum. *Clin Orthop* 359:18–26, 1999.

Cross-Reference

Musculoskeletal Imaging: THE REQUISITES, 3rd ed, pp 314–317.

Comment

Ossification of the posterior longitudinal ligament (OPLL) is a distinct clinical entity characterized by the development of ossifications, either in the form of a dense strip of bone or small plaques in the posterior longitudinal ligament. The majority of patients are middle-aged, and there is a 2:1 male to female predilection. Symptoms associated with this disorder have been related to cord impingement resulting in motor and sensory disturbances in either the lower or upper extremity. Patients may also present with pain in the neck, shoulder, or arm, and possibly neck stiffness. This case is an "Aunt Minnie" and shows typical features of this condition. The ossification of the posterior longitudinal ligament is depicted as a dense strip of bone bridging the posterior aspect of the vertebral bodies from the C2 level to C7 (it occurs most frequently from C3 to C5). There is diffuse narrowing of the diameter of the spinal canal by nearly 50%. The destructive process in C2 was a metastasis from lung cancer in this patient. The cause of OPLL is unknown although several factors have been suggested. The disorder frequently coexists in patients with diffuse idiopathic skeletal hyperostosis (DISH); however, there are distinct pathologic differences between the two entities.

Notes

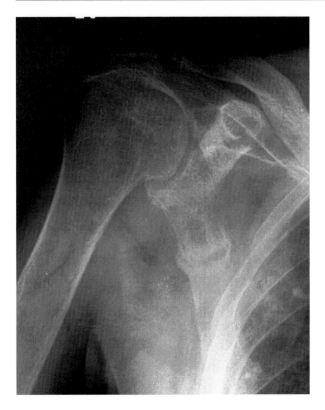 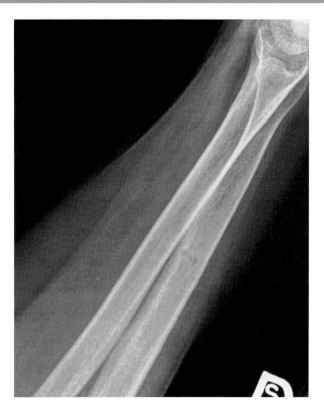

1. What is the underlying disorder?

2. What are the lesions in the bones? Can they progress?

3. What do these lesions represent?

4. What is the characteristic appearance of these lesions on bone scintigraphy? What is a "flare" response?

Looser's Zones

1. Osteomalacia.

2. Looser's zones. Yes, they can progress into a complete fracture.

3. Insufficiency stress fractures.

4. Bilateral, symmetric focal areas of increased activity. Transient increase in uptake after initiation of treatment reflecting osteoblastic activity associated with healing.

References

Akaki S, Ida K, Kanazawa S, et al: Flare response seen in therapy for osteomalacia. *J Nucl Med* 39:2095–2097, 1998.

Reginato AJ, Falasca GF, Pappu R, et al: Musculoskeletal manifestations of osteomalacia: Report of 26 cases and literature review. *Semin Arthritis Rheum* 28:287–304, 1999.

Cross-Reference

Musculoskeletal Imaging: THE REQUISITES, 3rd ed, pp 376–380.

Comment

Looser's zones are pseudofractures in the skeleton that occur late in the clinical course of osteomalacia. It is considered to be an insufficiency type of stress fracture that occurs without antecedent trauma. But they do occur at sites of increased bone stress and accelerated turnover. It has a characteristic appearance of a lucent area that is oriented perpendicular to the cortex and does not cross the entire diameter of the bone. Common locations include the lateral margin of the scapula, ribs, pubic rami, proximal femora medially, and the ulna posteriorly. They are typically bilateral and symmetric, differentiating them from other types of stress fractures. Sclerosis demarcates the intraosseous margins and callus formation manifests as new bone on the periosteum. Also unlike other stress fractures, these pseudofractures may remain unchanged for long periods. Bone scintigraphy and magnetic resonance imaging are more sensitive than radiography for early detection.

This patient has osteomalacia, a pathologic condition caused by the accumulation of uncalcified osteoid. Patients with osteomalacia complain of muscular weakness, nonspecific pain, and weak bones that become deformed with time. There are numerous causes of osteomalacia including dietary deficiency of calcium or vitamin D, deficient absorption of calcium or phosphorus (conditions that cause malabsorption and obstructive jaundice), enzyme deficiencies, renal diseases (acquired and congenital), tumors, and liver disease.

Notes

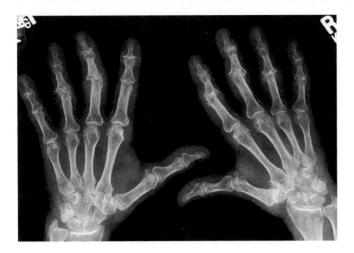 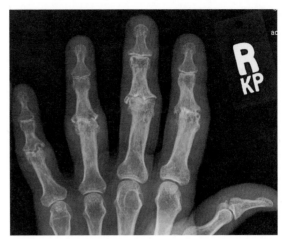

1. What is the diagnosis in this female patient? Which findings were most characteristic of this arthropathy?

2. What condition would you have to consider in the differential diagnosis if this patient was male?

3. What is Cronkhite-Canada syndrome and why would you consider this entity?

4. Does this patient have a risk of developing rheumatoid arthritis?

Erosive Osteoarthritis

1. Erosive osteoarthritis. Central erosions and soft tissue swelling indicating an inflammatory process.

2. Psoriatic arthritis.

3. Gastrointestinal polyposis, hyperpigmentation of the skin, and nail atrophy; a variant of erosive osteoarthritis may be seen as a feature of this syndrome.

4. Yes, 15% develop full-blown features of rheumatoid arthritis.

Reference

Belhorn LH, Hess EV: Erosive osteoarthritis. *Semin Arthritis Rheum* 22:298–306, 1993.

Cross-Reference

Musculoskeletal Imaging: THE REQUISITES, 3rd ed, pp 325–326.

Comment

Erosive osteoarthritis is an inflammatory form of osteoarthritis that affects predominantly postmenopausal middle-aged women. It combines certain clinical manifestations of a synovial inflammatory disease and the radiographic manifestations of osteoarthritis. Involvement is often limited to the hands, and the proximal and distal interphalangeal joints constitute preferred target sites. Early in the disease, patients present with a nonspecific synovial inflammatory arthropathy manifested by painful, swollen, and erythematous joints. The key radiologic features are bone proliferation and erosions. The proliferative changes are typical of osteoarthritis, as is its distribution. The articular erosions that develop tend to be centrally located, creating large defects in the cortex and subchondral bone. Osteophytes that develop at the margins of the joint result in a characteristic "gull-wing" appearance, although this finding may be seen in other arthritides. Ankylosis of the interphalangeal joint, not seen in noninflammatory osteoarthritis, can occur in the erosive form. Approximately 15% of patients with erosive osteoarthritis develop clinical, laboratory (elevated erythrocyte sedimentation rate and positive rheumatoid factor), and radiographic manifestations of rheumatoid arthritis. However, the exact relationship between these two conditions remains unclear.

Notes

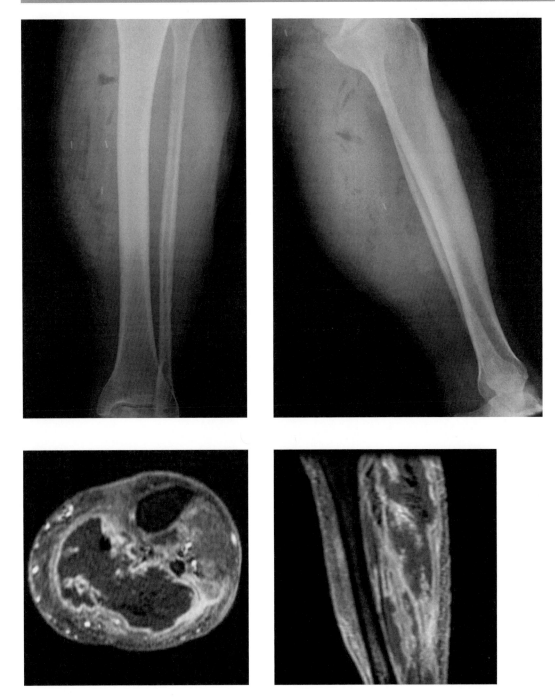

1. What is the diagnosis?

2. Is this an emergency?

3. Who is at risk for developing this process?

4. If the process is ascending and the clinicians request a magnetic resonance imaging examination, what should you do?

CASE 135

Necrotizing Fasciitis

1. Necrotizing fasciitis.

2. Yes, survival is directly linked to early diagnosis and surgical debridement.

3. Patients with impaired immunity (drug and alcohol abusers, diabetics, and patients who are HIV positive, undergoing chemotherapy, or on immunosuppressive medication).

4. If you have a magnetic resonance scanner available, expedite the examination STAT. The surgical exploration should not be delayed if a magnetic resonance scanner is not available and computed tomography is the next best test.

References

Fugitt JB, Puckett ML, Quigley MM, Kerr SM: Necrotizing fasciitis. *Radiographics* 24:1472–1476, 2004.

Schmid MR, Kossman T, Duewell S: Differentiation of necrotizing fasciitis and cellulites using MR imaging. *AJR Am J Roentgenol* 170:615–620, 1998.

Cross-Reference

Musculoskeletal Imaging: THE REQUISITES, 3rd ed, pp 545–547.

Comment

Necrotizing fasciitis is a rapidly progressive infection characterized by extensive necrosis of subcutaneous tissue and fascia and usually accompanied by severe systemic toxicity. It has a fatal outcome if diagnosis is not made immediately. In the early stages, the underlying muscle is spared and the clinical diagnosis of the infection may be difficult to differentiate from cellulitis. Cellulitis involves only the subcutaneous tissue and responds well to antibiotic therapy in the majority of cases. Necrotizing fasciitis is a surgical emergency. When performed early, adequate surgical debridement is associated with improved survival when compared to delayed exploration. On magnetic resonance imaging, necrotizing fasciitis demonstrates fluid collecting along the deep fascial sheaths characterized by high signal intensity on T2W images, and enhancement with contrast administration. Abscess-like delineation of necrotic tissue with rim enhancement is a poor prognostic finding as is generalized muscle edema. The administration of intravenous gadolinium helps to delineate abscesses, and the immediate extravasation of contrast in necrotic tissue is a marker for the aggressiveness of the infection. The diagnosis of necrotizing fasciitis on computed tomography relies on detection of soft tissue thickening and gas formation, which may be far advanced; otherwise, distinction from cellulitis is less reliable than with magnetic resonance imaging.

Notes

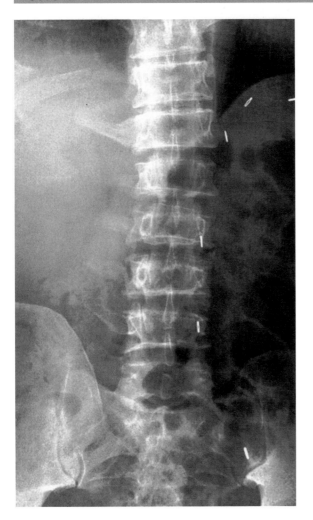 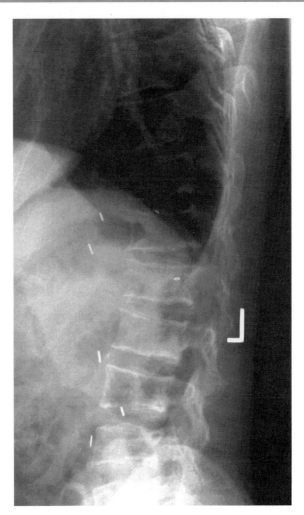

1. Describe the findings.

2. What factors determine the severity of these changes?

3. Estimate the minimum dose used in this patient.

4. What would magnetic resonance imaging of this spine show?

Radiation-Induced Hypoplasia

1. Left-sided hypoplasia of the pedicles and bodies of the T12-5 vertebrae, with flattening of the vertebral bodies and scalloping of the end plates.

2. Dose, age, field size, and the age of patient during the time of treatment.

3. At least 3000 cGy.

4. Decreased hematopoietic marrow and replacement with fatty marrow.

Reference

Makipernaa A, Heikkila JT, Merikanto J, et al: Spinal deformity induced by radiotherapy for solid tumours in childhood: A long-term follow up study. *Eur J Pediatr* 152:197–200, 1993.

Cross-Reference

Musculoskeletal Imaging: THE REQUISITES, 3rd ed, pp 533–534.

Comment

Radiation therapy is an important facet of medicine and is used for the treatment of a number of pediatric neoplasms. A field irradiated with a sufficient dose can suppress or arrest the growth of bones that are exposed. This consequence of treatment has great significance when the lesion is near or in the spine such as renal neoplasms, neuroblastoma, medulloblastoma, ependymomas, and astrocytomas. The key finding in this case is hypoplasia of the vertebral bodies, particularly on the left side of T12-L5. (Note the discrepancy between the heights of the T10 and T11 vertebrae compared to T12-L5). This is frequently associated with a lateral flexion curvature. A second type of scoliosis is rotatory scoliosis when the changes primarily affect the posterior elements. The dose is the most important factor that determines the changes in the bone. When the dose is less than 2000 cGy, little change is seen. Between 2000 to 3000 cGy, partial growth arrest may result in a "bone-in-bone" appearance and scoliosis of less than 20 degrees, and beyond 3000 cGy, flattening of the vertebral body, scalloping of the end plates, and growth cessation is pronounced, with scoliosis greater than 20 degrees. The disc spaces maintain a normal height. This patient had been treated with 4500 cGy for a Wilms' tumor involving the left kidney.

Notes

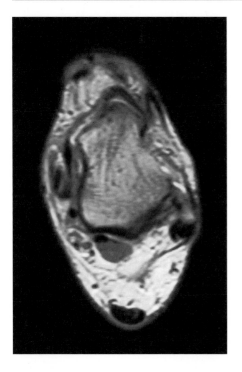
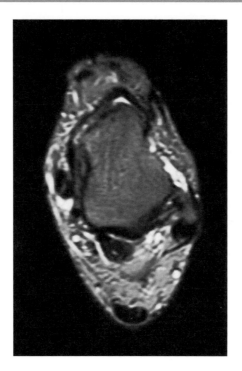
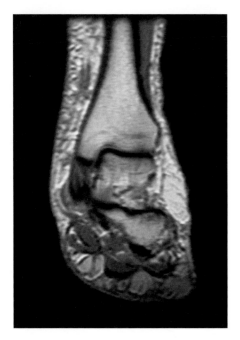

1. What is your diagnosis?

2. What is the most common imaging manifestation of this injury?

3. What is a potential consequence of this injury and who is at risk?

4. Are there any associated ligament injuries?

Posterior Tibial Tendon Tear

1. Tear of the posterior tibial tendon.

2. Tendon thickening with either linear or heterogenous intrasubstance signal abnormality.

3. Can lead to progressive pes planus deformity and weakened inversion; women in fifth or sixth decades of life.

4. Yes, the spring ligament complex (superomedial and inferomedial calcaneonavicular ligaments) and those of the sinus tarsi are frequently ruptured.

References

Balen PF, Helms CA: Association of posterior tibial tendon injury with spring ligament injury, sinus tarsi abnormality, and plantar fasciitis on MR imaging. *AJR Am J Roentgenol* 176:1137–1143, 2001.

Khoury NJ, el-Khoury GY, Saltzman CL, Brandser EA: MR imaging of posterior tibial tendon dysfunction. *AJR Am J Roentgenol* 167:675–682, 1996.

Cross-Reference

Musculoskeletal Imaging: THE REQUISITES, 3rd ed, pp 263–265.

Comment

The posterior tendon is the most frequently injured tendon in the medial aspect of the foot. Patients present with pain, local tenderness, and swelling. On magnetic resonance imaging, the posterior tibial tendon has an ovoid configuration and it inserts on the navicular, medial and intermediate cuneiforms, and bases of the 2-4 metatarsals. Its normal diameter is usually two to three times the size of the adjacent flexor tendons. There are three patterns of rupture of this tendon. A type 1 tear is characterized by longitudinal splitting of the tendon, producing a thickened morphology due to hemorrhage and fibrous tissue. The tendon may be four to five times its normal size and depict heterogeneous signal intensity changes. Type 2 tears are more severe, resulting in thinning or attenuation (atrophy) of the tendon. In type 3 tears, there is a complete tendon rupture with retraction and gap between the proximal and distal fibers. The gap usually fills with either fluid or hemorrhage. Initially, a significant number of patients are afflicted with tendinosis. Fusiform thickening of the tendon associated with degenerative signal intensity changes on T1W and T2W images are characteristic imaging features of this noninflammatory disorder. In these patients, the pathologic process is often insidious and symptoms may mimic arch instability.

Notes

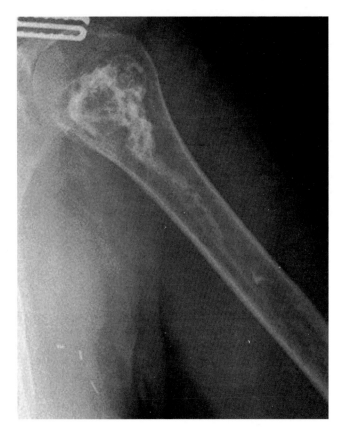 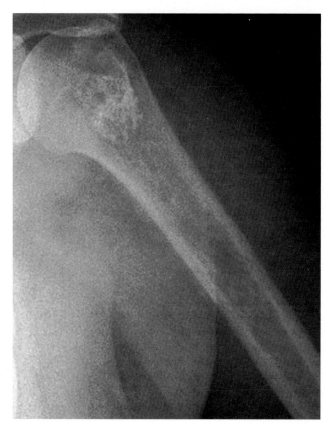

1. These radiographs were taken four years apart. What has happened?

2. Who is at risk for developing this complication?

3. What is the histology of the neoplasms?

4. Is this lesion common? When does this complication occur?

Sarcoma Associated with a Bone Infarct

1. Malignant transformation of a bone infarct.

2. Men in the fifth to seventh decades.

3. Malignant fibrous histiocytoma and osteosarcoma.

4. No, it is rare. After many years; there is a long latent period between bone infarction and malignant transformation.

References

Galli SJ, Weintraub HP, Proppe KH: Malignant fibrous histiocytoma and pleomorphic sarcoma in association with medullary bone infarcts. *Cancer* 41:607–619, 1978.

Mirra JM, Gold RH, Marafiote R: Malignant (fibrous) histiocytoma arising in association with a bone infarct in sickle-cell disease: Coincidence or cause-and-effect? *Cancer* 39:186–194, 1977.

Cross-Reference

Musculoskeletal Imaging: THE REQUISITES, 3rd ed, pp 472–474.

Comment

The radiographic appearance of a mature bone infarct is distinctive and is seldom a cause for concern. Infarcts are intramedullary lesions that have a characteristic serpentine rim of dense sclerosis surrounding a variably calcified central area. Occasionally, one must differentiate an infarct from an enchondroma but several observations, including internal or central calcifications and the lack of peripheral sclerosis in the latter, are sufficient to avoid confusion between these two entities.

An infarct can undergo two processes that may alter its appearance and both are rare. Cyst formation occurs most frequently in the humerus, followed by the tibia, femur, ilium, and calcaneus. These cysts may erode the endosteal cortex. Malignant transformation also may alter the appearance of an infarct. The majority of cases involve the femur, tibia, and humerus. The lesions are poorly differentiated, containing fibrous, osteoid, or cartilaginous tissue, and have a poor prognosis. The radiographic diagnosis is not challenging and this case of a malignant fibrous histiocytoma arising in association with an infarct in the proximal humerus is fairly typical. There is elevation of the periosteum and a change in the appearance of the infarction indicating infiltration of the marrow. In some patients, the sarcomatous proliferation may eventually obliterate all evidence of a preexistent infarction. This process is often accompanied by cortical destruction and a soft tissue mass.

Notes

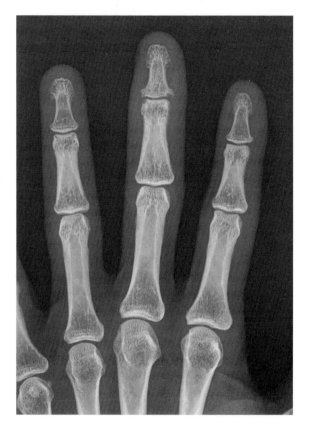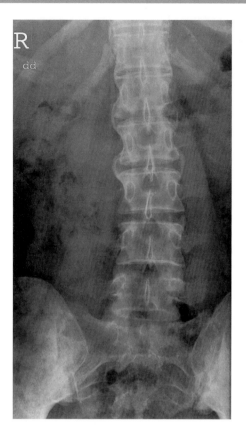

1. What characteristic signs in the hand did you notice?

2. What percentage of people with this disease develop arthritis? Who is at risk?

3. What percentage of people with the arthropathy develop sacroiliac joint abnormalities?

4. What differentiates the paravertebral ossification of this disease from syndesmophytes in patients with ankylosing spondylitis?

Psoriatic Arthropathy

1. Diffuse soft tissue swelling in the middle finger (sausage finger) and erosions with accompanying bony proliferation in the third distal interphalangeal joint ("Mickey Mouse" erosions).

2. Two percent to 6%, but as high as 25% in some populations. Patients with moderate to severe skin abnormalities; strongest association is with patients who demonstrate nail changes.

3. About 30% to 50%.

4. Psoriatic arthropathy does not involve the annulus fibrosus.

Reference

El-Khoury GY, Kathol MH, Brandser EA: Seronegative spondyloarthropathies. *Radiol Clin North Am* 34: 343–357, 1996.

Cross-Reference

Musculoskeletal Imaging: THE REQUISITES, 3rd ed, pp 321–324.

Comment

Psoriatic arthritis is a synovial inflammatory arthropathy that is considered a seronegative rheumatoid variant. It generally affects patients with moderate to severe skin disease, but its strongest correlation is in patients who demonstrate nail abnormalities such as pitting, ridging, splintering, and thickening. This arthropathy has five presentations: distal interphangeal joint polyarthritis, arthritis mutilans, rheumatoid arthritis–like symmetric polyarthritis, monoarthritis or asymmetric oligoarthritis, and sacroiliitis and spondylitis mimicking ankylosing spondylitis. The arthropathy may antedate skin changes in 20% of cases. The radiographic hallmark of this disease is bone proliferation, distinguishing it from rheumatoid arthritis (the prototypical non–bone-forming synovial inflammatory arthropathy). The joints of the hands and feet are common target sites. Key observations include soft tissue swelling that sometimes involves the entire digit (sausage finger), normal mineralization, bony erosions that begin at the margins of the joint and progress centrally, destroying the entire articular surface area ("pencil-in-cup" deformity), and resorption of the tufts of the distal phalanges. Bony proliferative changes may occur adjacent to these erosions but may also occur in the form of periostitis, joint ankylosis, and enthesopathy. In the axial skeleton, bilateral sacroiliitis is more frequent than unilateral involvement, and may be either symmetric or asymmetric. In the spine, asymmetric or unilateral paravertebral ossifications affect the lower thoracic and upper lumbar spine.

Notes

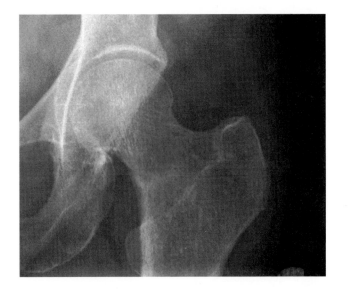

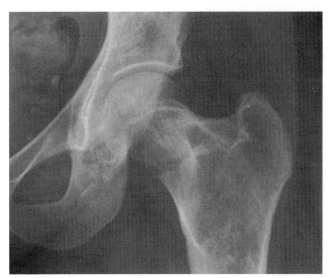

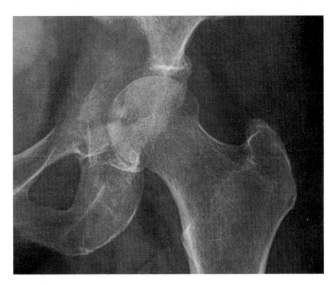

These three patients presented with hip pain.

1. What is the diagnosis?

2. What is the diagnosis?

3. What is the diagnosis?

4. What is the most common feature in the clinical history of patients with fatigue fractures?

Hip Pain

1. Compressive fatigue stress fracture of the femoral neck.

2. Fracture of the femoral neck. This patient fell.

3. Pathologic insufficiency fracture of the acetabulum in a metastasis from lung cancer.

4. New onset or increased intensity of a particular strenuous and repetitive activity.

Reference

Anderson MW, Greenspan A: Stress fractures. *Radiology* 199:1–12, 1996.

Cross-Reference

Musculoskeletal Imaging: THE REQUISITES, 3rd ed, pp 196–198 and 202–203.

Comment

This case illustrates three types of fractures in the left hip. A fatigue fracture is caused by abnormal stresses applied to normal bone, whereas an insufficiency fracture is caused by normal stresses on abnormal bone, such as through a neoplastic lesion or metastasis. When the cross-section of the bone is involved, a complete fracture occurs. Femoral stress fractures are classified as either compressive or tensile. Compressive stress fractures occur at the base of the femoral neck, near the calcar in the medial aspect of the bone. This type of stress fracture is by far more common than tensile stress fractures. Compressive stress fractures do not usually displace and can be treated with simple nonweight-bearing. Tensile stress fractures, however, tend to occur in older patients. The bone may have an underlying abnormality. A defect in the superior cortex of the femoral neck will progress to a complete fracture with displacement in 50% of patients if it is not treated appropriately. Once a fracture line is visible, internal fixation may be indicated. Fractures of the femoral neck may be difficult to identify if the patient is osteoporotic or if there is significant degenerative changes in the joint. In this situation, a magnetic resonance imaging examination is usually the follow-up study of choice because it allows direct inspection of the bone marrow.

Remember, patients who complain of hip pain may also have labral tears, arthritis, pigmented villonodular synovitis, osteochondromatosis, and impingement syndromes.

Notes

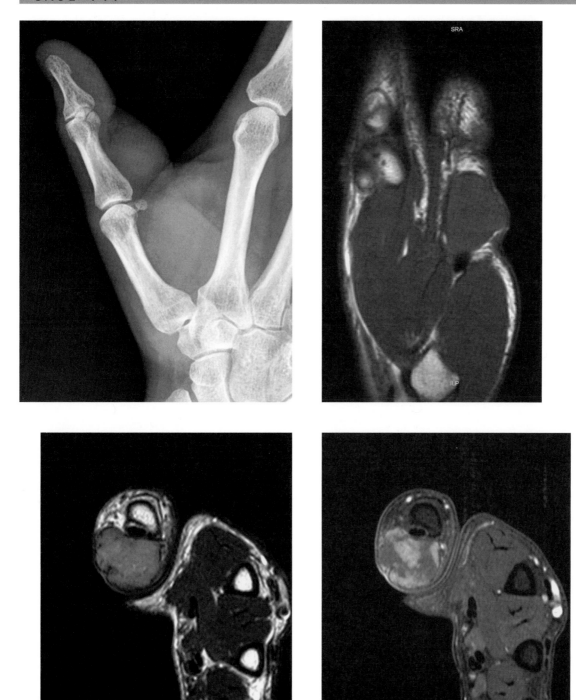

1. Do you think this patient has pain?

2. What percentage of patients with this lesion have osseous erosions?

3. Histologically, this lesion is identical to what other process?

4. What are the two forms of this disorder?

Giant Cell Tumor of Tendon Sheath

1. No, giant cell tumors of tendon sheath are painless masses.

2. Ten percent.

3. Pigmented villonodular synovitis (PVNS).

4. This patient has the localized nodular synovitis form, common in the digits. The diffuse florid synovitis form is less well defined and develops outside the joint, growing in an irregular multinodular pattern, and occurs about the knee and ankle.

References

Jelinek JS, Kransdorf MJ, Shmookler BM, et al: Giant cell tumor of the tendon sheath: MR findings in nine cases. *AJR Am J Roentgenol* 162:919–922, 1994.

Kitagawa Y, Ito H, Amano Y, et al: MR imaging for preoperative diagnosis and assessment of local tumor extent on localized giant cell tumor of tendon sheath. *Skeletal Radiol* 32:633–638, 2003.

Cross-Reference

Musculoskeletal Imaging: THE REQUISITES, 3rd ed, pp 506–507.

Comment

Giant cell tumor of the tendon sheath is a localized proliferative disorder of the synovium in the tendon sheath. It is characterized by a slow-growing, painless mass in the hand and occasionally in the feet. Patients are usually adults in their fourth or fifth decades of life and there is a female predominance. Radiographically, a dense focal soft tissue mass may be associated with osseous erosion with a well-defined sclerotic border, indicative of its slow growth, and occasionally cortical scalloping. Rarely, the degree of adjacent osseous erosion may mimic an intrinsic osseous lesion. When in the thumb or fingers, it is an obvious dense protruberance of the soft tissues. Calcifications are rare. If this lesion involves the joint, the pressure erosions of the bone may be seen on both sides of the joint. Histologically, it is identical to PVNS. However, this lesion hemorrhages much less than PVNS. On magnetic resonance imaging, the lesion is hypointense to muscle on T1W images and variably hypo- to hyperintense on T2W images, depending on the hemosiderin content. These lesions tend to have a polylobular morphology. They usually enhance after intravenous contrast administration owing to a rich capillary system.

Notes

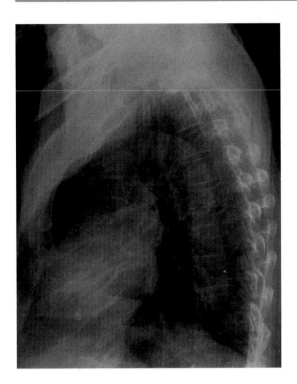 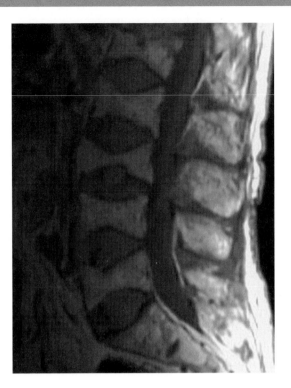

1. What is the condition and what complication did you observe?

2. What would you include in your differential diagnosis?

3. In the appendicular skeleton, what does cortical tunneling indicate?

4. How much heparin must be administered to induce this condition? Is it permanent?

C A S E   1 4 2

Osteoporosis with Sternal Stress Fracture

1. Osteopenia and biconcave vertebral bodies; insufficiency fracture of the sternum.

2. Senile osteoporosis, medication, endocrine disorders, nutritional deficiency states, alcoholism, marrow replacement processes, liver disease, anemia, and osteogenesis imperfecta.

3. Rapid bone loss.

4. More than 15,000 units per day. No.

Reference

Raymakers JA, Kapelle JW, van Beresteijn EC, Duursma SA: Assessment of osteoporotic spine deformity: A new method. *Skeletal Radiol* 19:91–97, 1990.

Cross-Reference

Musculoskeletal Imaging: THE REQUISITES, 3rd ed, pp 391–396.

Comment

Osteoporosis refers to a generalized decrease in bone mass caused by a deficiency of osteoid formation or from increased bone resorption. It can involve the entire skeleton (generalized), one segment of the skeleton (regional), or one or more focal areas (localized). Generalized osteoporosis can be caused by numerous conditions. The radiographic manifestations caused by many of these processes predominate in the axial skeleton and produce changes relatively early in the spine. Resorption of the horizontal trabeculae in the vertebral body causes a loss of bone density while increasing the conspicuity of the vertical trabeculation. Cortical thinning also occurs but the end plates remain prominent. Changes in the vertebral body contour can occur from compression fractures and protrusion of the intervertebral discs. Generalized height loss and a characteristic biconcave deformity (as seen in this patient) are common findings in senile and postmenopausal osteoporosis. Anterior wedging and diffuse compression fractures also are common manifestations and, in the thoracic spine, can contribute to significant kyphosis. Ultimately, it may contribute to the development of an insufficiency fracture of the sternum, which may go undetected until it becomes displaced. Bone pain can be associated with an acute loss of height of a vertebral body but it is often difficult, even with comparison radiographs, to determine the age of a vertebral body deformity.

Notes

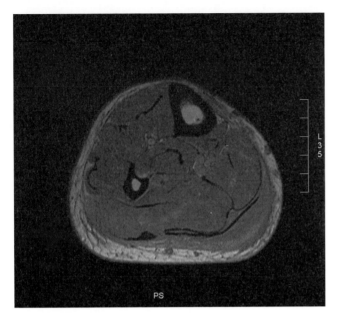 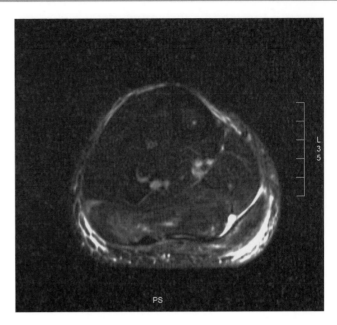

1. What are the findings on these proton-density and T2W images?

2. This patient ran a marathon two days ago and now has intense pain. What is the diagnosis?

3. Are the magnetic resonance imaging findings permanent?

4. Over the next few days, what will his serum values show?

Exercise-Induced Rhabdomyolysis

1. Intermediate to high signal intensity in the soleus and gastrocnemius muscles, subcutaneous fat edema, and intermuscular fluid accumulation posteriorly.

2. Exercise-induced rhabdomyolysis.

3. No, the signal intensity of the muscles will revert to normal within 1 to 2 weeks.

4. Elevated creatine phosphokinase and blood urea nitrogen.

References

May DA, Disler DG, Jones EA, et al: Abnormal signal intensity in skeletal muscle at MR imaging: Patterns, pearls, and pitfalls. *Radiographics* 20:S295–S315, 2000.

Shellock FG, Fukunaga T, Mink JH, Edgerton VR: Exertional muscle injury: Evaluation of concentric versus eccentric actions with serial MR imaging. *Radiology* 179:659–664, 1991.

Cross-Reference

Musculoskeletal Imaging: THE REQUISITES, 3rd ed, pp 33–40.

Comment

An increase in both extracellular and intracellular water content normally occurs in muscles after exercise, the majority of the increase being extracellular. Magnetic resonance imaging is sensitive to the alteration in T1 and T2 values that account for the increased signal intensity in the muscle on T2W images after strenuous exercise. Delayed onset muscle soreness is characterized by discomfort or pain after muscular exertion. The pain increases in intensity in the first 24 hours after exercise, peaks after 24 to 72 hours, then subsides to normal after approximately 7 days. Shellock and colleagues demonstrated statistically significant increases in T2 relaxation times in biceps muscles in patients with delayed onset muscle soreness, with the highest mean measurements occurring between days 3 and 5. Prolongation of relaxation times on magnetic resonance images is considered to be predominantly the result of accumulated edema, which develops shortly after severe exertional muscle injuries. Symptoms of pain and soreness localized to the insertion sites of the exercised muscles, and discernible swelling and distention of the arms was maximal from 3 to 10 days, correlating closely to peak T2 changes. Other investigators have also noted a high correlation between changes in muscle T2 relaxation time, pain, and elevation in serum creatine phosphokinase levels. This patient's creatine phosphokinase levels peaked at a level of 196,314 ti/IL on day 6.

Notes

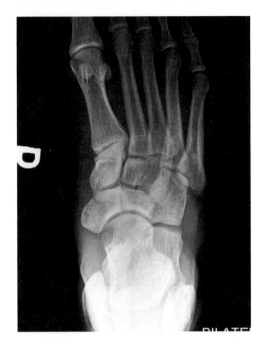
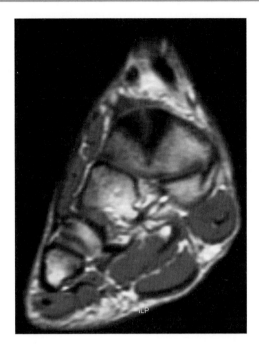
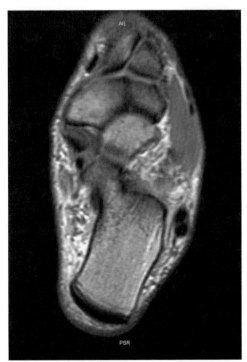
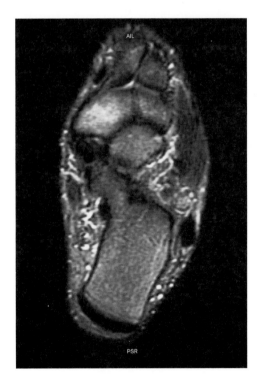

1. What is the diagnosis?

2. What is the classic clinical presentation?

3. What is the main complication of this injury?

4. What is the single most contributing factor to development of complications?

Navicular Stress Fracture

1. Navicular stress fracture.

2. Poorly localized pain over the course of several months.

3. Nonunion, which can occur in over 20% of cases.

4. Persistent weight-bearing. As soon as the diagnosis is made, cast immobilization with nonweight-bearing is the current recommendation.

Reference

Burne SG, Mahoney CM, Forster BB, et al: Tarsal navicular stress injury: Long-term outcome and clinicoradiological correlation using both computed tomography and magnetic resonance imaging. *Am J Sports Med* 33:1875–1881, 2005.

Cross-Reference

Musculoskeletal Imaging: THE REQUISITES, 3rd ed, pp 274–275 and 277.

Comment

Stress fractures of the navicular bone are uncommon when compared to the calcaneus and talus. However, they may occur with higher frequency in runners and basketball players. Symptoms are usually insidious and poorly localized to the medial arch of the foot. Characteristically, fractures are oriented in the sagittal plane and occur at the junction of the middle and lateral thirds of the navicular bone. As a result, this fracture may be difficult to identify on radiographs. Computed tomography and magnetic resonance imaging are both outstanding modalities for identifying this disorder, but the latter technique has the advantage of evaluating the marrow contents directly. A stress fracture appears as a linear or bandlike area of low signal intensity on all pulse sequences surrounded by a broader and less defined area of altered signal. If the foot is imaged within a few weeks of the onset of symptoms, however, the marrow edema is prominently seen as high signal intensity on fluid sensitive sequences. The potential for developing avascular necrosis of the lateral fragment of the navicular is a concern if the diagnosis if delayed. Ordinarily, navicular stress fractures respond equally well to conservative management and surgery, but they remain a source of morbidity in high caliber athletes.

Notes

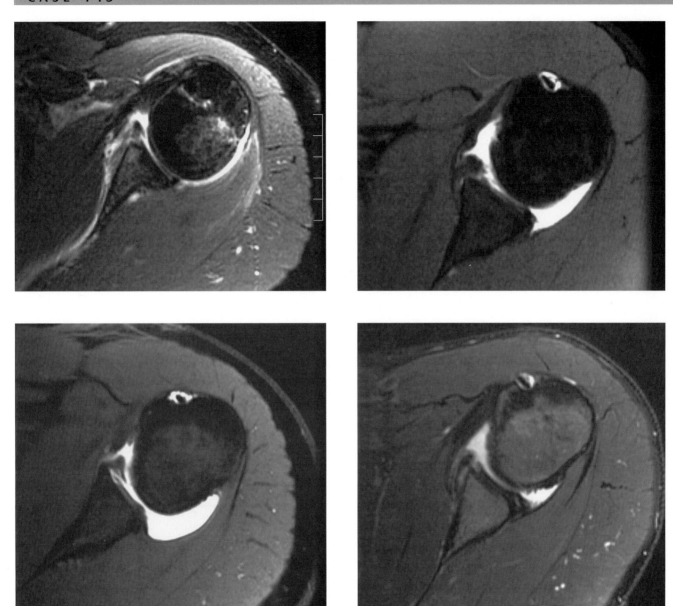

You are shown four axial MR images from four different patients with the same injury mechanism.

1. Name the finding and what it means.

2. Name the finding and what it means.

3. Name the finding and what it means.

4. Name the finding and what it means.

Anterior Shoulder Dislocation (Labrocapsular)

1. A Bankart lesion; avulsion of the anteroinferior labrum by the anterior limb of the inferior glenohumeral ligament with simultaneous rupture of the anterior periosteum.

2. Perthes lesion; the labrum is torn but remains attached to a stripped but intact periosteum.

3. Glenolabral articular disruption (GLAD) lesion; the anteroinferior labrum and a fragment of underlying cartilage have stripped as one unit.

4. Anterior labral periosteal sleeve avulsion (ALPSA) lesion; it represents an extended Perthes lesion with the labrum medially displaced.

Reference

Shankman S, Bencardino J, Beltran J: Glenohumeral instability: Evaluation using MR arthrography of the shoulder. *Skeletal Radiol* 28:365–382, 1999.

Cross-Reference

Musculoskeletal Imaging: THE REQUISITES, 3rd ed, pp 98–105.

Comment

Approximately 95% of dislocations of the glenohumeral joint are anterior. Osseous injuries such as a Hill-Sachs lesion, osseous Bankart lesion, and greater tuberosity fractures are important findings. Evaluation of soft tissue injuries, however, require additional imaging with magnetic resonance imaging to fully inspect the labrum, anterior capsule, and integrity of the subscapularis tendon and tendon of the long head of the biceps brachii. The Bankart lesion is described as an avulsion of the anteroinferior labrum by the anterior limb of the inferior glenohumeral ligament associated with a rupture of the anterior periosteum. There are many configurations for this injury. MR arthrography is particularly useful for delineating the various Bankart variants. Among the alphabet soup that has been reported in the literature are the Perthes lesion, GLAD lesion, ALPSA lesion, GOCD (glenoid osteochondral defect) lesion, HAGL (humeral avulsion of the inferior glenohumeral ligament) lesion, BAGL (HAGL lesion with a bony avulsion) lesion, and GLOM (glenolabral ovoid mass) lesion.

The attachment of the anterior capsule is generally stripped in many of these lesions. When the attachment is over 1 cm proximal to the base of the anterior labrum, it is considered pathologic and referred to as a type 3 anterior capsular insertion. A type 1 anterior capsule inserts at the labrum or its base. A type 2 anterior capsule indicates an attachment between type 1 and 3 insertions.

Notes

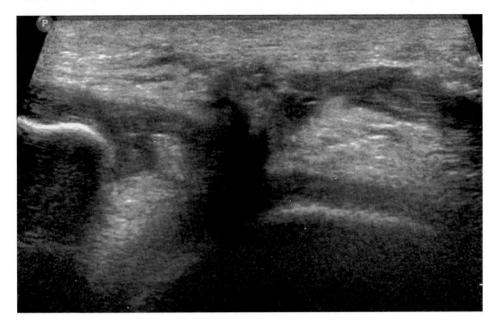

1. You are shown a longitudinal sonogram of the patellar tendon (right side is distal). What is the diagnosis?

2. How does this injury occur?

3. What are predisposing factors?

4. What transducer is best for high spatial resolution in this area?

Patellar Tendon Rupture

1. Complete rupture of the patellar tendon.

2. Rapid deceleration while running, or quadriceps failure while ascending or descending stairs.

3. Repeated microtrauma (tendinosis) and systemic diseases (renal disease, crystal diseases such as gout and CPPD, diabetes mellitus, RA, systemic lupus, hyperparathyroidism).

4. Generally 7 to 10 MHz transducers provide excellent images.

References

Carr JC, Hanly S, Griffin J, Gibney R: Sonography of the patellar tendon and adjacent structures in pediatric and adult patients. *AJR Am J Roentgenol* 176:1535–1539, 2001.

Yu JS, Petersilge C, Sartoris DJ, et al: MR imaging of injuries of the extensor mechanism of the knee. *Radiographics* 14:541–551, 1994.

Cross-Reference

Musculoskeletal Imaging: THE REQUISITES, 3rd ed, pp 216–217.

Comment

The extensor mechanism of the knee consists of the tendons of the quadriceps femoris muscles, patella, patellar tendon, patellar retinacula and extensor hood, and the insertion of the patellar tendon into the tibial tubercle. Normal tendons do not rupture under stress and are capable of withstanding up to 17.5 times the normal body weight. Abnormal tendons weakened by degeneration or repetitive microtrauma are susceptible to rupture. The common locations for these ruptures are at the enthesis of the tendon, and the inferior pole attachment of the patellar tendon is the most common location for failure of this tendon. Sonography is an effective means for evaluating the patellar tendon. It appears cylindrical on the transverse images and linear on longitudinal images, with well-defined margins and low to moderate internal echoes. The thickness does not exceed 4 mm and it is thinner more proximally than distally. It is demarcated by the hyperechoic subcutaneous fat anteriorly and fat in Hoffa's pad posteriorly. Tendon ruptures present with focal pain. They can be either complete or partial, and they may be preceded by tendinosis. A discrete hypoechoic focus indicates a tendon defect, and a complete tear causes frank discontinuity of the tendon margins. Posterior acoustic shadowing deep to the frayed free ends occurs as in this patient. Several bursae exist adjacent to the tendon including the prepatellar bursa that can distend with a tendon rupture. Contraction of the quadriceps musculature may produce a high riding patella, or patella alta. Therefore, complete tears are treated surgically to preserve the function of the extensor mechanism.

Notes

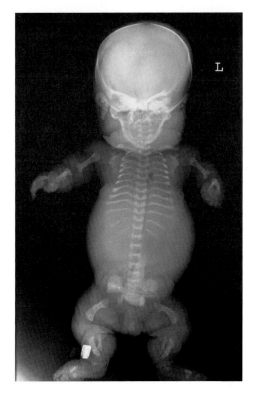 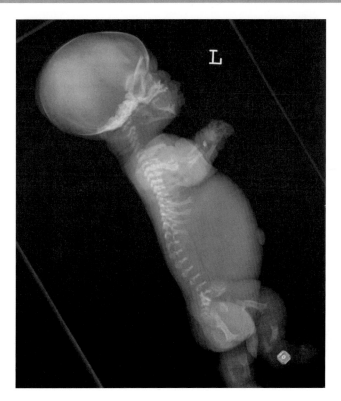

1. What is the diagnosis?

2. What is the life expectancy of this patient?

3. What do these patients succumb to?

4. What disorder closely mimics the clinical and radiographic appearance of this condition?

Thanatophoric Dwarfism

1. Thanatophoric dwarfism.

2. Most die within hours to days of birth. The longest reported life has been 7 months.

3. Respiratory arrest.

4. Homozygous achondroplasia.

Reference

Machado LE, Bonilla-Musoles F, Raga F, et al: Thanatophoric dysplasia: Ultrasound diagnosis. *Ultrasound Q* 17:235–243, 2001.

Cross-Reference

Musculoskeletal Imaging: THE REQUISITES, 3rd ed, p 633.

Comment

Thanatophoric dwarfism is a lethal short-limbed dwarfism characterized by very short limbs with a relatively normal-sized trunk in the newborn. The head is disproportionately large with bulging eyes. The thorax is small, and marked respiratory distress is evident if the child is born alive. Prenatal diagnosis may be established sonographically if fetal disproportion, polyhydramnios, and decreased fetal movement are observed. Radiographically, the diagnosis includes characteristic findings in the spine with diffuse platyspondyly with narrowing of the vertebral bodies most pronounced in the midline and narrow interpediculate distances. In the pelvis, the findings include short iliac bones in the craniocaudad dimension with horizontal acetabular roofs, small sciatic notch, and short and broad ischial bones. In the chest, the thorax is narrow with cupped anterior ribs, small scapulae, and long clavicles that are hooked. The extremity bones are markedly short with flared metaphyses and are bowed. The tubular bones of the hands and feet are broad. The skull is enlarged with a small foramen magnum, small face, and depressed nasal bridge. A "cloverleaf" skull is an occasional finding.

Notes

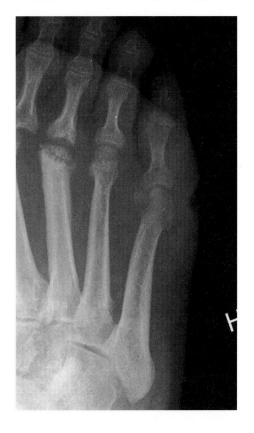

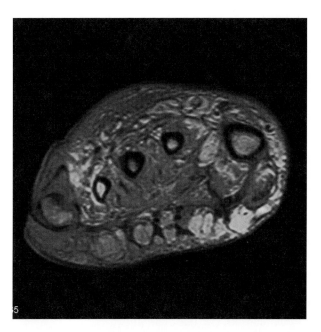

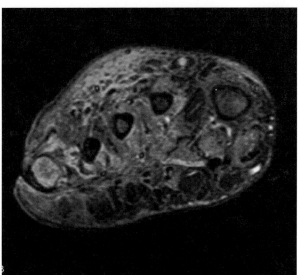

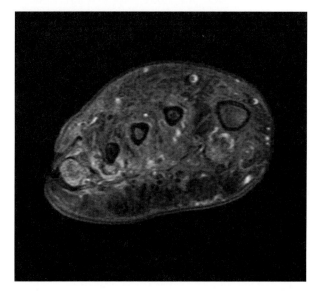

1. What are the radiographic findings?

2. What did you see on the T1W, short-τ inversion recovery, and fat-saturated contrast-enhanced images?

3. In the foot, how many plantar compartments are there and why is it important to inspect them in an infection of the foot?

4. What causes enhancement of the bone after intravenous administration of gadolinium? Is this a specific finding?

Diabetic Acute Osteomyelitis

1. Lateral ulcer, soft tissue swelling, and focal osteopenia of the fifth metatarsophalangeal joint.

2. Marrow edema that enhances, cellulitis around the ulcer, deep compartment myositis, and dorsal subcutaneous fat edema.

3. Three main compartments—medial, intermediate, and lateral; an infection may be contained by the intermuscular septae and spread proximally.

4. Hyperemia. No, it can be seen also in tumor, trauma, and neuropathic disease.

Reference

Ledermann HP, Morrison WB: Differential diagnosis of pedal osteomyelitis and diabetic neuroarthropathy: MR imaging. *Semin Musculoskelet Radiol* 9:272–283, 2005.

Cross-Reference

Musculoskeletal Imaging: THE REQUISITES, 3rd ed, pp 545–550.

Comment

Osteomyelitis implies an infection of bone and marrow and is most commonly caused by bacterial agents, although fungi, parasites, and viruses can also infect the bone and marrow. There are three routes (hematogenous spread, direct extension, and direct implantation) that cause infection in the bone. Direct extension from an adjacent soft tissue infection is the most common cause of acute osteomyelitis in a diabetic patient. In the hands and feet, skin ulceration is an important observation and requires close vigilance for an underlying infection. Furthermore, once the hands or feet become infected, the infection can spread through numerous structures and compartments, including the tendons, fascial planes, muscles, bones, and lymphatics. Infections caused by direct innoculation of the bone from a penetrating injury may be problematic because it may be associated with an unusual organism such as *Pseudomonas aeruginosa*. The radiographic features of acute osteomyelitis include osteopenia, focal bone lysis or destruction, and periostitis, in addition to surrounding soft tissue swelling and/or ulceration. Magnetic resonance imaging is useful for early detection of osteomyelitis because it allows direct inspection of the marrow. The use of gadolinium improves delineation of soft-tissue inflammatory masses, but does not distinguish osteomyelitis from other sources of marrow edema. It is therefore important to identify concomitant abnormalities such as an abscess, sinus tract, or skin ulceration.

Notes

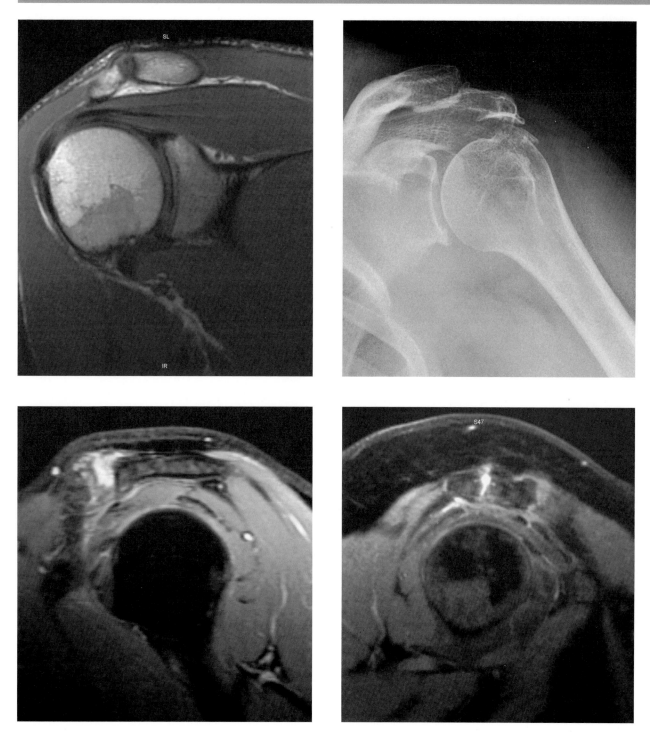

1. All four of these patients presented with chronic shoulder pain. List the principal observations in the order that you see them.

2. What is the aim of treatment?

3. What is the rotator cuff interval? What structure is normally seen here?

4. What does a posterosuperior glenoid tear and rotator cuff tear at the junction of the infraspinatus and supraspinatus tendons in a throwing athlete describe? What is the best way to demonstrate the abnormality?

Chronic Shoulder Pain—Impingement

1. Downsloping acromion, subacromial spur and deltoid enthesophyte, hooked acromion, and an unstable os acromiale.

2. Restoring the space between the humerus and the coracoacromial arch.

3. The region beneath the coracoacromial arch that is located between the subscapularis and supraspinatus tendons. The intra-articular portion of the tendon of the long head of the biceps muscle.

4. Internal (posterosuperior glenoid) impingement. Abducted, external rotation (ABER) position on magnetic resonance imaging.

Reference

Fritz RC: Magnetic resonance imaging of sport-related injuries to the shoulder: Impingement and rotator cuff. *Radiol Clin N Am* 40:217–234, 2002.

Cross-Reference

Musculoskeletal Imaging: THE REQUISITES, 3rd ed, pp 85–89.

Comment

Impingement syndrome of the shoulder is a painful condition characterized by sharp pain during the act of abduction and external rotation of the arm, or elevation and internal rotation. The pathogenesis of this syndrome is related to a loss of space between the proximal humerus and the structures that make up the coracoacromial arch. The region beneath the acromio-clavicular (AC) joint is also important in impingement. This leads to degeneration of the cuff, and it has been reported that up to 95% of rotator cuff tears are related to chronic impingement. The most vulnerable area of the rotator cuff is the critical zone of the supraspinatus tendon. Subacromial spurs cause mechanical trauma to the musculotendinous junction of the supraspinatus muscle. Impingement beneath the coracoacromial arch is frequently associated with a hooked acromion process. Impingement beneath a degenerated AC joint is caused by inferior osteophytosis. In this type of impingement, symptoms occur when the shoulder is abducted more than 120 degrees. An os acromiale is present in 8% of the population but when unstable, the anterior aspect of the acromion may efface the supraspinatus tendon. When the pseudoarthrosis itself hypertrophies and is associated with spurring, impingement may occur more posteriorly. On magnetic resonance imaging, effacement of the subacromial fat, subacromial bursal fluid, and any of these osseous abnormalities is diagnostic of impingement.

Notes

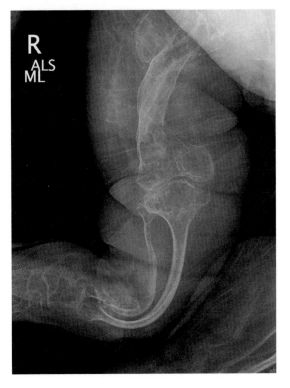
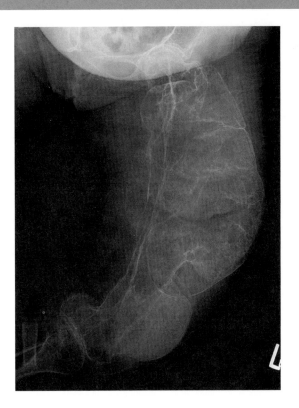

1. What is your diagnosis?

2. List the clinical manifestations of this disease.

3. What radiographic observations may be identified in the skull of patients with this condition?

4. At what age does otosclerosis occur in affected patients?

Osteogenesis Imperfecta

1. Osteogenesis imperfecta.

2. Skeletal fragility from osteoporosis, blue sclerae, dentinogenesis imperfecta, and premature otosclerosis.

3. Platybasia, basilar invagination, wormian bones, enlarged sinuses, and abnormal teeth.

4. Prior to age 40 years.

Reference

Sillence D: Osteogenesis imperfecta: An expanding panorama of variants. *Clin Orthop* 159:11–25, 1981.

Cross-Reference

Musculoskeletal Imaging: THE REQUISITES, 3rd ed, pp 622–625.

Comment

Osteogenesis imperfecta (OI) is an inherited disorder of connective tissue that affects the synthesis and quality of fibrillar collagen, producing a form of congenital osteoporosis. The incidence of OI is one in 20,000 to 60,000 births. There are two main forms: a congenital form (10%) and a tarda form that affects the majority of patients. Each form is further subdivided into two types. The congenital types, types II and III, are severe and characterized by multiple fractures at birth. Type II is incompatible with life and is fatal in the neonatal period. Type III is moderately severe and leads to significant deformities such as bowing of the bones and short-limbed dwarfism as seen in this patient. The congenital subtypes may be inherited as an autosomal recessive trait or occur as a spontaneous new mutation. The latent types, types I and IV, are inherited as an autosomal dominant and are milder by comparison. In these patients, the incidence of fractures varies, and only 20% of patients with these subtypes present with fractures at birth. In type I OI, the classic tarda form, the first fracture typically occurs in the second or third year of life. Radiographically, the classic findings include marked osteopenia, and slender and overconstricted tubular bones. The cortices may appear either thinned or thickened. Deformities from prior fractures may be dominant findings or bones may appear bowed secondary to microfractures. Excessive callus formation is a characteristic finding of the disease and may involve the entire length of the bone, although some fractures may heal with a pseudoarthrosis. Ligamentous laxity causes premature degenerative joint disease.

Notes

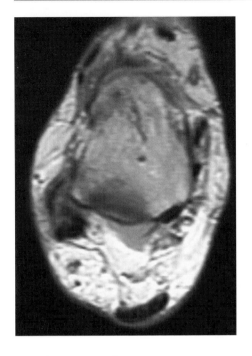
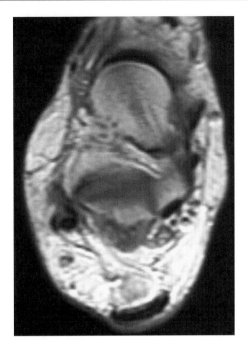

1. What is your diagnosis?

2. Where do most of these injuries begin?

3. What are predisposing factors that are contributory?

4. What is the mechanism of injury?

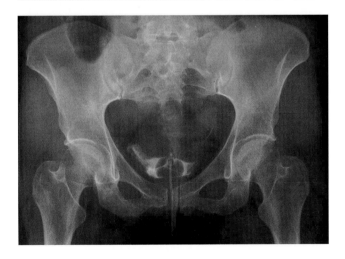
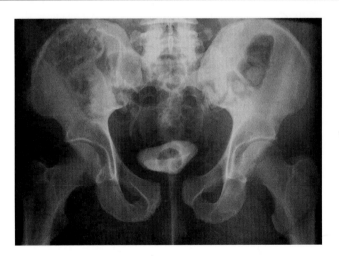

You are shown radiographs of two different patients.

1. What was the mechanism of injury on the first patient? And the second patient?

2. When present, does the orientation of the pubic fractures help to identify the force of injury?

3. Why is computed tomography indicated?

4. List some common complications seen with these injuries.

Peroneus Brevis Tendon Tear

1. Longitudinal tear of the peroneus brevis tendon.

2. Either just distal to the fibular tip or beyond the inferior extensor retinaculum.

3. Shallow or convex fibular groove, or laxity of the superior peroneal retinaculum.

4. Dorsiflexion with ankle inversion.

Reference

Khoury NJ, El-Khoury GY, Saltzman CL, Kathol MH: Peroneus longus and brevis tendon tears: MR imaging evaluation. *Radiology* 200:833–841, 1996.

Cross-Reference

Musculoskeletal Imaging: THE REQUISITES, 3rd ed, pp 265–267.

Comment

The majority of peroneal tendon tears are partial and oriented in the long axis of the tendon, splitting the tendon into two or more bundles. Note that in this patient portions of the peroneus brevis tendon straddle the peroneus longus tendon. Unsuspected tears can be a source of chronic pain and instability, and may require surgical repair. Tears of the peroneus brevis tendon can be caused by numerous mechanisms and have a high prevalence among young, athletic people as well as elderly people. When related to trauma, the mechanism of injury is forceful dorsiflexion with inversion of the foot. Magnetic resonance imaging is ideal for evaluating the peroneal tendons because it allows multiplanar assessment of these tendons, but also because it is highly sensitive for inflammatory changes in and about the tendon. The hallmark of acute tears of the peroneal tendons on magnetic resonance images is increased signal intensity within the substance of the tendon on T1W and T2W images, appearing as a linear area of altered signal. In this patient, the separated bundles of the peroneus brevis give a "Mickey Mouse ears" appearance. The tendon may also be thickened focally in a fusiform fashion depending on the length of the tear and chronicity of the injury. In chronic tears, the changes in signal intensity may be less intense on T2W images, although a thickened morphology usually persists and may be even more exaggerated than in the acute phase of the tear, owing to the development of fibrosis.

Notes

Pelvic Fractures

1. Lateral compression. Anteroposterior compression.

2. Yes, oblique fractures are lateral compression and vertical fractures are seen in anteroposterior and vertical shear injuries.

3. To evaluate the posterior structures including subtle sacral and iliac fractures, and integrity of the sacroiliac (SI) joints.

4. Pelvic hemorrhage, distant fractures, and neurologic injuries to the lumbosacral plexus.

Reference

Hunter JC, Brandser EA, Tran KA: Pelvic and acetabular trauma. *Radiol Clin North Am* 35:559–590, 1997.

Cross-Reference

Musculoskeletal Imaging: THE REQUISITES, 3rd ed, pp 183–188.

Comment

Pelvic ring fractures are broadly categorized into lateral compression, anteroposterior compression, and vertical shear injuries. About 50% of pelvic fractures are caused by a blow to the lateral side of the pelvis (lateral compression). These are classified into three types: type 1, the lateral force is to the posterior pelvis, producing unilateral or bilateral pubic rami fractures, crush injury of the sacrum, and central acetabular fractures (20%); type 2, the force is more anterior resulting in ipsilateral displacement of the innominate bone with either rupture of the SI joint (2A) or fracture of the iliac wing (2B) and ipsilateral pubis; and type 3, the force also is directed anteriorly, resulting in internal rotation of the innominate bone on the injured side and lateral displacement on the contralateral side, with disruption of the SI joint and posterior ligament complex (3A) or the ipsilateral iliac wing (3B) and bilateral pubic fractures.

There are three types of anterior compression injuries: type I, vertical pubic ramus fractures or mild pubic diastasis; Type II, "open book" injuries with pubic diastasis and disruption of anterior SI ligaments and posterior ligaments; and type III, further widening of pubic symphysis and SI joint. Vertical shear injuries are characterized by disruption of the hemipelvis through the symphysis or pubic rami with disruption of the ipsilateral sacroiliac joint or iliac bone.

Notes

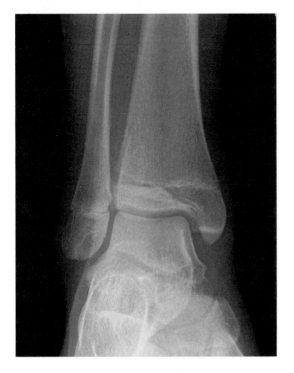
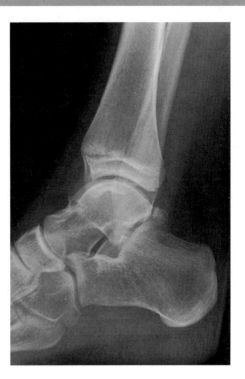

1. What is the mechanism of injury?

2. What determines whether the injury will result in a two-part or three-part fracture?

3. Would you consider this injury a Tillaux fracture?

4. What is Kump's bump? What is important about this area?

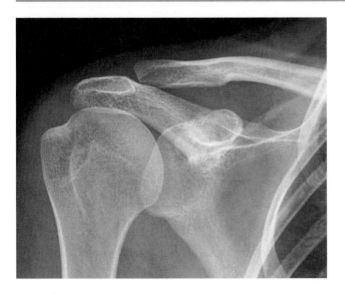
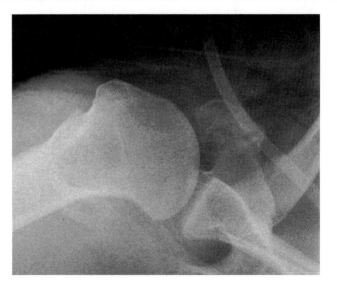

1. This patient had anterior shoulder pain for three months after an injury. What is the finding?

2. He had radiographs during the initial injury that showed no fracture. Can you explain this?

3. What other injury is difficult to diagnose in the scapula?

4. Is there an association with dislocations of the ipsilateral acromioclavicular joint?

Triplane Fracture

1. External rotation of the ankle often with plantar flexion of the foot.

2. Age of patient (fusion of the growth plate).

3. No, a Tillaux fracture is a Salter-Harris III fracture that involves the lateral aspect of the tibial epiphysis.

4. It is the superior convexity of the distal tibial growth plate in the anteromedial quadrant of the physis. This is where fusion begins.

Reference

Brown SD, Kasser JR, Zurakowski D, Jaramillo D: Analysis of 51 tibial triplane fractures using CT with multiplanar reconstruction. *AJR Am J Roentgenol* 183: 1489–1495, 2004.

Cross-Reference

Musculoskeletal Imaging: THE REQUISITES, 3rd ed, pp 255–257.

Comment

A triplane fracture refers to a fracture of the distal tibia that occurs in skeletally immature patients. The lateral one half of the distal tibial epiphysis and physeal plate, and posterior tibial metaphysis are involved. "Triplane" indicates that fractures occur in all three geometric planes. The fracture planes include a sagittally oriented fracture through the epiphysis, a transverse fracture through the anterolateral aspect of the physeal plate, and a coronally oriented oblique fracture through the posterior aspect of the metaphysis. There are two types of triplane fractures and the appearance of the fracture is dependent upon fusion of the medial portion of the growth plate. When the physeal plate is unfused, these fractures result in three fragments. Older adolescents, owing to a partially fused growth plate, develop a two-fragment triplane fracture because the medial mallelus remains attached to the tibial shaft.

Computed tomography is advocated for delineating the extent of injuries in patients with triplane fractures. It accurately identifies the number of fracture fragments and the degree of displacement of the epiphysis, and reformatted images allow determination of any distraction of the growth plate. Articular incongruity that exceeds 2 mm requires reduction. Radiographically, these fractures mimic Salter-Harris type IV fractures because they represent a combination of a Salter-Harris II fracture of the posterior tibial metaphysis and a Salter-Harris III fracture of the medial aspect of the distal tibial epiphysis.

Notes

Coracoid Fracture

1. Subacute fracture of the coracoid process.

2. An axillary view either was not obtained or was suboptimal.

3. Acromion process fractures.

4. Yes, that is why you should inspect the coracoid process closely in all cases of acromioclavicular joint separation.

References

Goss TP: The scapula: Coracoid, acromial, and avulsion fractures. *Am J Orthop* 25:106–115, 1996.

Wang KC, Hsu KY, Shih CH: Coracoid process fracture combined with acromioclavicular dislocation and coracoclavicular ligament rupture: A case report and review of the literature. *Clin Orthop Relat Res* 300: 120–122, 1994.

Cross-Reference

Musculoskeletal Imaging: THE REQUISITES, 3rd ed, pp 73–74.

Comment

The anteroposterior radiograph of the right shoulder barely shows a faint lucency near the base of the coracoid process. In the axillary view, a transverse fracture of the coracoid process near its base is present with some callus formation. Coracoid process fractures have this characteristic orientation through its base. It may be caused by a direct impaction against the tip of the coracoid, an anterior glenohumeral joint dislocation, or separation of the acromioclavicular joint. Occasionally, the ossification center of the coracoid process may be avulsed, which mimics this fracture. Fractures of the coracoid process are difficult to visualize with conventional radiographs. Axillary views and transscapular Y views are considered essential projections for depicting fractures of the coracoid process. When "missed," a fracture may result in a nonunion.

Occasionally, computed tomography may be required for diagnosis. It is an optimal modality for evaluating fractures of the scapula because it allows unimpeded inspection of this bone. Magnetic resonance imaging allows simultaneous inspection of the bone marrow and the ligamentous structures of the shoulder girdle but is best reserved as a follow-up examination after the osseous injuries have been ascertained acutely.

Notes

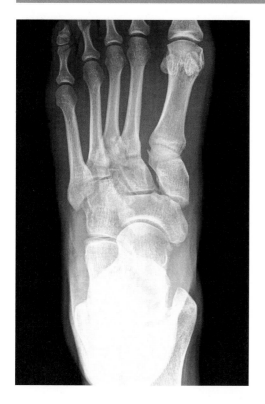
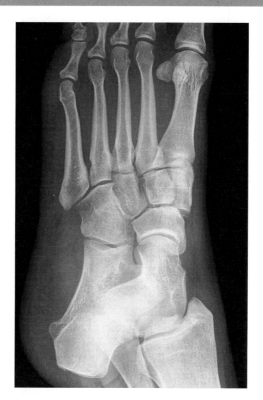
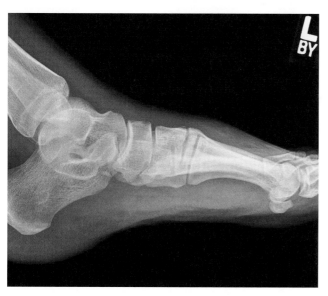

1. What is the mechanism of injury?

2. Name the different types that may occur in this injury. What type does this patient have?

3. If you suspect this injury but the initial radiographic series is equivocal, what simple maneuver can you do to stress the foot?

4. What vascular structure may be simultaneously injured?

Lisfranc's Fracture/Dislocation

1. Forced plantar flexion of the forefoot.

2. Homolateral, partial incongruity, and divergent Lisfranc's fracture/dislocation. Partial incongruity with subluxation of the medial cuneiform.

3. Perform a standing lateral view to look for dorsal displacement of the base of the metatarsal bones.

4. The dorsalis pedis artery.

Reference

Norfray JF, Geline RA, Steinberg RI, et al: Subtleties of Lisfranc fracture-dislocations. *Am J Roentgenol* 137: 1151–1156, 1981.

Cross-Reference

Musculoskeletal Imaging: THE REQUISITES, 3rd ed, pp 275–277.

Comment

Tarsometatarsal fracture/dislocations are referred to as Lisfranc's injuries. Transverse metatarsal ligaments connect the bases of the second through fifth metatarsal bones, but this ligament does not exist between the first and second metatarsal bones. Instead, the base of the second metatarsal bone is attached to the medial cuneiform by an oblique ligament (Lisfranc's ligament). Avulsion fractures of the second metatarsal base frequently occur at the enthesis of this ligament. It may occur with subluxation of the medial cuneiform medially, as in this patient. Because there is greater support on the plantar surface by the plantar ligaments and tendons, most dislocations occur dorsally but this may require a standing stress view to become evident. Soft tissue swelling in the dorsum of the midfoot should increase your index of suspicion. If the space between the first and second metatarsal bases appears widened, then the diagnosis is clear.

Lisfranc's injuries may have several patterns. A homolateral (convergent) pattern occurs when there is displacement of all five metatarsal bases, and the direction of displacement is nearly always laterally. A partial incongruity pattern occurs when there is a fracture of the first metatarsal base with displacement of the shaft medially, or when there is lateral displacement of the base of the second to fifth metatarsal bones. A divergent pattern occurs when the first metatarsal base displaces medially without a fracture and the second metatarsal, or a combination of the second to fifth metatarsals, displaces laterally. Treatment is aimed at restoring the anatomy. If displacement is less than 2 mm, closed reduction is adequate. More significant fracture/dislocations require open reduction and internal fixation. If reduction is difficult, evaluation with magnetic resonance imaging or computed tomography is advocated to exclude entrapment of either a tendon or fracture fragment.

Notes

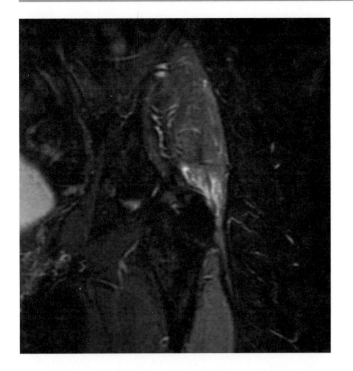
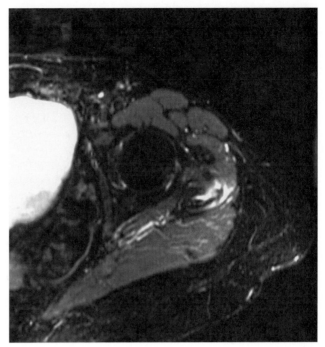
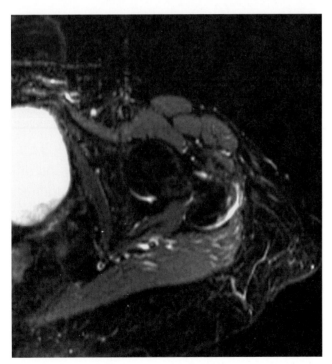

1. What is the likely diagnosis?

2. What is the reported accuracy of magnetic resonance imaging for this diagnosis?

3. Is fluid in the trochanteric bursa specific for this entity?

4. What nerve may supply this bursa?

Gluteus Medius Muscle Tear

1. Partial tear of the gluteus medius tendon insertion.

2. About 91%.

3. No; although it occurs with regularity, bursal fluid may also occur with tendinosis and tendonitis.

4. Branches of the inferior gluteal nerve.

References

Cvitanic O, Henzie G, Skezas N, et al: MRI diagnosis of tears of the hip abductor tendons (gluteus medius and gluteus minimus). *AJR Am J Roentgenol* 182: 137–143, 2004.

Kingzett-Taylor A, Tirman PF, Feller J, et al: Tendinosis and tears of gluteus medius and minimus muscles as a cause of hip pain: MR imaging findings. *AJR Am J Roentgenol* 173:1123–1126, 1999.

Cross-Reference

Musculoskeletal Imaging: THE REQUISITES, 3rd ed, pp 194 and 198.

Comment

Tendinopathy of the hip abductors and gluteus medius and minimus muscles are common findings on magnetic resonance imaging in patients with hip pain, groin pain, or buttock pain. Tendinopathy of the gluteus medius and minimus muscles is also a frequent cause of greater trochanteric pain syndrome, a common regional pain syndrome that can mimic other important conditions that cause hip pain such as osteonecrosis of the femur and stress fractures of either the femur or acetabulum.

Partial tears of the gluteus medius muscle insertion on the greater trochanter are more common than complete tears, but the latter tend to be retracted. These patients present with pain with resistance to hip internal rotation or abduction. Patients typically are middle-aged women and the duration of symptoms tends to be long-standing, averaging over one year. On magnetic resonance imaging, the characteristic finding is edema at the insertion manifested by high signal intensity on T2W images, located superior to the greater trochanter. When completely disrupted, there is retraction of the muscle resulting in a free end of the tendon. In most series, tendinosis and tendonitis (calcific tendonitis) are as frequent as tears. Fluid in the trochanteric bursa often coexists with pathology of the gluteus medius tendon.

Notes

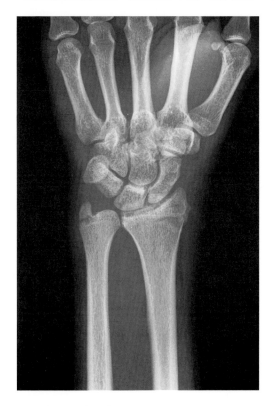 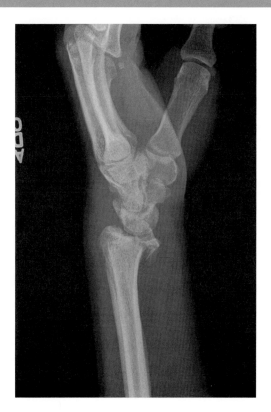

1. What is the diagnosis?
2. Is age a predictive factor in distal radius fracture configuration?
3. What are the goals for reduction of a distal radius fracture?
4. Describe the Frykman classification.

Smith's Fracture

1. Smith's fracture of the distal radius.

2. Yes.

3. Maintenance of radial length, 0 to 10 degree palmar tilt, 14 degree ulnar inclination, and articular congruity.

4. Type 1 is extra-articular. Type 3 is intra-articular to the radiocarpal joint. Type 5 is intra-articular to the distal radioulnar joint. Type 7 is intra-articular to both the radiocarpal joint and distal radioulnar joint. Types 2, 4, 6, and 8 denote the presence of an ulnar styloid fracture concomitant to the preceding type.

Reference

Louis DS: Barton's and Smith's fractures. *Hand Clin* 4:399–402, 1988.

Cross-Reference

Musculoskeletal Imaging: THE REQUISITES, 3rd ed, pp 138–140.

Comment

Distal radius fractures are extremely common injuries. They are 10 times more likely to occur than carpal fractures and have a wide spectrum of appearances. A Smith's fracture is similar to a Colles fracture except for volar displacement and/or angulation; hence these fractures are frequently referred to as *reverse Colles fractures*. The mechanism is likely related to a fall on the dorsum of the hand. The fracture can be intra- or extra-articular. The lateral view is the key to diagnosis, showing that the distal radial fragment displaces anteriorly with palmar angulation of the articular surface. The Thomas classification describes three types. Type 1 is transverse extra-articular, type 2 is volar intra-articular, and type 3 is oblique juxta-articular. These fractures are frequently associated with ulnar styloid fractures and may also be associated with injury to the extensor tendons.

Notes

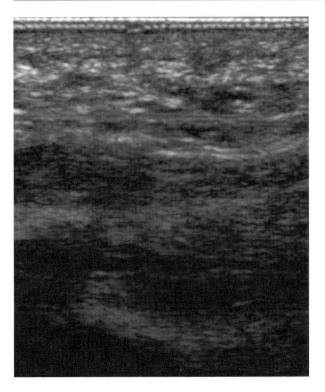 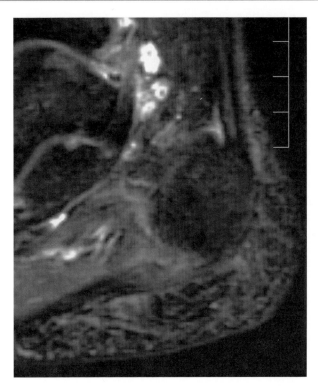

You are shown a longitudinal (right side is distal) sonogram of the heel and a sagittal inversion recovery magnetic resonance image.

1. What is the diagnosis?

2. Identify the findings in the ultrasound image. In the Magnetic resonance image.

3. Name the components of the plantar fascia. Which segment(s) is/are affected by fasciitis?

4. What differentiates acute plantar fasciitis from chronic fasciitis?

C A S E 1 5 8

Plantar Fasciitis

1. Acute plantar fasciitis.

2. Hypoechoic thickening of the insertion of the central cord. Thickened plantar fascia with perifascicular and intrafascial edema.

3. Medial, central, and lateral cords. Nearly all affect the central cord but may extend to involve the lateral cord.

4. The presence of edema in and about the aponeurosis.

References

Cardinal E, Chhem RK, Beauregard CG, et al: Plantar fasciitis: Sonographic evaluation. *Radiology* 201: 257–259, 1996.

Yu JS: Pathologic and post-operative conditions of the plantar fascia: Review of MR imaging appearances. *Skeletal Radiology* 29:491–501, 2000.

Cross-Reference

Musculoskeletal Imaging: THE REQUISITES, 3rd ed, pp 279–280.

Comment

Plantar fasciitis is a painful condition that has been attributed to repeated mechanical stresses that cause chronic microtears of the calcaneal attachment of the plantar aponeurosis. It is the most common cause of inferior heel pain. Plantar fasciitis is a straightforward diagnosis. The hallmark of plantar fasciitis is marked thickening (typically two- to threefold increase) of the calcaneal attachment of the central cord of the plantar aponeurosis. The normal thickness of the plantar fascia should not exceed 4 mm and it is hyperechoic, appearing nearly isoechoic to the adjacent fat of the heel pad and low in signal intensity on all magnetic resonance imaging pulse sequences.

The sonographic manifestation of plantar fasciitis is a proximally thickened, hypoechoic fascia. On magnetic resonance imaging, the insertion will demonstrate signal alterations in the aponeurosis consistent with edema. Perifascial edema causes indistinctness of the margins of the fascia. Edema in the subcutaneous fat is usually evident as well. Inversion recovery images may be more sensitive to changes in the adjacent bone marrow than conventional spin-echo imaging and are useful in excluding stress fractures. When the condition is more chronic or if the patient responds to a course of conservative therapy, regional soft tissue edema will diminish and the signal alterations in the fascia will dissipate. In a majority of patients with chronic plantar fasciitis, an enthesophyte will develop at the enthesis of the plantar fascia after a few months.

Notes

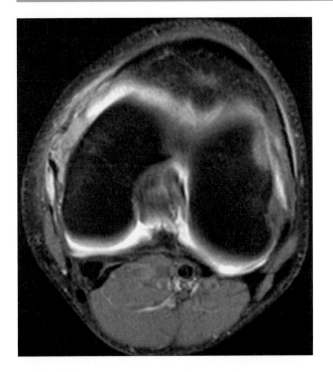

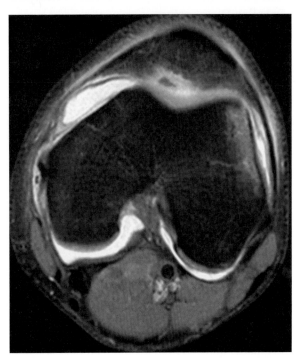

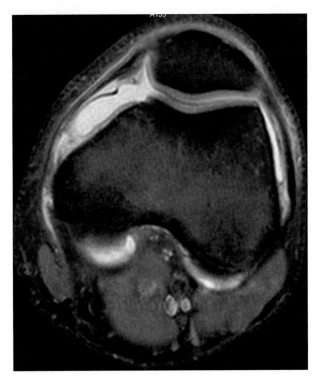

1. List the injuries you see.

2. What cartilagenous abnormality should you look for?

3. How often is the patellar tilt abnormal?

4. What must be present for an intra-articular dislocation to occur?

Lateral Patellar Dislocation

1. Lateral patellar dislocation with bone contusion of the lateral femoral condyle and medial patella, complete rupture of the medial patellofemoral ligament, strain of medial patellar retinaculum and injury to anterior fibers of the medial collateral ligament.

2. Osteochondral defects of either the patella or the lateral femoral condyle.

3. In over 40% of cases.

4. A complete quadriceps tendon tear.

Reference

Elias DA, White LM, Fithian DC: Acute lateral patellar dislocation at MR imaging: Injury patterns of medial patellar soft-tissue restraints and osteochondral injuries of the inferomedial patella. *Radiology* 225: 736–743, 2002.

Cross-Reference

Musculoskeletal Imaging: THE REQUISITES, 3rd ed, pp 216–217.

Comment

True patellar dislocations are relatively less common than subluxation of the patella, which is caused by tracking abnormalities of the extensor mechanism. A lateral patellar dislocation is the most common type of patellar dislocation and occurs when there is forced internal rotation of the femur on a fixed, externally rotated tibia with the knee in flexion. The pull of the quadriceps muscles on the patella causes it to displace out of the trochlea. When there is significant displacement, the medial retinaculum and medial patellofemoral ligament tears, which allows impaction between the medial patellar facet and the lateral surface of the lateral femoral condyle. If this occurs with sufficient force to produce bone contusions, a characteristic "kissing" bone contusion pattern is created, as demonstrated by this patient. Magnetic resonance imaging has played an important role in identifying unsuspected osteochondral or pure chondral defects of the hyaline cartilage of the patella or trochlea in patients who have persistent anterior knee pain after a dislocation of the patella.

Notes

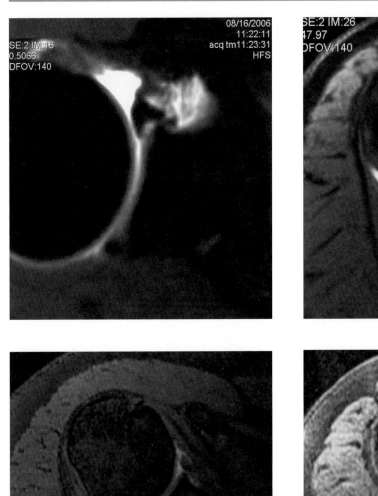

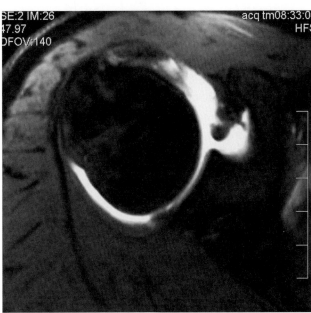

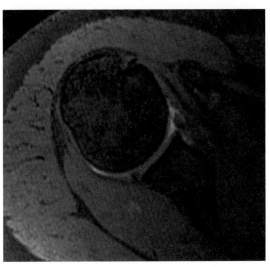

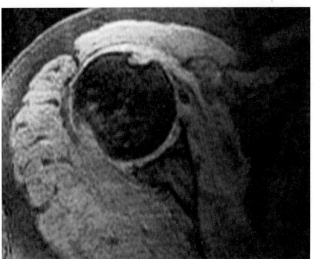

You are shown images from four different patients.

1. Identify the finding. Is this normal?

2. Identify the finding. Is this normal?

3. Identify the finding. Is this normal?

4. Identify the finding. Is this normal?

C A S E   1 6 0

Glenoid Labrum (Anterosuperior Position)

1. Sublabral foramen. Yes.

2. Sublabral sulcus. Yes.

3. Buford complex. Yes.

4. Intra-articular dislocation of the biceps tendon. No.

Reference

De Maeseneer M, Van Roy F, Lenchik L, et al: CT and MR arthrography of the normal and pathologic anterosuperior labrum and labral-bicipital complex. *Radiographics* 20:S67–S81, 2000.

Cross-Reference

Musculoskeletal Imaging: THE REQUISITES, 3rd ed, pp 83–85 and 96.

Comment

The normal glenoid labrum varies in morphology and fixation to the glenoid rim. Small clefts may occur as a normal variant. The peripheral margin of the majority of the labrum is fixed to the glenoid periosteum, and usually to the joint capsule and underlying glenoid articular cartilage. A sublabral foramen is a variant where there is absence of fixation of the labrum in the anterosuperior aspect of the rim (between 1- and 3-o'clock positions). A sublabral sulcus is a cleft between the superior labrum and the glenoid. This can mimic a superior labral tear. A Buford complex is the absence of the anterosuperior labrum associated with a thickened, cordlike middle glenohumeral ligament. All three of these appearances are variations of normal and have no clinical significance. However, when there is a defect in the attachment of the subscapularis tendon on the lesser tuberosity, the intracapsular portion of the tendon of the long head of the biceps muscle can dislocate anterior to the glenoid rim and mimic a Buford complex or labral tear.

Notes

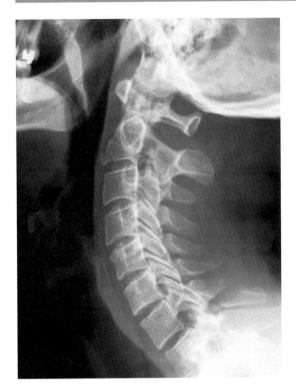 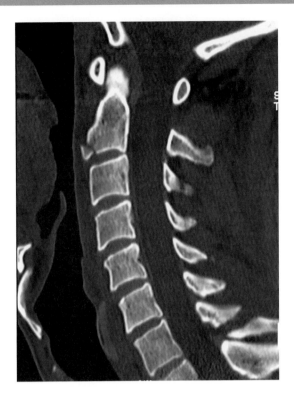

1. What is the mechanism of injury? How many people suffer cord compression?

2. Where is the point of failure?

3. Is this fracture stable or unstable, and how do you tell?

4. What is a common associated injury?

Hyperextension Teardrop (C2) Fracture

1. Sudden hyperextension. About 20%.

2. Avulsion of the anteroinferior aspect of the vertebral body by the anterior longitudinal ligament.

3. Stable; isolated vertebral body fractures are stable because the posterior elements and posterior longitudinal ligament are intact. It is considered unstable when there is also a fracture of the posterior arch.

4. Hangman's fracture.

Reference

Rao SK, Wasyliw C, Nunez DB, Jr: Spectrum of imaging findings in hyperextension injuries of the neck. *Radiographics* 25:1239–1254, 2005.

Cross-Reference

Musculoskeletal Imaging: THE REQUISITES, 3rd ed, pp 170–171.

Comment

Hyperextension injuries of the cervical spine are relatively common. They are caused by a superiorly directed force upon the mandible or a posteriorly directed force upon the forehead. Acutely, the radiographic findings include prevertebral soft tissue swelling, widening of the anterior disc space, and a small triangular fracture from the anterior and inferior aspect of the vertebral body, which represents an avulsion fracture at the attachment site of the anterior longitudinal ligament. Most hyperextension fractures occur at C1 and C2. Posterior retrolisthesis at the level of ligamentous disruption can narrow the spinal canal and compress the cord. Vascular compromise can cause central cord syndrome. In both situations, magnetic resonance imaging is indicated to evaluate the spinal cord. When the majority of the force is absorbed by the posterior elements, you may see fractures involving the pedicle, lamina, articular pillar, and spinous process (did you notice C7?). Fractures of the pedicle below C2 occur nearly exclusively with hyperextension injuries. The problem with pedicle fractures is that 80% of them are missed on conventional radiographs so you must carefully inspect the computed tomography images.

Notes

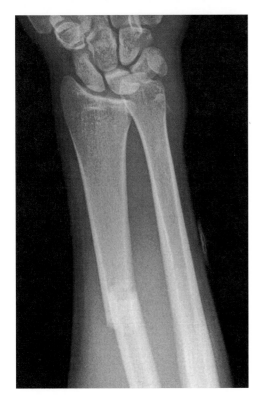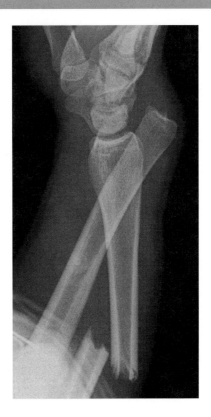

1. What is this injury called?

2. What is the mechanism of injury?

3. List some of the potential complications of this injury.

4. What fracture-dislocation injury of the forearm is frequently associated with an injury to the radial nerve or its branches?

Galeazzi's Fracture-Dislocation

1. Galeazzi's fracture-dislocation, which is a fracture of the distal radius with dislocation of distal radioulnar joint.

2. Either a fall on an outstretched hand with pronation of the forearm or a direct blow.

3. Angulation, delayed union, or nonunion of fracture. Entrapment of the extensor carpi ulnaris tendon can be a rare complication.

4. Monteggia's fracture-dislocation is associated with this complication in 20% of cases.

References

Bado JL: The Monteggia lesion. *Clin Orthop* 50:71–86, 1967.

Rogriguez-Merchan EC: Pediatric fractures of the forearm. *Clin Orthop Relat Res* 432:65–72, 2005.

Cross-Reference

Musculoskeletal Imaging: THE REQUISITES, 3rd ed, pp 131–133.

Comment

A Galeazzi's fracture-dislocation represents one of a common group of injuries of the forearm that affects both bones. It is defined as a fracture of the diaphysis of the radius associated with a subluxation/dislocation of the ulnar head. A Monteggia's lesion is another complex injury, comprised of a fracture of the ulnar shaft associated with a dislocation of the radial head. Bado classified this injury complex into four types. A type I Monteggia's lesion, the most common type (accounts for 60% of fracture-dislocations in this group), is characterized by anterior angulation of the ulnar fracture and an anterior dislocation of the radial head. Posterior angulation of the ulnar fracture and posterior dislocation of the radial head characterize a type II Monteggia's lesion (10% to 15%). A type III Monteggia's lesion (6% to 20%) is characterized by a fracture of the proximal ulna occurring distal to the coronoid process of the ulna and lateral dislocation of the radial head. The least common type is a type IV Monteggia's fracture (5%), which is characterized by a fracture of the proximal ends of both the radius and ulna and an anterior dislocation of the radial head. The mechanism of injury and direction of an impaction force dictate the type of fracture seen. The Essex-Lopresti fracture is the other type of forearm injury that you should know, characterized by a fracture of the radial head and disruption of the distal radioulnar joint.

Notes

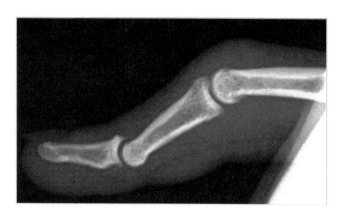

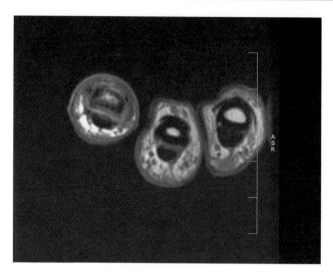

1. What is the diagnosis?
2. How is it caused?
3. What will happen if the injury is not treated?
4. What is the appropriate treatment?

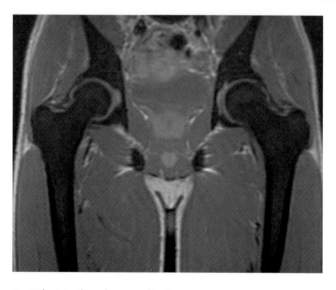

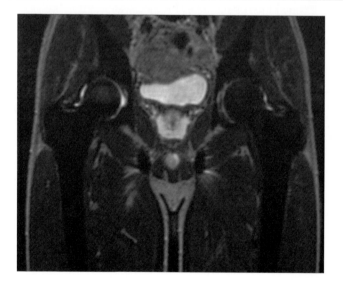

1. What is the abnormality?
2. What is your differential diagnosis?
3. What other organs are affected in the primary (idiopathic) form of this condition?
4. What are common diseases associated with the secondary form of this condition?

CASE 163

Boutonnière Deformity

1. Boutonnière deformity.

2. Avulsion of the central extensor slip allows flexion of the proximal interphalangeal joint between the lateral slips.

3. Volar migration of the lateral slips will result in a permanent deformity.

4. Splint the finger with the proximal interphalangeal joint fully extended.

Reference

Peterson JJ, Bancroft LW: Injuries of the fingers and thumb in the athlete. *Clin Sports Med* 25:527–542, 2006.

Cross-Reference

Musculoskeletal Imaging: THE REQUISITES, 3rd ed, pp 162–163.

Comment

The boutonnière (buttonhole) deformity is an important injury of the finger. It is allowed to occur owing to the anatomy of the extensor mechanism at the level of the proximal interphalangeal (PIP) joint. Recall that the central slip inserts on the dorsal lip of the middle phalanx whereas the lateral slips course around the central slip insertion producing a buttonhole configuration. The boutonnière injury is caused by a rupture of the central slip of the extensor mechanism. This avulsion can be purely tendinous or associated with a small bony fragment. This allows unrestricted flexion of the PIP joint, which protrudes through the buttonhole created by the lateral extensor slips, and hyperextension of the distal interphalangeal joint. The lateral slips migrate volarly and this may be a gradual process, "locking" the deformity in place. The diagnosis requires careful inspection of the radiograph. It is important to establish the diagnosis so that the finger can be splinted in extension, in contradistinction to other injuries in this area of the finger. If there is a sizable bone fragment, open or closed fixation may be required. Magnetic resonance imaging is useful in chronic cases to determine if there has been significant retraction of the tendon.

Notes

CASE 164

Hemosiderosis

1. The bone marrow has low signal intensity on both T1W and T2W images.

2. Hemochromatosis, and hemosiderosis from transfusions and iron overload.

3. In primary hemochromatosis, other involved sites are the liver, spleen, pancreas, heart, and kidneys.

4. Thallasemia, sickle cell disease, and other chronic hemolytic anemias.

Reference

Emy PY, Levin TL, Sheth SS, et al: Iron overload in reticuloendothelial systems of pediatric oncology patients who have undergone transfusions: MR observations. *AJR Am J Roentgenol* 168:1011–1015, 1997.

Cross-Reference

Musculoskeletal Imaging: THE REQUISITES, 3rd ed, pp 539–542.

Comment

Hemosiderin deposition owing to chronic hemolytic anemias or transfusions can alter the bone marrow characteristics on magnetic resonance imaging. Recall that the elements of the marrow change as a person ages. The basic components of the bone marrow are lipoid (yellow) marrow, hematopoietic (red) marrow, and trabecular bone. One is born with an abundance of hematopoietic marrow but as the skeleton matures, the red marrow converts to yellow marrow, which has high signal intensity on T1W and lower signal intensity on T2W images. The pattern of conversion is orderly, beginning at the epiphysis, followed by the diaphysis, and then the metaphysis of the bones: distal end of the bone to proximal end, distal appendicular skeleton to proximal, and last in the axial skeleton. The mature distribution is reached at around age 30, with hematopoietic marrow seen in the axial skeleton, and the proximal humerus and femoral metaphyses. The key finding to this case is that the marrow signal intensity is very low on both the T1W and T2W images. There are only a few processes that can cause such diffuse involvement of the marrow space. Gaucher's disease may give a similar appearance when severe on T1W images.

Notes

Challenge

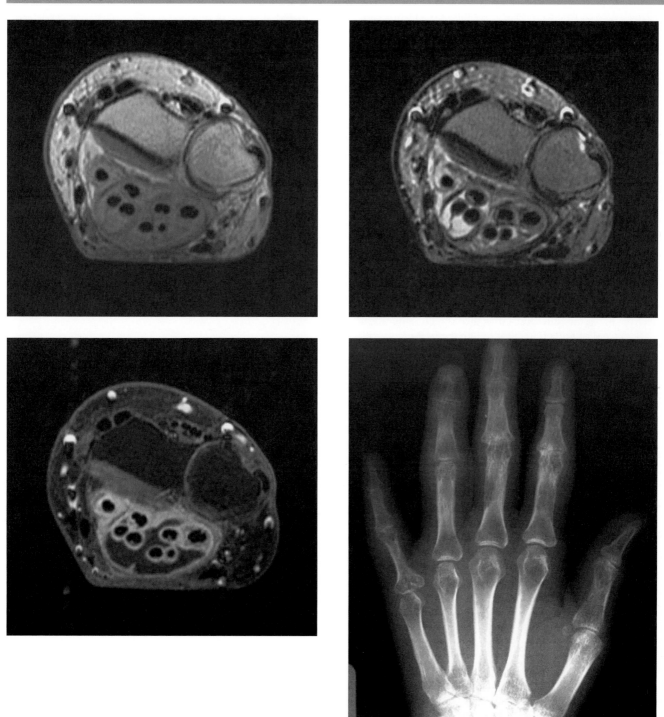

1. The radiograph was obtained 3 years after the magnetic resonance images. What is the diagnosis?
2. Characterize the different arthropathies.
3. What is Löfgren's syndrome? What is the differential diagnosis for this condition?
4. How do patients with myopathy present? What are the magnetic resonance imaging characteristics?

CASE 165

Chronic Sarcoidal Arthropathy/Tenosynovitis

1. Sarcoidal arthropathy and flexor tenosynovitis.

2. Acute synovial inflammatory polyarthritis (small and medium joints) of short duration (4 to 6 weeks); chronic polyarthritis (lasting months to years) producing irreversible joint destruction and disability; and tenosynovitis, bursitis, and tendonitis.

3. Arthralgia, erythema nodosum, and bilateral hilar lymph node enlargement. Rheumatoid arthritis.

4. Resemble polymyositis with weakness, elevated creatine kinase and aldolase levels, and abnormal electromyographic evaluation. Proximal muscle atrophy and discrete enhancing nodules with a low signal intensity spiculated central region.

Reference

Moore SL, Teirstein AE: Musculoskeletal sarcoidosis: Spectrum of appearances at MR imaging. *Radiographics* 23:1389–1399, 2003.

Cross-Reference

Musculoskeletal Imaging: THE REQUISITES, 3rd ed, pp 562–564.

Comment

Sarcoidosis is an inflammatory disorder of unknown etiology that is characterized by noncaseating granulomas in tissues. Skeletal involvement occurs in about 5% of people affected. Osseous lesions typically involve the small tubular bones of the hands and feet with classic "lacy" lytic patterns or cyst lesions. Involvement of long bones often is radiographically occult and requires magnetic resonance imaging for detection. Lesions are depicted as round low signal intensity lesions on T1W with high signal intensity with sharp margination on T2W images. Less commonly, areas of osteosclerosis may occur in the tubular bones of the hand and feet (acro-osteosclerosis). Rarely, this process can become widespread in the skeleton, mimicking blastic metastasis.

Löfgren's syndrome is a well-recognized manifestation presenting with pain, swelling, and stiffness. Radiographs may show periarticular osteoporosis in the first 6 months of symptoms provoking the diagnosis of rheumatoid arthritis. In addition to Löfgren's syndrome, the symptoms of granulomatous arthritis are noted in another 10% to 35% of patients, manifested by synovitis of the knee, ankle, shoulder, or wrist, and dactylitis of the fingers. Tenosynovitis, tendonitis, and bursitis are nonspecific and required synovial or soft tissue biopsy to establish the cause. This patient shows distension of the flexor tendon sheath with fluid and synovial enlargement.

A biopsy showed noncaseating granulomas. The radiograph a few years later shows characteristic findings in the fingers.

Notes

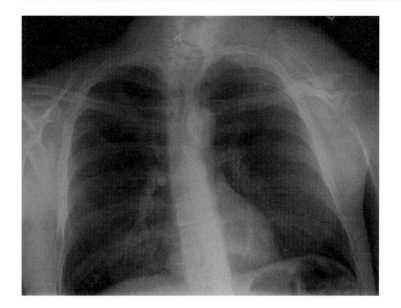
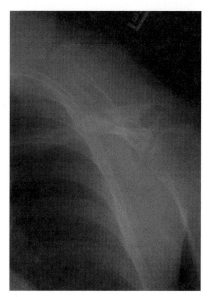
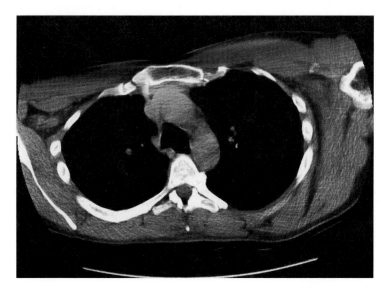

1. What is the diagnosis?

2. What are associated problems that may be seen in this injury?

3. What is the most severe consequence of this injury?

4. What is meant by a "locked scapula"?

Scapulothoracic Dissociation

1. Lateral scapulothoracic dissociation.

2. Injuries to the muscles of the shoulder girdle, brachial plexus, and subclavian artery and vein.

3. Avulsion of the brachial plexus.

4. Intrathoracic dislocation of the scapula.

References

Brucker PU, Gruen GS, Kaufman RA: Scapulothoracic dissociation: Evaluation and management. *Injury* 36:1147–1155, 2005.

Rubenstein JD, Ebraheim NA, Kellam JF: Traumatic scapulothoracic dissociation. *Radiology* 157:297–298, 1985.

Cross-Reference

Musculoskeletal Imaging: THE REQUISITES, 3rd ed, pp 73–75.

Comment

Scapulothoracic dissociation is a rare severe injury that occurs from high-energy trauma. These injuries are associated with complex multisystem problems including the muscles, vessels, and brachial plexus. The scapula may be dislocated from the shoulder girdle either laterally or intrathoracically. Intrathoracic dislocations are the result of a direct blow to the scapula or an outward pull of the arm causing the inferior angle of the scapula to become inserted between two ribs. This injury is treated by abduction of the arm and direct manipulation of the scapula, followed by immobilization for six weeks. In lateral scapular dislocations, such as in this patient, the scapula is laterally displaced from a severe rotational or traction force. This is particularly conspicuous on a well-centered chest radiograph, with asymmetry of the shoulders. It is usually associated with neurovascular disruption, effectively representing a forequarter-closed amputation with a poor prognosis of recovery. Arteriography and immediate vascular repair of the subclavian artery and vein is recommended. In addition to displacement of the scapula, you should recognize other associated injuries including fracture of the clavicle and scapula, dislocation of the sternoclavicular or acromioclavicular joint, and presence of an extrapleural hematoma.

Notes

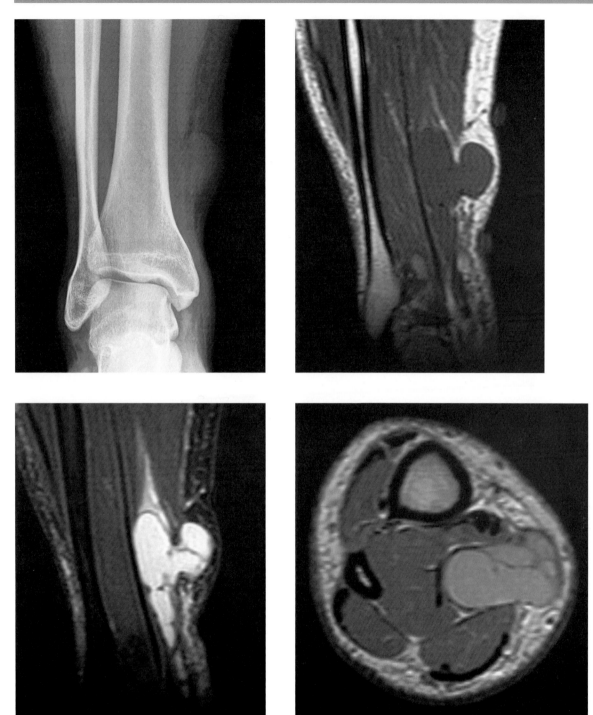

1. What is the differential diagnosis?

2. This 29-year-old patient has an enlarging, painful mass. What is the likely diagnosis and why?

3. Is sharp margination an indication of tumor isolation?

4. What is the prognosis?

Synovial Cell Sarcoma

1. Synovial cell sarcoma and myositis ossificans, and occasionally myonecrosis, abscess, and liposarcoma.

2. Synovial cell sarcoma; the age, location, calcification, and symptoms all suggest this diagnosis.

3. This observation should not mislead you. This tumor is an aggressive lesion with characteristic tumor microinvasion beyond the pseudocapsule.

4. Poor. Pulmonary metastasis is common at presentation and local recurrence despite local aggressive therapy occurs in 25% of patients.

Reference

Morton MJ, Berquist TH, McLeod RA, et al: MR imaging of synovial sarcoma. *AJR Am J Roentgenol* 156:337–340, 1991.

Cross-Reference

Musculoskeletal Imaging: THE REQUISITES, 3rd ed, p 506.

Comment

Synovial cell sarcoma is a soft tissue tumor named for its predominant histologic differentiation: tumor cells that resemble synovioblastic cells. The majority of lesions (90%) do not originate from a joint, although they are frequently found near a joint. It represents 5% of malignant soft tissue sarcomas but is one of the most common soft tissue sarcomas in young people between 15 and 35 years of age. It is most frequently located in the lower extremities, particularly around the knee joint. The most common symptom is a painful swelling or mass for several years, since the tumor grows slowly. Rarely, pain alone will be the presenting symptom. At the time of diagnosis, tumors are between 3 cm to 5 cm with sharp margins. They may appear encapsulated but local extension beyond the margin is typical. Radiographically, the mass may show calcification 30% of the time. The adjacent bone is eroded or shows periostitis in 20% of cases. On magnetic resonance imaging, the mass appears multilocular and the T1W signal intensity is isointense to muscle, but high on T2W images, with occasional fluid-fluid levels. Sometimes, they are very bright on fluid sensitive sequences, mimicking a fluid cavity. They show either a well-defined or infiltrative margin usually without reactive edema. Enhancement distinguishes synovial cell sarcomas from a benign cystic process.

Notes

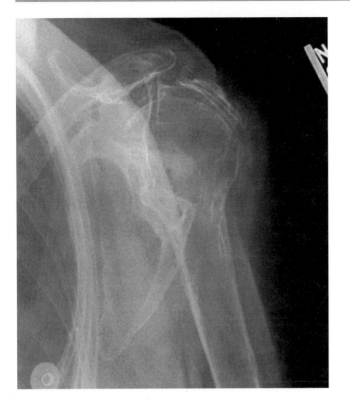 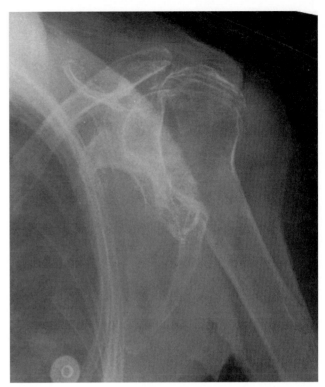

1. What observation did you make?

2. Can this abnormality be the result of prior trauma?

3. What do you expect to find in the contralateral shoulder?

4. What can you see on magnetic resonance imaging?

Glenoid Hypoplasia

1. Severe hypoplasia of the glenoid neck (dentate anomaly) with a complete rotator cuff tear.

2. Only if the glenoid ossification center was previously injured from a fracture.

3. Glenoid hypoplasia that appears symmetric with the left shoulder.

4. Subluxation, labral pathology (enlargement, detachment, tear), abnormal accumulation of fibrocartilage, and hypertrophy of the middle glenohumeral ligament.

References

Theodorou SJ, Theodorou DJ, Resnick D: Hypoplasia of the glenoid neck of the scapula: Imaging findings and report of 16 patients. *J Comput Assist Tomogr* 30:535–542, 2006.

Trout TE, Resnick D: Glenoid hypoplasia and its relationship to instability. *Skeletal Radiol* 25:37–40, 1996.

Cross-Reference

Musculoskeletal Imaging: THE REQUISITES, 3rd ed, p 75.

Comment

Glenoid hypoplasia, or dysplasia of the scapular neck, is an uncommon entity that affects men and women with equal frequency. There often is a familial tendency, suggesting a hereditary trait. It represents anomalous development of the scapula with hypoplasia or dysplasia of the glenoid neck and is generally a bilateral and symmetric process. The glenoid fossa develops in a broad, irregular fashion resulting in a widened inferior glenohumeral joint, and the articular surface becomes notched. Patients present with shoulder pain and limited range of motion, and instability is more common than previously suspected. The radiographic findings are classic and diagnostic. Hypoplasia of the humeral head and neck, varus deformity of the proximal portion of the humerus, and enlargement and bowing of the acromion and the clavicle are associated deformities.

Only one other process may mimic the appearance of glenoid hypoplasia. An injury to the brachial plexus occurring at birth may produce radiographic abnormalities that are similar to this anomaly, but these patients also have upper extremity paralysis, with atrophic musculature that provides a differentiating finding.

Notes

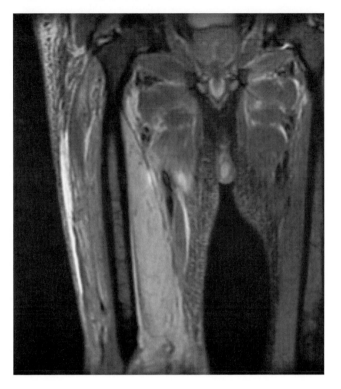
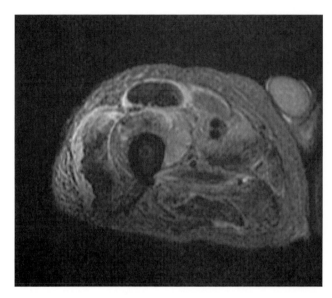

1. This patient has intense pain, no fever, and a normal white blood cell count. What other information would you like to know?

2. What is the diagnosis?

3. What is the classic presentation?

4. Does this patient need a biopsy for diagnosis?

Diabetic Muscle Infarction

1. Does the patient have diabetes? (Answer is yes, long-standing insulin dependent).

2. Diabetic muscle infarction.

3. Abrupt pain and swelling, with a palpable mass in a poorly controlled diabetic patient.

4. In most patients, the diagnosis can be made when the characteristic clinical presentation is combined with typical magnetic resonance imaging results.

References

Kattapuram TM, Suri R, Rosol MS, et al: Idiopathic and diabetic skeletal muscle necrosis: Evaluation by magnetic resonance imaging. *Skeletal Radiol* 34:203–209, 2005.

Umpierrez GE, Stiles RG, Kleinbart J, et al: Diabetic muscle infarction. *Am J Med* 101:245–250, 1996.

Cross-Reference

Musculoskeletal Imaging: THE REQUISITES, 3rd ed, pp 39–40.

Comment

Diabetic muscle infarction is a rare complication of long-standing diabetes mellitus occurring in patients with poorly controlled disease. It is frequently misdiagnosed clinically as abscess, neoplasm, or myositis, and is often biopsied. Patients usually present with abrupt thigh or calf pain and swelling, but do not have fever and have a normal white blood cell count. Serum enzymes are normal or mildly elevated. The involved area may be palpable, with induration of the surrounding tissue. The painful lesion persists for weeks, occasionally with exacerbations of symptoms, spontaneously resolving over several weeks to months. Recurrent episodes are reported in half of the patients. Muscles frequently affected are the vastus muscles, thigh adductors, and biceps femoris, but calf muscles may be involved as well.

Magnetic resonance imaging studies show diffuse enlargement of involved muscle groups and partial loss of normal fatty intermuscular septa. Identification of subfascial fluid is noted in 75% of cases and edema in the subcutaneous fat in 90%. Affected muscles are best depicted with T2W and inversion-recovery images, appearing diffusely hyperintense when compared with adjacent normal muscles. Gadolinium-enhanced images show enlarged, enhancing muscles or small, focal, rim-enhancing fluid collections representing devitalized tissue. Histologic features of diabetic muscle infarction consist of large areas of muscle necrosis and edema. Regenerating muscle fibers and lymphocytic interstitial infiltration may be present.

Notes

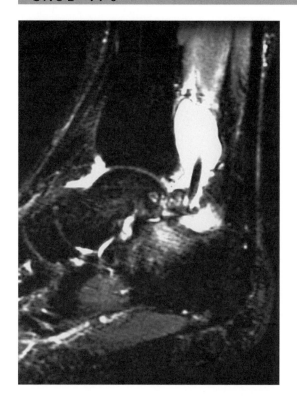
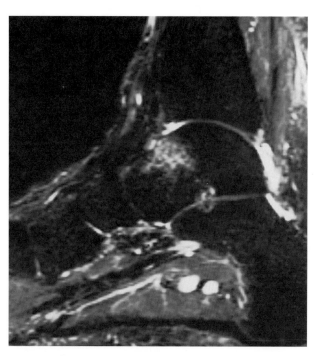
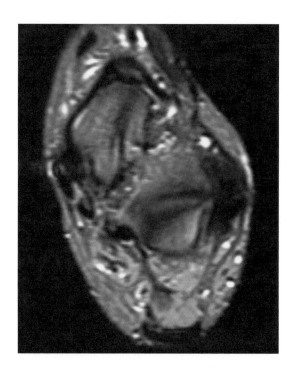
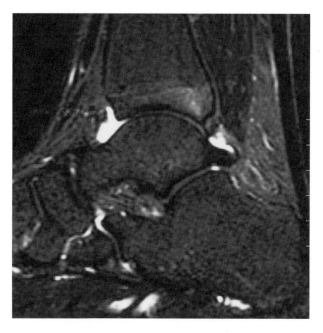

All of these patients have chronic pain.

1. What is the most likely diagnosis in the first patient? What attaches to the os trigonum?

2. What is the diagnosis in the second patient?

3. What do you see and what does the third patient likely have?

4. What is the diagnosis in the fourth patient?

Ankle Impingement Syndromes

1. Os trigonum syndrome with tenosynovitis of the flexor hallucis longus tendon. Posterior talofibular and posterior talocalcaneal ligaments.

2. Bone marrow edema of the talus from anterior ankle impingement.

3. Hypertrophy of the anterior talofibular ligament; anterolateral ankle impingement.

4. Edema in posterior tibia plafond from posterior ankle impingement.

References

Niek van Dijk C: Anterior and posterior ankle impingement. *Foot Ankle Clin* 11:663–683, 2006.

Robinson P, White LM: Soft-tissue and osseous impingement syndromes of the ankle: Role of imaging in diagnosis and management. *Radiographics* 22:1457–1469, 2002.

Cross-Reference

Musculoskeletal Imaging: THE REQUISITES, 3rd ed, pp 268–269.

Comment

There are many different causes of ankle pain. Impingement syndromes describe a group of pain-producing disorders stemming from conditions that are caused by abnormal osseous or ligamentous morphology including congenital anomalies, as well as those that are acquired such as osteophytosis, ligament hypertrophy, and arthrofibrosis. Anterior ankle impingement is characterized by pain with dorsiflexion and may be caused by anterior tibial osteophytes and traction spurs on the dorsal talar neck. In anterolateral ankle impingement, pain with dorsiflexion occurs owing to soft tissue fibrosis, synovitis, and cartilage injury in the anterolateral tibiotalar joint. There is often hyalinization of the anterolateral soft tissues, which becomes a firm mass. Posterior impingement occurs from either trauma or overuse and may be caused by posterior osteophytes or an unstable os trigonum. The os trigonum syndrome is a condition characterized by chronic pain with tenderness and soft tissue swelling in the posterior ankle. It commonly affects people who perform activities that subject their ankle to extreme plantar flexion (e.g., ballet). Pain is produced by disruption of the cartilaginous synchondrosis between the os trigonum and the lateral talar tubercle, which then can produce compression of the adjacent synovial and capsular tissues against the posterior tibia. With repeated entrapment, the soft tissue becomes chronically inflamed and fibrosed, particularly the tendon of the flexor hallucis longus (FHL) muscle.

Notes

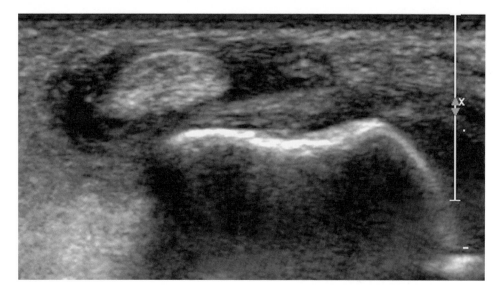

You are shown a transverse sonogram of the dorsum of the metacarpophalangeal (MP) joint with the hand in the clenched-fist position.

1. What is the diagnosis?

2. What is a common association with this disorder?

3. Which finger is most commonly affected with this disorder? In which direction?

4. Can this be a manifestation of arthritis?

Boxer's Knuckle

1. Dislocation of the common extensor tendon of the finger with respect to the metacarpal bone.

2. Capsular tears of the MP joint.

3. The long finger. Dislocation in the ulnar direction.

4. Yes, inflammatory arthropathies such as rheumatoid arthritis.

References

Hame SL, Melone CP: Boxer's knuckle: Traumatic disruption of the extensor hood. *Hand Clin* 16:375–380, 2000.

Lopez-Ben R, Lee DH, Nicolodi DJ: Boxer knuckle (injury of the extensor hood with extensor tendon subluxation): Diagnosis with dynamic US—report of three cases. *Radiology* 228:642–646, 2003.

Cross-Reference

Musculoskeletal Imaging: THE REQUISITES, 3rd ed, p 32.

Comment

A *boxer's knuckle* is an eponym that describes an injury to the sagittal bands of the extensor hood of the finger, the aponeurotic sheet that overlies the MP joint. This is a severe injury that occurs when the hand in the clenched-fist position strikes an object. The sagittal bands are transversely oriented ligaments that assist in the stabilization of the extensor tendon during joint motion. They arise from the palmar plate and the intermetacarpal ligament at the neck of the metacarpal bone. When ruptured, patients present with pain, swelling, loss of full joint extension, and either ulnar or radial subluxation of the extensor tendon. If the hand is swollen, the subluxation may not be detectable on clinical inspection. The extensor tendon normally appears as a hyperechoic oval structure that resides in the dorsal depression of the metacarpal head. The ulnar and radial sagittal bands exert tensile forces in opposite directions during flexion, keeping the extensor tendon in apposition with the metacarpal bone. If one of the sagittal bands ruptures, there is unopposed tension on the remaining sagittal band displacing the tendon. The long finger is the most commonly affected, owing to the normal 10 to 15 degree ulnar inclination that predisposes the radial sagittal band to rupture.

Notes

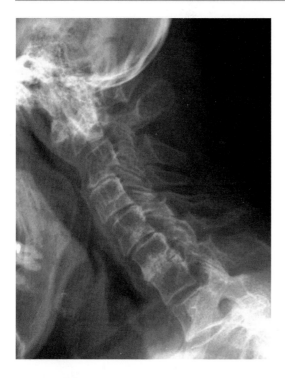

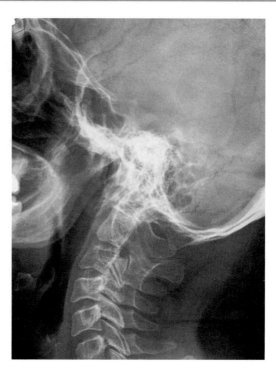

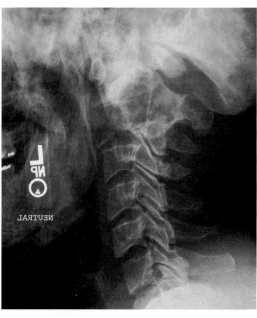

1. You are shown lateral C-spine radiographs of three different patients. What is the diagnosis of the first patient and the most likely cause?

2. What is the diagnosis of the second patient?

3. What is the diagnosis of the third patient? Can you tell what the underlying disorder is?

4. Define atlantoaxial subluxation. When do patients with rheumatoid arthritis become symptomatic?

Cranial Settling, Platybasia, and Basilar Invagination

1. Cranial settling most likely from rheumatoid arthritis.

2. Platybasia.

3. Basilar invagination. Fibrous dysplasia.

4. Predental space exceeds 2.5 mm. At about 9 mm.

Reference

Riew KD, Hilibrand AS, Plumbo MA, et al: Diagnosing basilar invagination in the rheumatoid patient: The reliability of radiographic criteria. *J Bone Joint Surg* 83:194–200, 2001.

Cross-Reference

Musculoskeletal Imaging: THE REQUISITES, 3rd ed, pp 296–298.

Comment

When the odontoid process and the transverse ligaments are destroyed, as in rheumatoid arthritis, the atlas may shift in any direction. Destruction of the lateral masses may result in cranial settling or lateral subluxation (torticollis) if asymmetrically eroded. The first patient clearly shows evidence of cranial settling. This is a process that is characterized by inferior migration of the atlas relative to the odontoid process and collapse of the occipitoatlantal and atlantoaxial articulations. A clue to the diagnosis of cranial settling is recognition that the anterior arch of C1 (which normally articulates with the odontoid process) articulates with the base of the odontoid or the body of C2.

Platybasia is a condition in which the base of the skull is abnormally flattened. It may be a developmental anomaly or caused by softening of the bones of the skull base. It is characterized by a cranial basal angle exceeding 136 degrees (formed by a line drawn from the nasion to the center of the sella turcica and then to the anterior margin of the foramen magnum). It is often seen with basilar invagination, which is the inward and upward migration of the cervical spine through the foramen magnum. The tip of the dens protrudes above McRae's line, which defines the opening of the foramen magnum.

Notes

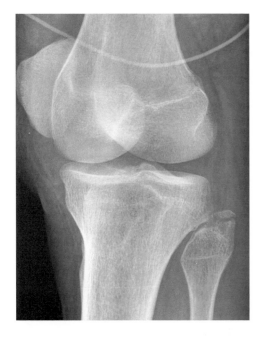
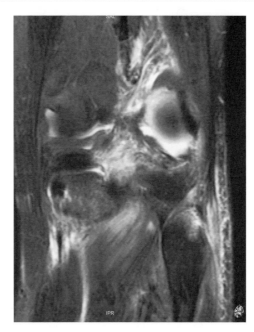
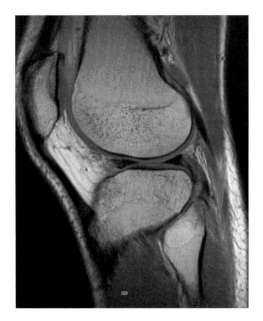
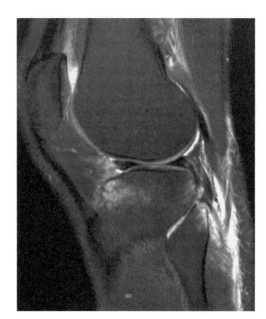

1. What is the finding and what is it called?

2. What does it imply?

3. Are there any other associated injuries to the knee?

4. Where does the lateral collateral or conjoined tendon insert?

Arcuate Fracture of Fibular Head

1. Avulsion fracture of the fibular styloid; arcuate sign.

2. Insufficiency of the arcuate complex may lead to posterolateral instability.

3. Yes, tears of the cruciate and collateral ligaments and the menisci.

4. On the lateral aspect of the fibular head.

Reference

Huang GS, Yu JS, Munshi M, et al: Avulsion fracture of the head of the fibula (the "arcuate" sign): MR imaging findings predictive of injuries to the posterolateral ligaments and posterior cruciate ligament. *AJR Am J Roentgenol* 180:381–387, 2003.

Cross-Reference

Musculoskeletal Imaging: THE REQUISITES, 3rd ed, pp 217–220.

Comment

Injuries that affect the ligaments in the posterolateral aspect of the knee are important because they may lead to posterolateral instability, characterized clinically by posterior subluxation and external rotation of the tibial plateau relative to the femur. The most common mechanism of injury is a direct blow to an extended knee with a force directed to the anteromedial surface of the proximal tibia while the tibia is externally rotated. The fibular styloid is the site of attachment for the arcuate, fabellofibular, and popliteofibular ligaments, often termed the arcuate complex. Identification of an avulsion fracture of the fibular styloid, termed the arcuate sign, may reflect an injury to these ligaments. This avulsion has a characteristic appearance, with an elliptical fragment of bone with its long axis oriented horizontally on an anteroposterior radiograph of the knee. The avulsion is not as readily evident on a lateral radiograph, as the bone fragment is often superimposed with the cortex of the posterior tibial plateau. On magnetic resonance imaging, marrow edema is more prevalent in the fibular head than the tiny avulsion fracture. The importance of this injury is its association with injuries to other vital structures of the knee, including tears of the cruciate ligaments, collateral ligaments, and/or menisci.

Notes

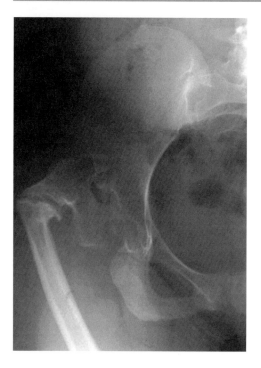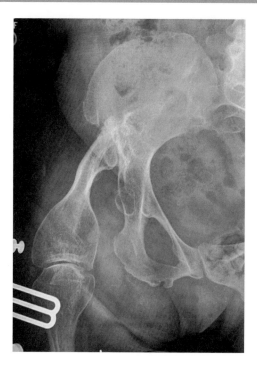

1. What are the main observations in these two patients?

2. What do you call these entities?

3. What percentage of patients have bilateral disease?

4. Classification of this disorder is based on what observations?

Proximal Focal Femoral Deficiency

1. Focal dysgenesis of the proximal femur.

2. Proximal focal femoral deficiency.

3. Less than 10%.

4. Presence of the head of the femur, development of the acetabulum, length of femoral shortening, and relationship of the femur to the acetabulum at skeletal maturity.

Reference

Resnick D: Additional congenital or heritable anomalies and syndromes. In Resnick D (ed): *Diagnosis of Bone and Joint Disorders*, 3rd ed. Philadelphia, WB Saunders, 1995, pp 4282–4285.

Cross-Reference

Musculoskeletal Imaging: THE REQUISITES, 3rd ed, p 607.

Comment

Proximal focal femoral deficiency is a spectrum of congenital disorders that is characterized by segmental length discrepancy of the femur caused by defective formation of the proximal femur. The etiology is unknown but occurs early in embryologic development, either from a disturbance in cellular nutrition or blood flow. There is an increased incidence in children of diabetic mothers. The majority of cases are unilateral. The segmental defect usually is isolated to the femur although on rare occasions it has been reported to occur in association with tibial agenesis and aplasia of the cruciate ligaments of the knee.

There are four types. In type A, there is a varus deformity of the femoral neck, osseous connection between the components of the femur, and adequate development of the acetabulum. In type B, a pseudoarthrosis forms at the femoral neck and there may be moderate dysplastic changes of the acetabulum. In type C, there is severe dysplasia of the acetabulum, a tapered proximal shaft and variable connection between the femoral diaphysis and poorly formed femoral head. In type D, the most severe deformity, there is absence of the acetabulum, enlargement of the obturator foramen, and absence of the proximal femur. Magnetic resonance imaging and ultrasound have been gaining acceptance over radiography and arthrography for early assessment of the condition since these modalities allow imaging of nonossified cartilaginous structures.

Notes

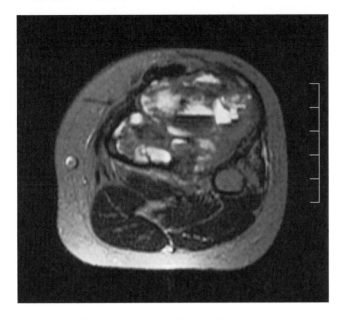 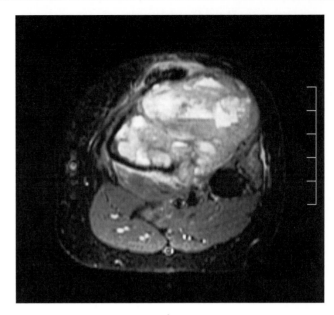

1. What is the incidence of this finding?

2. Are you able to arrive at a specific diagnosis based on your observation?

3. What is the most likely cause of the fluid-fluid level?

4. Is this finding compatible with benignity?

Lesions with Fluid-Fluid Levels

1. Nearly 3% of bone or soft tissue tumors show a fluid-fluid level.

2. No, fluid-fluid levels in bone or soft tissue tumors cannot be considered diagnostic of any particular tumor.

3. Prior hemorrhage within the lesion.

4. No, because it may be seen in osteosarcoma (classic and telangiectatic), malignant fibrous histiocytoma, and soft tissue sarcomas.

References

Keenan S, Bui-Mansfield LT: Musculoskeletal lesions with fluid-fluid level: A pictorial essay. *J Comput Assist Tomogr* 30:517–524, 2006.

Van Dyck P, Banhoenacker FM, Vogel J, et al: Prevalence, extension and characteristics of fluid-fluid levels in bone and soft tissue tumors. *Eur Radiol* 16:2644–2651, 2006.

Cross-Reference

Musculoskeletal Imaging: THE REQUISITES, 3rd ed, p 418.

Comment

A fluid-fluid level is one of the most common observations during the evaluation of tumors of the bone and soft tissues. This may be noted on either computed tomography or magnetic resonance imaging. These levels become apparent when a fluid collection containing substances of different density is allowed to settle, and when the plane of imaging is perpendicular to the fluid level. Frequently but not always, fluid-fluid levels indicate prior hemorrhage. This finding can be observed in a wide variety of lesions: osseous and soft tissue masses, neoplastic or non-neoplastic lesions, malignant or benign neoplasms, and primary or metastatic malignancies. It may also be seen in tumoral calcinosis, with calcium-fluid levels. When a fluid-fluid level is detected, in conjunction with clinical history, the differential diagnosis for a lesion can often be limited to a few choices. Fluid-fluid levels were first reported to occur in aneurysmal bone cysts. However, fluid-fluid levels have more recently also been associated with malignant neoplasms such as telangiectatic osteosarcoma, conventional osteosarcoma, and malignant fibrous histiocytoma of bone; benign neoplasms such as chondroblastoma, giant cell tumor of bone, fibrous dysplasia, simple bone cyst, and osteoblastoma; and soft tissue tumors including soft tissue hemangioma, synovial sarcomas, and other soft tissue sarcomas.

Notes

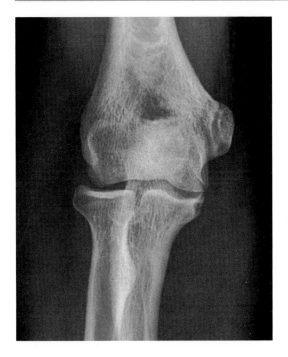

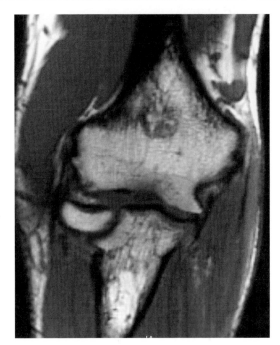

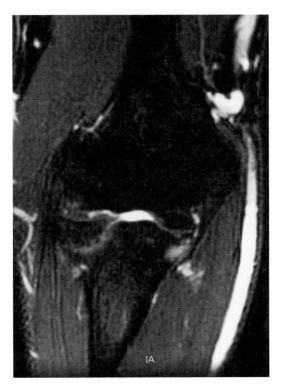

1. How did this patient injure his elbow?

2. What is the injury that you see?

3. What are some potential associated injuries?

4. How are most people with this injury treated?

Avulsion of the Ulnar Collateral Ligament

1. He is likely a throwing athlete and sustained a valgus injury.

2. Avulsion of the sublime tubercle, the insertion of the anterior band of the ulnar collateral ligament.

3. Contusion of the capitellum and radial head, and osteochondral defect of the capitellum.

4. Immobilization. Surgery is usually reserved for high-caliber athletes.

Reference

Ouellette H, Kassarjian A, Tretreaut P, Palmer W: Imaging of the overhead throwing athlete. *Sem Musculoskelet Radiol* 9:316–333, 2005.

Cross-Reference

Musculoskeletal Imaging: THE REQUISITES, 3rd ed, pp 125–128.

Comment

The ulnar collateral ligament (UCL) comprises three bands: the anterior, posterior, and oblique bands. The anterior band is the largest of the three and primary stabilizer against valgus forces on the elbow. It originates from the inferior aspect of the medial epicondyle and inserts on the sublime tubercle at the medial aspect of the coronoid process of the ulna. Repetitive tension on the UCL during the acceleration phase of the throwing cycle may result in ligamentous attenuation, inflammation, and progressive laxity. With repetitive stress, the anterior band of the UCL may eventually tear, either at the sublime insertion or proximally near the epicondylar origin. Occasionally, a small avulsion fracture of the sublime tubercle may occur instead of a ligamentous tear such as in this patient. Radiographically, indirect signs of UCL injury include heterotopic ossification in the course of the UCL, and abnormal widening of the medial joint space on stress views. Lysis of bone at the sublime tubercle insertion is an important observation. Magnetic resonance imaging is indicated in any athlete in which this injury is suspected. The components of the UCL appear as linear low signal intensity structures. The presence of discontinuity, morphologic change, or edema heralds the presence of pathology. On MR arthrography, extracapsular leakage of contrast indicates complete disruption.

Notes

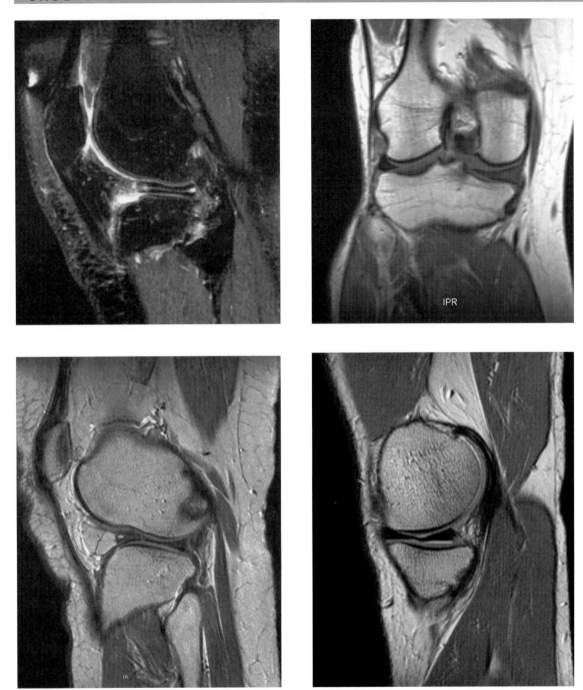

These four patients all have a normal variation of a meniscus.

1. What is the normal variant in the first patient? What is the leading hypothesis for the development of this congenital variant?

2. What is the normal variant in the second patient? Which side is more common, lateral or medial meniscus?

3. What is the normal variant in the third patient?

4. What is the normal variant in the fourth patient?

Meniscal Variants

1. Discoid lateral meniscus (torn). Abnormal inferior fascicular attachment of the posterior horn, which contributes to discoid growth.

2. Discoid medial meniscus (degenerated). Lateral.

3. Meniscal ossicle (with radial tear).

4. Normal meniscal flounce.

References

Yu JS, Cosgarea AJ, Kaeding CC, Wilson D: Meniscal flounce MR imaging. *Radiology* 203:513–515, 1997.

Yu JS, Resnick D: Meniscal ossicle: MR imaging appearance in three patients. *Skeletal Radiol* 23:637–639, 1994.

Cross-Reference

Musculoskeletal Imaging: THE REQUISITES, 3rd ed, pp 224–232.

Comment

There are several normal variants that occur in the meniscus of the knee. The importance of these observations on magnetic resonance imaging is that they either mimic a true disorder or may predispose the meniscus to premature degeneration or tear. A discoid meniscus is a morphologic variant, seen in 3% of knees, characterized by poor constriction of the central portion of the meniscus and thickening of its free end. Most experts believe that it represents a developmental defect due to abnormal peripheral attachments. Owing to the thickened morphology, there is an abnormal extension of fibrocartilage between the femoral condyle and tibial plateau that is more susceptible to trauma. The aim of treatment is resection of this unstable free-end segment. Clinically, patients present with symptoms of a meniscal tear. A discoid meniscus is suspected when a bow tie is present on three or more consecutive sagittal sections. A meniscal ossicle is a rare variant often mistaken for intra-articular bodies on radiographs. Magnetic resonance imaging is definitive, depicting the area of ossification within the meniscus. A meniscal flounce is a fold in the meniscus of no significance but it can mimic a tear owing to blunting of the free end on certain images.

Notes

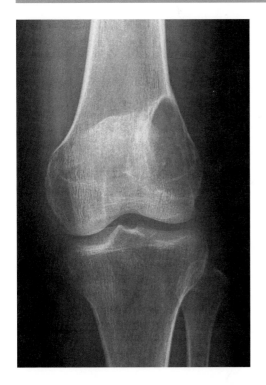

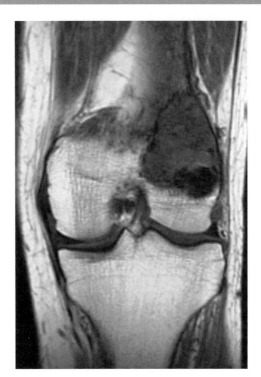

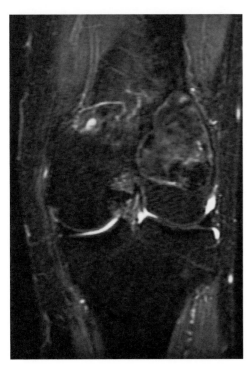

1. What is the most likely diagnosis? Based on the radiograph, what else did you consider?

2. What "discordant" finding did you use to make the diagnosis? Is this always reliable?

3. When involving the long bones, where are they located?

4. Are these neoplastic?

Solid Variant of Aneurysmal Bone Cyst

1. Solid variant of aneurysmal bone cyst. Bone cyst (aneurysmal or simple), giant cell tumor, nonossifying fibroma, chondromyxoid fibroma, fibrous dysplasia, and osteosarcoma.

2. Cystic-appearing mass on radiograph but solid on magnetic resonance imaging. No, because many lesions are not aneurysmal, and some are periosteal in location.

3. The metaphysis and diaphysis are preferred regions of the bone but no location is exempt.

4. No, they do not recur after resection or metastasize. But they can be mistaken for osteosarcoma.

Reference

Ilaslan H, Sundaram M, Unni KK: Solid variant of aneurysmal bone cysts in long tubular bones: Giant cell reparative granuloma. *AJR Am J Roentgenol* 180:1681–1687, 2003.

Cross-Reference

Musculoskeletal Imaging: THE REQUISITES, 3rd ed, pp 516–520.

Comment

A solid variant of an aneurysmal bone cyst (ABC), also known as giant cell reparative granuloma, is a rare, non-neoplastic lesion. Histologically, the lesion is characterized predominantly with spindle cell, fibroblastic proliferation, with minor foci of reactive osteoid formation and osteoclast-like giant cells. There is neither cellular atypia nor mitotic figures present. Amorphous lacelike calcifications typical of ABC are also present. They are most common in the mandible and in short tubular bones of the hands and feet, but when in long bones they may be mistaken for a malignancy, particularly osteosarcoma. They may occur anytime but most patients are young and there is a slight female predominance. In long bones, the femur is most commonly involved (33%), followed by the ulna and tibia (23% each). Radiographically, they present as eccentrically located, expansile lesions with variably aggressive features, and occasionally present as a subperiosteal lesion. One third of lesions are not aneurysmal at all, particularly when in the surface of the bone. On magnetic resonance imaging, most lesions are slightly hyperintense to muscle on T1W images and heterogeneous with areas of low signal intensity on T2W images, and they appear solid. Edema in the bone or soft tissues may occur in 50% of cases and is more typical of smaller lesions. Treatment is local curettage and bone grafting. Recurrence has not been reported.

Notes

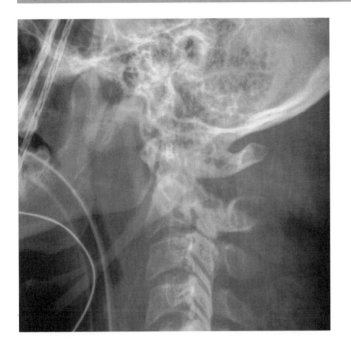

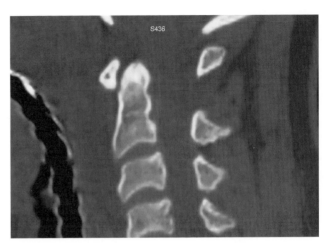

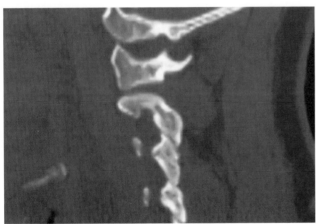

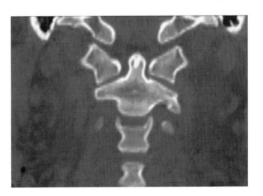

1. How common is this injury and what is its usual outcome?

2. What is the proposed mechanism of injury?

3. How is the diagnosis confirmed on the radiograph?

4. Is this injury more common in children or adults, and why?

Craniocervical Dislocation

1. Rare; nearly universally lethal (brainstem injury).

2. Extreme hyperextension of the neck with a second distractive force acting on the head.

3. By a Powers ratio greater than 1.

4. More common in children because their condyles are smaller and the articular relationship of the condyles with the lateral masses of C1 is more horizontal.

Reference

Bellabarba C, Mirza SK, West GA, et al: Diagnosis and treatment of craniocervical dislocation in a series of 17 consecutive survivors during an 8-year period. *J Neurosurg Spine* 4:429–440, 2006.

Cross-Reference

Musculoskeletal Imaging: THE REQUISITES, 3rd ed, pp 167–169.

Comment

The injury sustained by this patient is rare, and few patients survive this type of dislocation. It is caused by either significant distractive force applied to the head when the neck is hyperextended or a shearing injury to the face or the occipital region of the skull. Both mechanisms can cause rupture of the tectorial membrane and alar ligaments of the occipitoatlantoaxial joints and usually require a high-velocity force such as those sustained during a motor vehicle accident. The diagnosis usually is relatively straightforward and based on observations obtained from the lateral radiograph of the cervical spine, but it is very subtle on this examination that shows only soft tissue swelling anterior to C1. The Powers ratio defines a normal relationship between the base of the skull and the atlas. In this ratio, the length of a line drawn from the basion to the spinolaminar line of C1 divided by the length of a line drawn from the opisthion to the posterior margin of the anterior arch of C1 is determined. If the ratio is less than 1, no dislocation exists. In this patient, the ratio was 1:1. Note that the occipital condyles do not articulate with the lateral masses of C1. The treatment, if a patient survives this injury, is surgical stabilization by occipito-C2 arthrodesis followed by halothoracic immobilization for at least 12 weeks.

Notes

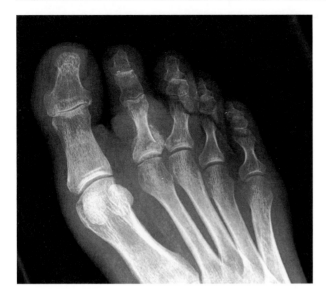

1. There is no history of trauma. What is the differential diagnosis?

2. The patient later presented with a mass after 5 months. What do you think the diagnosis is?

3. What is Nora's lesion?

4. What is distinctive about this process on magnetic resonance imaging?

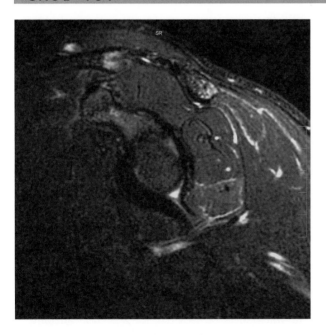 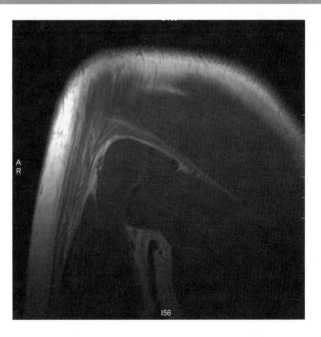

1. The sagittal image was from a study performed 2 years prior to the coronal image shown. What did you observe in the first study? And the second?

2. What is the cause of these findings in the absence of trauma? Any thoughts on etiology?

3. Is the process usually reversible?

4. What is the most common etiology of isolated teres minor involvement?

Florid Reactive Periostitis

1. Infection, neoplasm, and florid reactive periostitis.

2. Florid reactive periostitis.

3. Bizarre parosteal osteochondromatous proliferation, a progressed state of florid reactive periostitis.

4. The adjacent cortex, medullary cavity, and soft tissues appear normal.

References

Dhondt E, Oudenhoven L, Khan S, et al: Nora's lesion, a distinct radiological entity? *Skeletal Radiol* 35: 497–502, 2006.

Porter AR, Tristan TA, Rudy FR, Eshbach TB: Florid reactive periostitis of the phalanges. *AJR Am J Roentgenol* 144:617–618, 1985.

Cross-Reference

Musculoskeletal Imaging: THE REQUISITES, 3rd ed, pp 412–415.

Comment

Florid reactive periostitis, also known as parosteal or nodular fasciitis, is an unusual bone-producing lesion that may be confused with an infectious or neoplastic process. It most typically involves the small bones of the hands and feet. Clinically, patients present with soft tissue swelling of the affected part, sometimes accompanied by pain, tenderness, and redness. Radiographically, the condition is characterized by periosteal reaction, which begins as a minimal periostitis and is associated with swelling. It may mimic an infection in the first 1 to 2 weeks. Subsequently, the periosteal reaction progresses to a florid state to involve both sides of an intact phalanx. Occasionally, it can become an ossified mass resembling an osteochondroma; this is referred to as bizarre parosteal osteochondromatous proliferation (BPOP). Histologically, lesions contain hypercellular cartilage with calcification and ossification with maturing cancellous bone and a spindle cell stroma without atypia. Magnetic resonance imaging shows low signal intensity on T1W images and high signal intensity on fluid sensitive sequences. The cortex, medullary cavity, and adjacent soft tissues appear normal, excluding a neoplastic or infectious process. Treatment is local excision.

Notes

Quadrilateral Space Syndrome

1. Interstitial muscle edema in the posterior deltoid and teres minor muscles (high T2 signal intensity). The patient developed atrophy of these muscles with volume loss and fat replacement (high T1 signal intensity).

2. Quadrilateral space syndrome from axillary nerve compression. Fibrous bands are likely but any space-occupying process can cause it.

3. In the acute phase, decompression of the quadrilateral space may alleviate the progression of atrophy.

4. Chronic traction injury of the teres minor nerve.

References

Linker CS, Helms CA, Fritz RC: Quadrilateral space syndrome: Findings at MR imaging. *Radiology* 188: 675–676, 1993.

Wilson L, Sundaram M, Piraino DW, et al: Isolated teres minor atrophy: Manifestation of quadrilateral space syndrome or traction injury to the axillary nerve? *Orthopedics* 29:447–450, 2006.

Cross-Reference

Musculoskeletal Imaging: THE REQUISITES, 3rd ed, p 87.

Comment

Quadrilateral space syndrome refers to an isolated axillary nerve compressive neuropathy that is one of the causes of shoulder pain. The axillary nerve and posterior humeral circumflex artery course through the quadrilateral space in the posterior aspect of the shoulder. The quadrilateral space is demarcated by the teres major (superior margin) and teres minor muscles (inferior margin), long head of the triceps muscle (medial margin), and the humeral neck (lateral margin). Clinically, the syndrome is characterized by pain that localizes poorly but is exacerbated by abduction and external rotation. Paresthesia in the lateral shoulder and upper posterior arm and weakness may be present. Atrophy of the teres minor and posterior deltoid muscles are late findings. In the absence of trauma, the syndrome is usually caused by fibrous bands although any space-occupying process in the quadrilateral space may elicit the syndrome. Magnetic resonance imaging is the preferred method for diagnosis.

The incidence of isolated teres minor atrophy is about 5%, usually seen in elderly men over the age of 60 years who have other shoulder pathology such as rotator cuff tears and glenohumeral joint instability. This noncompressive cause of atrophy is likely related to humeral decentering, which produces traction of the teres minor nerve from the axillary nerve, and not to quadrilateral space syndrome.

Notes

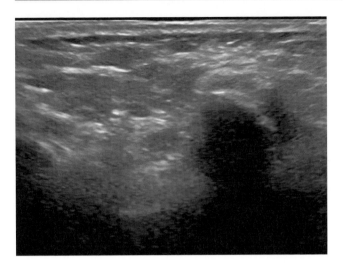 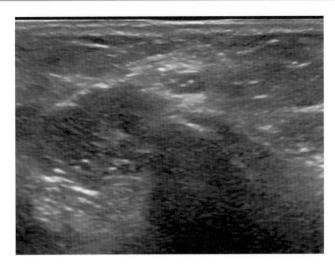

You are shown transverse sonograms (right side is anterior) of the ulnar nerve at the level of the medial epicondyle of the elbow in a neutral position and with the elbow flexed.

1. What is the normal appearance of the ulnar nerve?

2. What happened in the sonogram performed with flexion? Is it permanent?

3. What is snapping triceps syndrome? What is its significance?

4. What is the abnormality in the congenital type?

Ulnar Nerve Dislocation

1. Oval hypoechoic structure posterior to the medial epicondyle (shown by large area of acoustic shadowing) surrounded by hyperechoic perineural fat.

2. Dislocaton of the ulnar nerve. No, it reduces with elbow extension.

3. Medial dislocation of the medial head of the triceps muscle over the medial epicondyle during elbow flexion. It can coexist with ulnar nerve dislocation and produce similar symptoms.

4. Absence of the cubital tunnel retinaculum.

References

Finlay K, Ferri M, Friedman L: Ultrasound of the elbow. *Skeletal Radiol* 33:63–79, 2004.

Jacobson JA, Jebson PJ, Jeffers AW, et al: Ulnar nerve dislocation and snapping triceps syndrome: Diagnosis with dynamic sonography—report of three cases. *Radiology* 220:601–605, 2001.

Cross-Reference

Musculoskeletal Imaging: THE REQUISITES, 3rd ed, p 131.

Comment

The ulnar nerve lives within the medial olecranon groove. On ultrasound, the appearance on transverse imaging is that of an oval or round hypoechoic structure, interspersed by multiple, discrete, and slightly echogenic foci. These echogenic foci represent the nerve fascicles. The ulnar nerve has a uniform thickness measuring 2 mm by 3 mm. Dislocation of the ulnar nerve is an important cause of medial elbow pain. It is manifested by abnormal movement of the ulnar nerve out of the cubital tunnel and over the medial epicondyle during elbow flexion. The strength of sonography is in the ability to directly detect the dislocation of the nerve with dynamic imaging. The nerve position can be followed through the range of motion, and is often associated with a snapping sensation felt through the transducer. When magnetic resonance imaging is performed with the elbow extended, the ulnar nerve lies in its anatomic position, and the transient pathology may escape detection. Dislocation of the ulnar nerve over the medial epicondyle may cause irritation of the nerve due to friction as it passes over the bone, and it places the nerve at risk for direct injury. When associated with ulnar neuritis, the cross-sectional area increases. An area greater than 0.075 cm² at the level of the cubital tunnel indicates cubital tunnel syndrome.

Notes

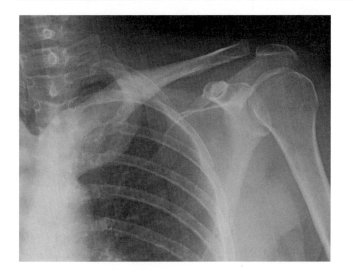

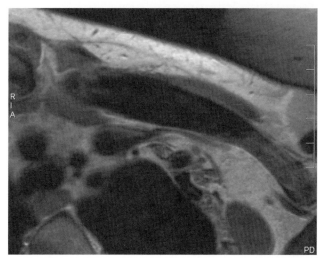

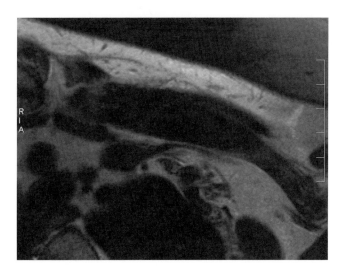

1. Do you think this patient has pain?

2. What is the differential diagnosis?

3. Which conditions are associated with sternoclavicular joint narrowing?

4. What is SAPHO?

Condensing Osteitis of the Clavicle

1. Yes, but it followed by periods of remission.

2. Condensing osteitis of the clavicle and sternocostoclavicular hyperostosis. Occasionally, chronic osteomyelitis.

3. Chronic osteomyeltis and sternocostoclavicular hyperostosis.

4. A cutaneous disorder of the hands and feet, where sterile pustules erupt in the palms and soles in association with skeletal hyperostosis (synovitis, acne, pustulosis, hyperostosis, and osteomyelitis).

References

Greenspan A, Gerscovich E, Szabo RM, Matthews JG: Condensing osteitis of the clavicle: A rare but frequently misdiagnosed condition. *AJR Am J Roentgenol* 156:1011–1015, 1991.

Habib PA, Huang GS, Mendiola JA, Yu JS: Anterior chest pain: Musculoskeletal considerations. *Emerg Radiol* 11:37–45, 2004.

Cross-Reference

Musculoskeletal Imaging: THE REQUISITES, 3rd ed, pp 75–76.

Comment

Osteitis condensans is a painful condition that affects women between the ages of 20 and 50 years, although it can occur in patients who are much younger. It is caused by stressful activities focused on the sternocostoclavicular joint such as heavy lifting or rigorous athletic activity. The radiographic evaluation demonstrates eburnation, mild enlargement of the inferomedial aspect of the clavicle, osteophytosis, and surrounding soft tissue swelling; however, joint space narrowing is conspicuously absent. Bone scintigraphy shows increased uptake of the radionuclide substance. Magnetic resonance imaging typically reveals hypointense areas on T1W images corresponding to sclerosis with variable signal intensity on T2W images as well as marrow edema.

The differential diagnosis includes sternocostoclavicular hyperostosis and chronic osteomyelitis. Sternocostoclavicular hyperostosis is a clinical syndrome of pain, swelling, tenderness, and heat that affects people in the fourth to sixth decades of life. Hyperostosis and soft tissue ossification of the clavicle, anterior portion of the upper ribs, and sternum characterize this disorder. Eventually, there is severe limitation of motion due to extensive ossification. It is more common in men than women and in older people. Chronic osteomyelitis of the clavicle is most common as a result of an invasive procedure of the chest, or following septic arthritis of the sternocostoclavicular joint.

Notes

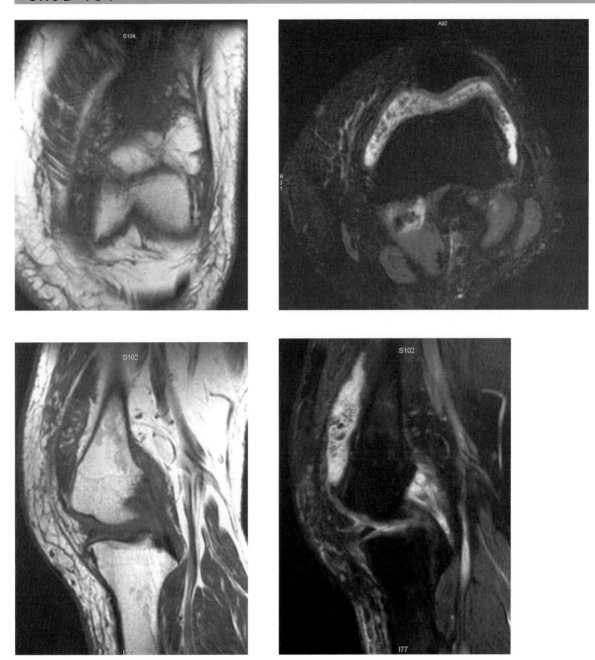

1. What is the diagnosis?

2. What is the characteristic presentation of the condition?

3. Is this a bilateral process?

4. How is it diagnosed and treated?

C A S E 1 8 4

Lipoma Arborescens

1. Lipoma arborescens.

2. Slow and progressive swelling of the knee with effusion and eventual development of osteoarthritis.

3. It is reported as bilateral in 20% of cases.

4. Diagnosis by magnetic resonance imaging; synovectomy.

References

Ryu KN, Jaovisidha S, Schweitzer M, et al: MR imaging of lipoma arborescens of the knee joint. *AJR Am J Roentgenol* 167:1229–1232, 1996.

Vilanova JC, Barcelo J, Villalon M, et al: MR imaging of lipoma arborescens and the associated lesions. *Skeletal Radiol* 32:504–509, 2003.

Cross-Reference

Musculoskeletal Imaging: THE REQUISITES, 3rd ed, p 477.

Comment

Lipoma arborescens, or diffuse articular lipomatosis, is a rare, benign intra-articular lesion of unknown etiology. It is characterized by villous proliferation of the synovium and diffuse replacement of the subsynovial tissue by mature adipose cells. Although described in several different joints, it is most commonly seen in the suprapatellar bursa when in the knee. It forms part of the differential diagnosis for a slowly progressive, chronically swollen knee with intermittent effusion. The average length of symptoms is 2 to 7 years (the longest reported is 30 years), but occasionally it may present with sudden onset. Generally, this is a painless process until the onset of osteoarthritis. Mechanical symptoms such as locking and crepitus may occur, likely related to entrapment of the fat projections. Arthroscopically, the lesion appears as a synovial lesion with numerous fatty-appearing globules and villous projections. Lesions are treated with synovectomy, which is considered curative; therefore, magnetic resonance imaging is recommended to document the full extent of involvement. It is also useful in differentiating this lesion from other lesions associated with chronic effusions such as rheumatoid arthritis, pigmented villonodular synovitis, synovial hemangioma, and synovial chondromatosis. On magnetic resonance imaging, lipoma arborescens closely resembles other collections of subsynovial fat, the only difference being its large size. The lesion does not demonstrate enhancement with administration of intravenous gadolinium. Rarely, it is associated with osseous erosion.

Notes

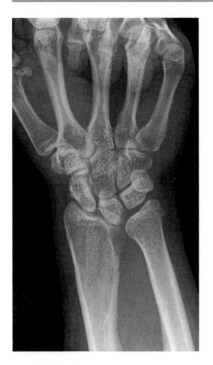
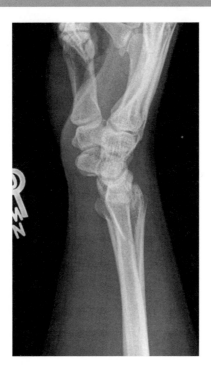
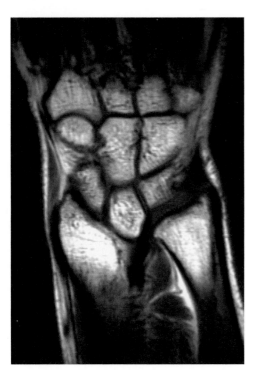

1. What is the differential diagnosis?

2. Based on the magnetic resonance image, what is the essential abnormality?

3. List the characteristic radiographic findings.

4. This patient has the idiopathic form. Who is affected?

Idiopathic Madelung Deformity

1. Dyschondrosteosis, idiopathic Madelung deformity, and Turner syndrome.

2. Anomalous ligaments contribute to bowing of the distal end of the radius while the ulna continues to grow in a straight direction.

3. Variable bowing of radius, lunate subsidence, marked ulnar tilting of radius, hypertrophy of short radiolunate ligament and, if the bowing is dramatic, subluxation of distal radioulnar joint and palmar carpal displacement.

4. Females.

References

Cook PA, Yu JS, Wiand W, et al: Madelung deformity in skeletally immature patients: Morphologic assessment using radiographs, CT, and MR imaging. *J Comput Assist Tomogr* 20:505–511, 1996.

McCarroll HR, Jr, James MA, Newmeyer WL, III, et al: Madelung's deformity: Quantitative assessment of x-ray deformity. *J Hand Surg* 30-A:1211–1220, 2005.

Cross-Reference

Musculoskeletal Imaging: THE REQUISITES, 3rd ed, pp 637 and 645–646.

Comment

Madelung deformity can occur as an isolated finding or as part of a syndrome, most commonly dyschondrosteosis. The differential diagnosis is limited since the Madelung deformity is not typically seen in other mesomelic dwarfs. Other distinct clinical manifestations differentiate between idiopathic Madelung deformity, dyschondrosteosis, and Turner syndrome. Radiographically, the disorder is characterized by variable bowing of the distal radius in an ulnar and volar direction, giving rise to a relatively elongated and dorsally dislocated ulna. A pyramidal-shaped carpus, or lunate subsidence, is a typical feature along with an abnormal lunate tilt of the radial articular surface. Anomalous ligaments contribute to the deformity in the volar aspect of the wrist. Palmar carpal displacement owing to absence of the volar part of the lunate fossa is seen with severe bowing deformity of the radius. Treatment is aimed at restoring functional motion and is most commonly treated surgically with a combination of radial osteotomy and insertion of a trapezoidal wedge.

Notes

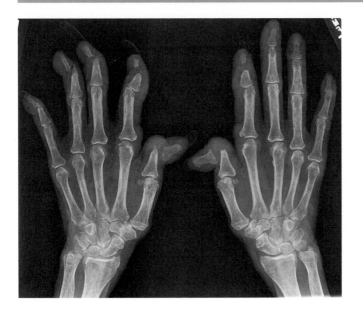 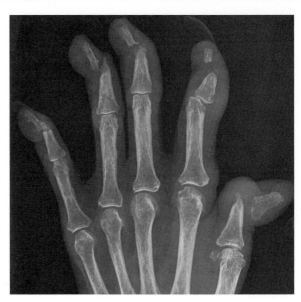

1. This patient has numerous red nodules in the hand, forearms, and elbow. What is your diagnosis?

2. What causes erosions at the distal interphalangeal (DIP) joints and interphalangeal (IP) joints of the thumb?

3. What is the radiographic differential diagnosis?

4. What other associated lesion may occur in these patients? Where does it commonly occur?

Multicentric Reticulohistiocytosis

1. Multicentric reticulohistiocytosis.

2. Proliferation and infiltration of histiocytes and giant cells from the synovial tissues into the bone.

3. The findings are typical of advanced multicentric reticulohistiocytosis. Early in the disease you may consider gout, psoriasis, erosive osteoarthritis, scleroderma, and occasionally rheumatoid arthritis.

4. Xanthomas related to hypercholesterolemia. Eyelids.

Reference

Gold RH, Bassett LW, Seeger LL: The other arthritides: Roentgenologic features of osteoarthritis, erosive osteoarthritis, ankylosing spondylitis, psoriatic arthritis, Reiter's disease, multicentric reticulohistiocytosis, and progressive systemic sclerosis. *Radiol Clin North Am* 26:1195–1212, 1988.

Cross-Reference

Musculoskeletal Imaging: THE REQUISITES, 3rd ed, p 331.

Comment

Multicentric reticulohistiocytosis is a disease characterized by proliferation of histiocytes in the skin, mucosa, subcutaneous tissues, synovia, periosteum, and bone. It has no known cause. It has an onset in the fifth decade of life and is more common in women. Two thirds of those affected present with initial polyarthritis followed by development of firm yellow to red nodules in the skin within months. In the rest, the arthropathy follows the skin eruptions. The joint manifestations are symmetric and involve the IP joints of fingers and thumb, knee, shoulder, wrist, hip, ankle, feet, elbow, spine, and temporomandibular joints. Clinically, stiffness, swelling, and tenderness are typical symptoms. Radiographically, joint disease begins with marginal erosions that spread centrally, producing separation of the joint surfaces. Two important distinctions from rheumatoid arthritis are notable: There is a lack of osteopenia and a high frequency of involvement of the DIP joints. In some cases, the early radiographic changes may mimic gouty arthritis. Progression to arthritis mutilans is common with resorption of the phalanges, foreshortening of the fingers, and telescoping of the digits. Generally, the skin nodules are not radiographically detectable but demonstrate low signal intensity on T1W and high signal intensity on T2W images on magnetic resonance imaging.

Notes

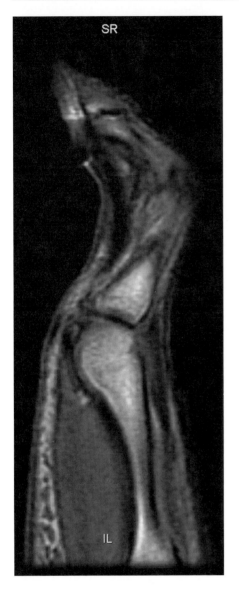
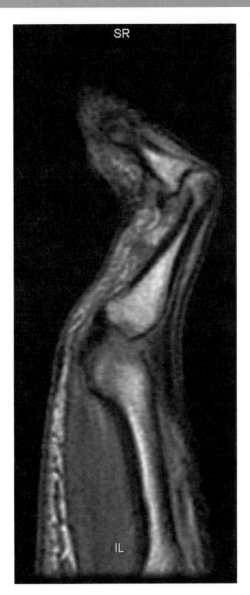

1. What is the injury?

2. Who is at risk for this type of injury?

3. What should be done?

4. How is this injury different from a "Jersey finger"?

Pulley Injury of the Finger

1. Rupture of the A4, A3, and distal part of the A2 pulleys resulting in bowstringing of the flexor tendon.

2. Rock climbers.

3. In high-level climbers, the ruptured pulleys should be reconstructed either with a free tendon or retinaculum graft.

4. A "Jersey finger" is a rupture of either the flexor digitorum profundus or superficialis tendon insertion. In a pulley injury, the tendon is intact but displaced.

Reference

Martinoli C, Bianchi S, Cotton A: Imaging of rock climbing injuries. *Semin Musculoskelet Radiol* 9:334–345, 2005.

Cross-Reference

Musculoskeletal Imaging: THE REQUISITES, 3rd ed, pp 162–163.

Comment

The flexor tendons of the fingers are held closely adjacent to the cortical surfaces of the proximal and middle phalanges by fibrous envelopes called the annular pulley system. These fibrous bands prevent divergence of the tendons from the finger midline axis in both the anteroposterior and lateral directions and provide the points where the force of the tendons is exerted during flexion movements. Because flexion occurs at the interphalangeal joints, these bands are of different thickness along the finger length and include several segments. There are five in all: A1 extends from the palmar plate of the metacarpophalangeal joint, A2 is at the proximal end of the proximal phalanx, A3 is small and located over the proximal interphalangeal joint, A4 lies in the middle of the middle phalanx, and A5 is located over the distal interphalangeal joint. Three additional cruciform bands crisscross between them: the A2 and A3 pulleys (C1), A3 and A4 pulleys (C2), and A4 and A5 pulleys (C3). In rock climbing, the hand holds required in climbing exert force on the fingers while flexed at either the proximal or distal interphalangeal joints. This increases the tension on the pulleys by as much as 40%, occasionally overwhelming the integrity of the connective tissue.

Notes

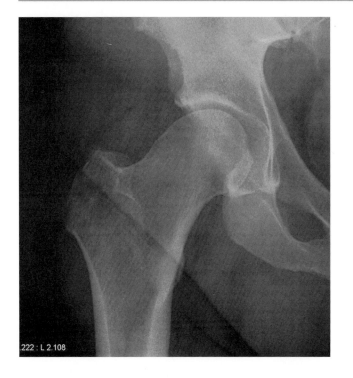
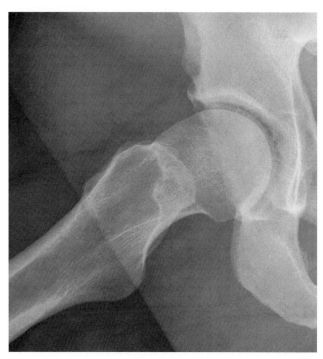
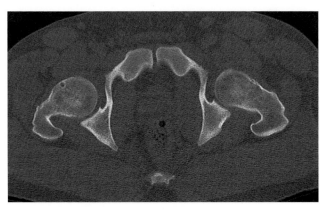
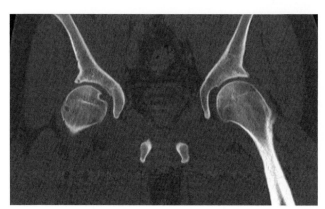

1. What is the diagnosis?

2. Who are affected by this condition and how do they present?

3. What is the hypothesized cause of the deformity?

4. What is the classic triad on magnetic resonance arthrography?

Femoroacetabular Impingement

1. Cam-type impingement of the hip.

2. Young athletic males with hip pain.

3. Abnormal separation of the common physis of the femoral head and greater trochanter during development.

4. Abnormal α angle, an anterior-superior acetabular cartilage lesion, and an anterior-superior labral tear.

References

Ganz R, Parvizi J, Beck M, et al: Femoroacetabular impingement: A cause for osteoarthritis of the hip. *Clin Orthop Relat Res* 417:112–120, 2003.

Kassarjian A: Hip MR arthrography and femoroacetabular impingement. *Semin Musculoskelet Radiol* 10:208–219, 2006.

Cross-Reference

Musculoskeletal Imaging: THE REQUISITES, 3rd ed, pp 204–207.

Comment

Femoroacetabular impingement is a recently recognized cause of hip pain and is caused by abnormal contact between the femur and the acetabular rim. Several predisposing factors have been reported including Legg-Calve-Perthes disease, slipped capital femoral epiphysis, coxa magna, hip dysplasia, and prior fractures. Recently, some patients with no known predisposing abnormality have been described. Although radiographs initially appear normal, close inspection of the hip joint shows subtle abnormalities of femoroacetabular impingement. There are two types, cam-type impingement and pincer-type impingement. In cam-type impingement, the main finding is abnormal contour of the proximal femur with a normal acetabulum. The anterior-superior head-neck junction, normally concave, is either flattened or convex (pistol grip deformity). In the computed tomography image, the anterior-superior head-neck junction is offset producing a bony protruberance. In pincer-type impingement, the proximal femur is normal in contour but the acetabulum is abnormal. This can include retroversion, anterior and/or lateral overcoverage, and acetabular protrusion. Cartilage lesions are often seen along the posterior aspect of the acetabulum because of a contrecoup type of injury as the femur abnormally contacts the acetabular rim. Labral degeneration and tears are most common in the anterosuperior labrum. Treatment for femoroacetabular impingement is dependent on the type and is still emerging. It includes osteoplasty of the proximal femur, debridement of labral and cartilage pathology, resection of excess along the acetabulum, and periacetabular rotational osteotomy.

Notes

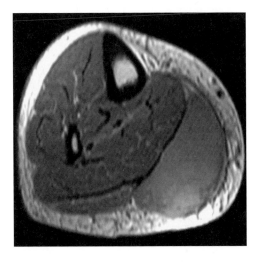 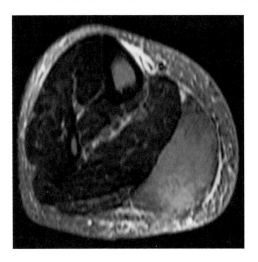

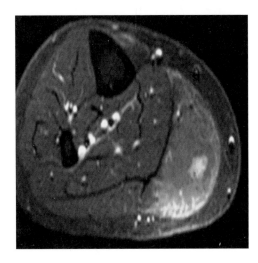

1. What is the differential diagnosis?

2. Histologically, what does the identification of Reed-Sternberg giant cells indicate? Is it common in the bone?

3. Where is the source of the majority of musculoskeletal manifestations of lymphoma? How long does it take?

4. Which is least common in the muscle—primary lymphoma, disseminated disease, or direct extension?

Skeletal Muscle Lymphoma

1. Skeletal lymphoma, fibrosarcoma, fibromatosis, and possibly acute myositis ossificans. Infection (myositis) is not a consideration because there is no inflammation.

2. Hodgkin's lymphoma. It is rare.

3. Secondary hematogenous dissemination from nodal disease. Average is about 5 years.

4. Primary skeletal lymphoma is rare, accounting for 1.5% of non-Hodgkin's lymphoma and 0.3% of Hodgkin's lymphoma.

Reference

Ruzek KA, Wenger DE: The multiple faces of lymphoma of the musculoskeletal system. *Skeletal Radiol* 33:1–8, 2004.

Cross-Reference

Musculoskeletal Imaging: THE REQUISITES, 3rd ed, pp 491–493.

Comment

Lymphoma is a disorder characterized by the proliferation of cells native to the lymphoid tissue, namely lymphocytes, histiocytes, and their precursors. It has a wide spectrum of musculoskeletal manifestations involving the bone, muscle, and soft tissues. The disease can arise in lymphoreticular tissue anywhere in the body and spread through hematogenous dissemination to distant sites. The majority of cases of musculoskeletal lymphoma develop from secondary hematogenous dissemination from nodal disease, a process that takes an average of about 57 months.

Primary bone lymphoma, that is, lymphoma that originates in the bone, accounts for less than 5% of malignant tumors. Over half present in patients older than 40 years, and the vast majority are non-Hodgkin's lymphoma. Although nodal disease is the most common soft tissue manifestation of lymphoma, it occasionally presents as a focal mass or as a diffuse infiltrative process affecting the skin, subcutaneous tissue, and muscle. Primary skeletal lymphoma is rare. It may present as a focal mass or diffuse infiltration of a muscle with low signal intensity on T1W images, high signal intensity on T2W images, and heterogeneously diffuse enhancement. Muscular enlargement is typical with preservation of morphology, particularly intermuscular septation. This case is difficult but the recognition of infiltration and enlargement of the medial gastrocnemius muscle is important. Equally important is the lack of inflammatory findings.

Notes

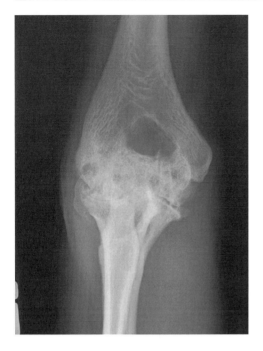
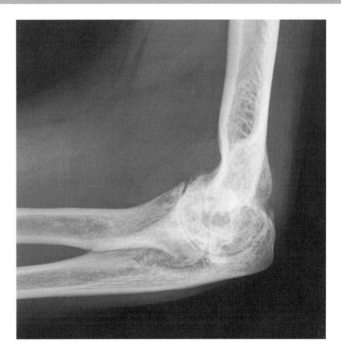
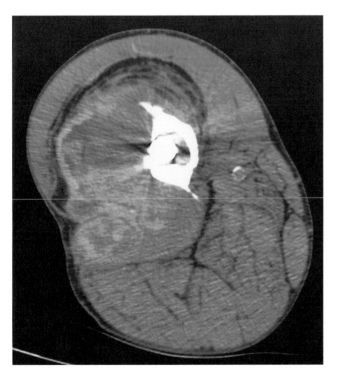

1. List your differential diagnosis for the elbow joint.

2. Does the computed tomography image of the thigh narrow the diagnosis? What is the process?

3. Regarding the thigh lesion, where are they common?

4. Explain why these patients may develop a leg length discrepancy.

Hemophiliac Arthropathy

1. Hemophilia, septic arthritis, and, occasionally, juvenile rheumatoid arthritis and chronic rheumatoid arthritis.

2. Yes. There is a hemophiliac pseudotumor, which is an intraosseous or subperiosteal hemorrhage that gives the appearance of an expansile lytic tumor.

3. Ilium and tibia.

4. Hemorrhage into the physeal (growth) plate.

References

Kerr R: Imaging of musculoskeletal complications of hemophilia. *Semin Musculoskelet Radiol* 7:127–136, 2003.

Kilcoyne RF, Lundin B, Pettersson H: Evolution of the imaging tests in hemophilia with emphasis on radiography and magnetic resonance imaging. *Acta Radiol* 47:287–296, 2006.

Cross-Reference

Musculoskeletal Imaging: THE REQUISITES, 3rd ed, pp 565–568.

Comment

Hemophilia is an X-linked genetic disorder caused by a deficiency of coagulation factor VIII, resulting in a coagulopathy. In hemophilia, recurrent intra-articular hemorrhages occur frequently. The knee and elbow are particularly vulnerable to repeated injuries. When repeated intra-articular hemorrhages occur, the irritating effect of the blood within the joint causes the development of a chronic synovitis. Increased blood flow from chronic synovitis is responsible for periarticular osteopenia and accelerated bone growth. The hypertrophied synovial membrane (pannus) causes degeneration of the articular cartilage and erosion of the cortex and subchondral bone. In acute hemorrhages, the joint capsule may become distended with blood and diminish the range of motion. This effusion appears more radiodense than nonhemorrhagic effusions, which is a useful observation in narrowing the differential possibilities (note the lateral view of the elbow). An acute hemorrhage may mimic a septic joint. Soft tissue swelling and warmth about the joint are common findings, and fever, increased erythrocyte sedimentation rate, and elevated leukocytosis may be present. In chronic cases, the deposition of hemosiderin in the tissues may lead to areas of increased density in the joint, which mimic calcification on radiographs. About 1% to 2% of patients develop osseous pseudotumors. These lesions may arise as a subperiosteal hematoma from tears of the periosteal vessels, or from within the bone, which can destroy the trabeculae and cortex and be associated with a soft tissue mass. In small bones, the osseous pseudotumor may become expansile.

Notes

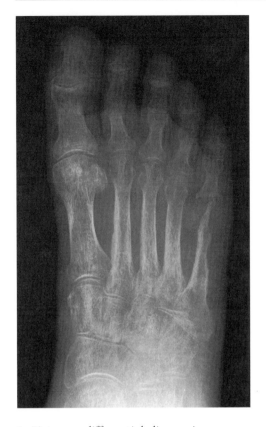

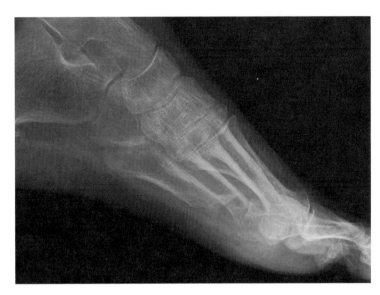

1. List your differential diagnosis.

2. Does the appearance of the fifth metatarsal bone help narrow the above considerations?

3. What is a Dupuytren's contracture and what associations does it have?

4. What is Gorham's disease?

Plantar Fibromatosis

1. Plantar fibromatosis, Gorham's syndrome, hereditary osteolysis, metastasis, any aggressive primary bone neoplasm, and soft tissue sarcoma.

2. Yes, the tapering of the bone suggests slow extraosseous process.

3. Fibromatosis of the palmar fascia; plantar fibromatosis (Ledderhose disease) and penile fibromatosis (Peyronie's disease).

4. "Disappearing" bone disease is characterized by proliferation of hemangiomatous and lymphangiomatous tissue.

Reference

Quinn SF, Erickson SJ, Dee PM, et al: MR imaging of fibromatosis: Results in 26 patients with pathologic correlation. *AJR Am J Roentgenol* 156:539–542, 1991.

Cross-Reference

Musculoskeletal Imaging: THE REQUISITES, 3rd ed, pp 465–468.

Comment

Fibromatoses comprise a group of soft tissue lesions that may occur either as a superficial nodular mass or as a deep infiltrative soft tissue mass that may mimic a malignancy. Histologically, this pathologic process is characterized by fibroblastic proliferation within the muscles and/or connective tissue. Clinically, a majority of patients present with a small nodule beneath the skin; however, deeper lesions tend to be more insidious and may not be detected until they elicit a mass effect on the adjacent musculature or neurovascular structure. The recurrence rate for simple excision is high, ranging from 60% to 100%.

This patient has plantar fibromatosis, known as Ledderhose disease, which occurs when proliferative fibrous tissue involves the plantar fascia. It can be highly aggressive and infiltrate the surrounding muscles, producing pressure erosions, cortical destruction, and bone lysis. Pathologic fractures are not uncommon. On magnetic resonance imaging, fibromatosis may have a variety of appearances, reflecting the tissue composition and cellularity. On T1W images, lesions are iso- to slightly hyperintense in comparison to the signal intensity of muscle. Areas of low signal intensity represent dense clusters of collagen. On T2W images, a wide spectrum of signal intensity has been observed and correlates with the extent of fibrosis and cellular concentration. In comparison to the signal intensity of muscle, lesions may appear homogeneously low in signal intensity (abundant fibrous tissue), iso- to slightly hyperintense, or heterogeneously bright (extensive cellularity).

Notes

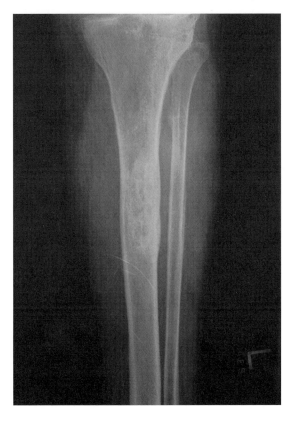
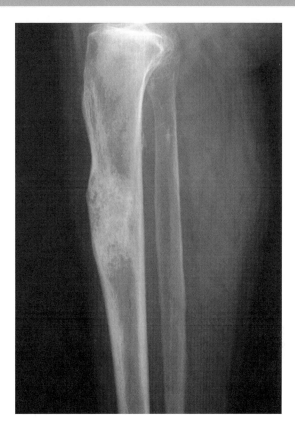

1. Describe the finding in this 23-year-old woman.

2. What is the differential diagnosis?

3. Is this patient a characteristic patient?

4. Is this a malignant lesion?

Osteofibrous Dysplasia

1. Cortically based expansile sclerotic lesion in the anterior cortex of the proximal tibial diaphysis with scattered lucencies. A smaller lesion in the fibula causes periostitis.

2. Osteofibrous dysplasia, fibrous dysplasia, adamantinoma, chronic infection.

3. Yes, most patients with osteofibrous dysplasia are children or young adults.

4. No, but there is debate whether osteofibrous dysplasia progresses to adamantinoma, a malignant lesion with a 60% 5-year survival. Histologically, there are some differences between the two lesions and most consider osteofibrous dysplasia to be a variant of fibrous dysplasia.

References

Kahn LB: Adamantinoma, osteofibrous dysplasia and differentiated adamantinoma. *Skeletal Radiol* 32: 245–258, 2003.

Seeger LL, Yao L, Eckardt JJ: Surface lesions of bone. *Radiology* 206:17–33, 1998.

Cross-Reference

Musculoskeletal Imaging: THE REQUISITES, 3rd ed, pp 425–428.

Comment

Osteofibrous dysplasia, also known as ossifying fibroma of long bones, is one of the fibro-osseous lesions that affect the tibia and fibula principally in the first through third decades of life. There is no gender predilection. The most common presenting symptom is either pain or mass. These lesions are eccentrically located in the diaphysis of the tibia and may contribute to pseudoarthrosis if located in the distal tibia. The fibula is also involved in 20% of cases. Radiographic appearance is similar to monostotic fibrous dysplasia of long bones. It may appear as a cortically based geographic lesion with a sclerotic border that may expand the bone. It may be predominantly lytic or contain osseous matrix, such as in this case. When lytic, it is radiographically indistinguishable from adamantinoma. Histologically, these lesions depict a combination of woven bone trabeculae with prominent osteoblastic rimming and a loose, slightly myxoid stroma, which is less collagenized than in instances of intramedullary fibrous dysplasia. It differs from adamantinoma by the lack of epithelial cells, which are abundant in the latter. There are published patient series that suggest that there is some common histogenetic relationship with adamantinoma.

Treatment is aimed at resection. Nearly 50% of tumors recur after resection but overall, the prognosis is good even with recurrence.

Notes

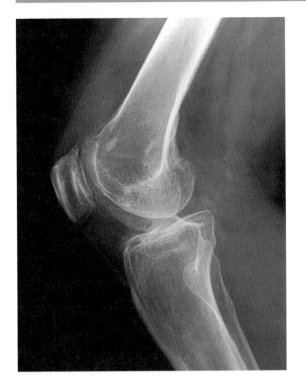

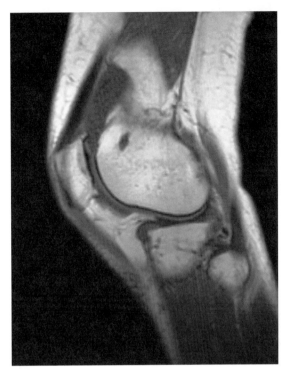

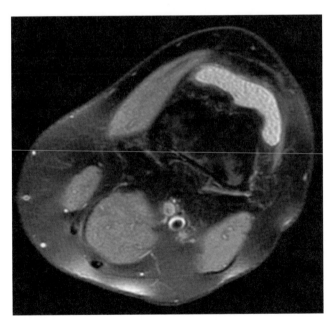

1. What is your differential diagnosis?

2. Describe your findings.

3. What are the two types?

4. Describe the Klippel-Trenaunay-Weber syndrome.

Synovial Hemangioma

1. Synovial hemangioma, less likely hemophilia. The appearance is nearly pathognomonic on the radiograph (notice the phleboliths).

2. Lobulated intra-articular mass with intermediate T1W signal intensity and marked hyperintensity on T2W images, reflecting the pooling of blood within the vascular spaces.

3. Pedunculated and diffuse.

4. Varicose veins, arteriovenous malformations, soft tissue and osseous hypertrophy, and cutaneous hemangiomas.

References

Greenspan A, Azouz EM, Matthews J, II, Decarie JC: Synovial hemangioma: Imaging features in eight histologically proven cases, review of the literature, and differential diagnosis. *Skeletal Radiol* 24:583–590, 1995.

Sheldon PJ, Forrester DM, Learch TJ: Imaging of intraarticular masses. *Radiographics* 25:105–119, 2005.

Cross-Reference

Musculoskeletal Imaging: THE REQUISITES, 3rd ed, pp 478–479.

Comment

Synovial hemangiomas are rare, intra-articular vascular tumors. These intra-articular lesions tend to occur in adolescent or young women, causing pain, swelling, and a diminished range of motion. There are two pathologic types. One type presents as a pedunculated synovial mass with symptoms of locking and pain. The other pattern is more diffuse and associated with synovial proliferation. The latter type may present with intermittent pain, hemarthrosis, and occasionally increased limb length. Associated cutaneous and soft tissue hemangiomas are commonly seen with the diffuse form.

The radiographic features of a synovial hemangioma may become similar to hemophilia with repeated episodes of hemorrhage. Joint space narrowing secondary to cartilage destruction, epiphyseal overgrowth, and synovial proliferation are common findings. In the past, the diagnosis was suggested when a villonodular pattern was depicted on arthrography, and this is true with magnetic resonance imaging. Conventional radiographs depict phleboliths or bony erosions in 50% of cases. Angiography shows fine-caliber, smooth walled vessels with contrast pooling in dilated vascular spaces. Today, magnetic resonance imaging is preferred because it is capable of showing the extent of the lesion, deposition of hemosiderin, and severity of joint destruction. Fluid-fluid levels are occasional findings in cavernous-type lesions.

Notes

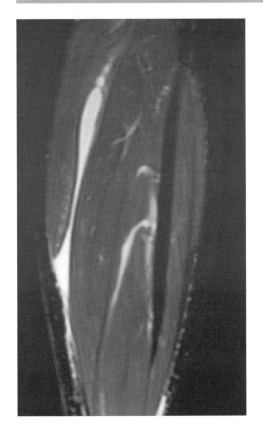
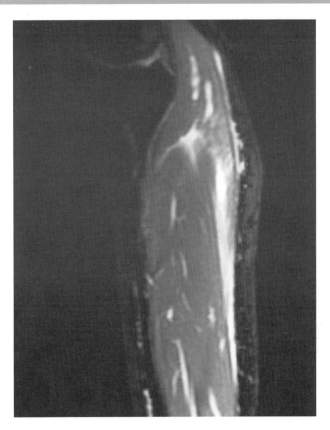
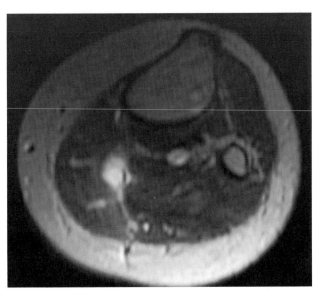
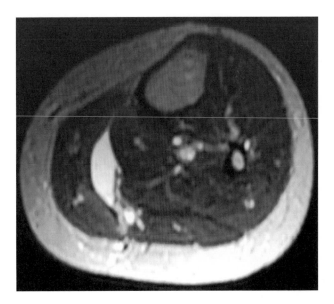

1. You are shown fat-saturated T2W coronal and sagittal images, and two routine axial T2W images of the calf. What is the diagnosis?

2. Where is the location of the injury?

3. What other injuries are common with this finding?

4. Is absence of this muscle abnormal?

Tennis Leg (Plantaris Muscle Tear)

1. Rupture of the plantaris muscle.

2. At the myotendinous junction. There is controversy whether the tendon itself can tear.

3. Anterior cruciate ligament tears and medial gastrocnemius muscle tears.

4. No, 7% to 10% of the population does not have a plantaris muscle.

References

Delgado GJ, Chung CB, Lektrakul N, et al: Tennis leg: Clinical US study of 141 patients and anatomic investigation of four cadavers with MR imaging. *Radiology* 224:112–119, 2002.

Helms CA, Fritz RC, Garvin GJ: Plantaris muscle injury: Evaluation with MR imaging. *Radiology* 195:201–203, 1995.

Cross-Reference

Musculoskeletal Imaging: THE REQUISITES, 3rd ed, pp 260–262.

Comment

Tennis is a popular sport and injuries may occur either from overuse or acute trauma. In the leg, the most common sites for muscle strain are the adductor muscles (groin pull), hamstrings, and the calf. The term "tennis leg" has been applied to an injury to either the muscle or tendon of the medial head of the gastrocnemius muscle or the plantaris muscle. The plantaris muscle is a thin, small muscle that lies just deep to the lateral head of the gastrocnemius muscle in the proximal portion of the lower leg. The plantaris tendon is long and located between the medial gastrocnemius and soleus muscles and medial to the Achilles tendon more distally. A complete tear of the plantaris tendon occurring at the myotendinous junction has a characteristic appearance on magnetic resonance imaging. The muscle body retracts proximally. More distally in the lower leg, a tubular fluid collection accumulates in between the medial gastrocnemius and soleus muscles. This fluid collection and the absence of the plantaris tendon are evidence of a tear. This injury may be associated with a tear of the anterior cruciate ligament as well as an injury to the medial gastrocnemius in two thirds of cases.

Notes

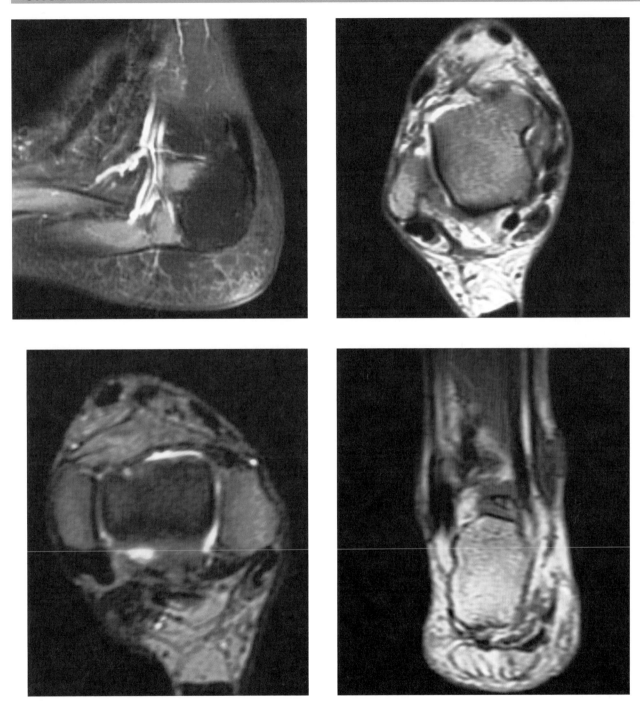

1. What do these four patients have in common? Name them.

2. What is the classic symptom? What is the most common cause?

3. Where is the transverse interfascicular septum and what does it separate?

4. How is this disorder treated?

Tarsal Tunnel Syndrome

1. Lesions in the tarsal tunnel. Patient 1, varicosities; patient 2, accessory flexor digitorum longus muscle; patient 3, tophaceous gout; and patient 4, schwannoma.

2. Burning type paresthesia and pain in the plantar aspect of the foot and toes. Idiopathic; in 50% of cases, no definable cause is determined.

3. Connective tissue band between the medial surface of the calcaneus and the abductor hallucis muscle; medial and lateral plantar nerves (branches of posterior tibial nerve).

4. Surgical decompression of the flexor retinaculum or resection of causative lesion.

References

Rosenberg ZS, Beltran J, Bencardino JT: MR imaging of the ankle and foot. *Radiographics* 20:S153–S179, 2000.

Zeiss J, Ebraheim N, Rusin J: Magnetic resonance imaging in the diagnosis of tarsal tunnel syndrome: Case report. *Clin Imaging* 14:123–126, 1990.

Cross-Reference

Musculoskeletal Imaging: THE REQUISITES, 3rd ed, p 270.

Comment

The tarsal tunnel refers to a space in the foot that extends from the level of the medial malleolus to the tarsal navicular. The floor comprises the tibia, talus, sustentaculum tali, and calcaneus. Its roof is formed by the flexor retinaculum, the deep fascia of the lower extremity, and the abductor hallucis muscle. The tendons of the posterior tibial, flexor digitorum longus, and flexor hallucis longus muscles are separated from the neurovascular bundle by fibrous septations. The septae are attached to the neurovascular bundle, causing it to be relatively immobile. The posterior tibial nerve, accompanied by an artery and vein, bifurcates into the medial and lateral plantar nerves beneath the flexor retinaculum, and these nerves are separated by the transverse interfascicular septum.

Tarsal tunnel syndrome refers to an entrapment neuropathy of the posterior tibial nerve or one of its branches. Pain, paresthesia, sensory deficits, and weakness are characteristic symptoms of this syndrome. Magnetic resonance imaging is the preferred method for diagnosing this condition since this imaging technique allows unimpeded visualization of the tarsal tunnel and its contents. Intrinsic (accessory muscles, lipoma, varicosities, synovial hypertrophy, fibrosis) and extrinsic (foot deformities, hypertrophied muscles, accessory ossicles) lesions can cause this syndrome, but 50% of patients have an idiopathic etiology.

Notes

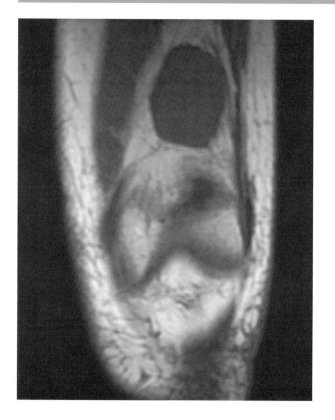

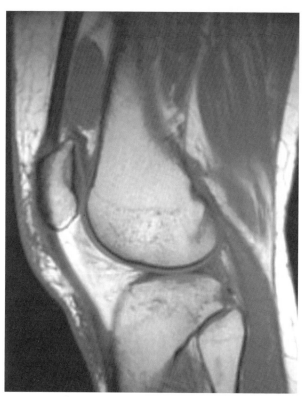

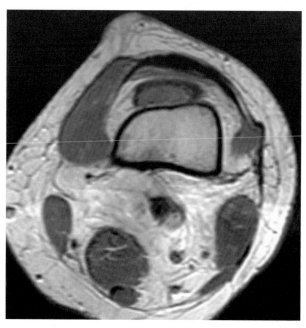

1. What conditions would you consider?

2. Is this lesion malignant?

3. What is its histologic "cousin"?

4. Why is pigmented villonodular synovitis (PVNS) not a good diagnosis?

CASE 196

Focal Nodular Synovitis

1. Focal nodular synovitis and intra-articular chondroma. Gout occasionally can mimic this lesion on T1W but appears lower in signal intensity on T2W images.

2. No, it does not metastasize and there is little risk of recurrence after excision.

3. Pigmented villonodular synovitis (PVNS).

4. No hemorrhagic joint effusion, no obvious hemosiderin in the lesion, and only a small focal region of synovium involved.

Reference

Huang GS, Lee CH, Chan WP, et al: Localized nodular synovitis of the knee: MR imaging appearance and clinical correlates in 21 patients. *AJR Am J Roentgenol* 181:539–543, 2003.

Cross-Reference

Musculoskeletal Imaging: THE REQUISITES, 3rd ed, pp 503–507.

Comment

Focal nodular synovitis, also termed synovial giant cell tumor, is a benign lesion characterized by localized synovial proliferation. It is found predominantly in the tendon sheaths or joints of the fingers and toes. Rarely, however, focal nodular synovitis involves a large joint, such as the knee or ankle. Histologically, focal nodular synovitis consists of a well-defined soft tissue, mass with varying amounts of histiocytic mononucleated giant cells, collagen strands, and xanthomatous cells covered by a smooth lining of synovial tissue, and these features are similar to those of PVNS. It is important to make a distinction between the two entities because their clinical presentations differ, as do their responses to treatment. In the knee, Hoffa's fat pad is the most common location followed by the suprapatellar bursa and intercondylar notch. The most common symptom is restriction of knee motion. The majority of lesions are radiographically occult. On magnetic resonance imaging, lesions may appear either as a small ovoid lesion or as a large polylobulated soft tissue mass with iso- or hyperintense signal intensity relative to skeletal muscle on T1W images and variable signal intensity on T2W images. Hemosiderin deposition is variable. Focal nodular synovitis is treated by simple excision and the risk of recurrence is negligible.

Notes

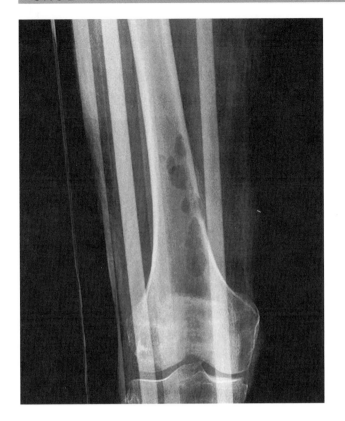 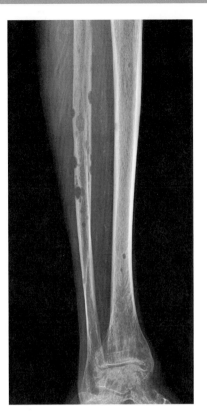

1. What is the differential diagnosis?

2. What should the multifocality of lesions suggest to you?

3. Are pathologic fractures common?

4. What determines the therapeutic management? What is the 5-year survival?

Angiosarcoma

1. Angiosarcoma and hemangioendothelioma, and rarely hemangioma, eosinophilic granuloma, myeloma, and metastasis.

2. The origin of the tumor is vascular. This patient has angiosarcoma.

3. They are relatively uncommon with angiosarcomas.

4. A number of factors including patient age, size and location of tumor, solitary versus multifocal, and the presence of extra-osseous disease. Less than 20%.

References

Seeger LL, Yao L, Eckardt JJ: Surface lesions of bone. *Radiology* 206:17–33, 1998.

Wenger DE, Wold LE: Malignant vascular lesions of bone: Radiologic and pathologic features. *Skeletal Radiol* 29:619–631, 2000.

Cross-Reference

Musculoskeletal Imaging: THE REQUISITES, 3rd ed, pp 480 and 488.

Comment

Angiosarcoma of bone, also known as malignant hemangioendothelioma or hemangioendothelial sarcoma, is a rare vascular neoplasm of bone. It is most common in the fourth and fifth decades of life and has a slight male predominance. It may be either low grade or a highly lethal tumor. It may present as a solitary lesion or multifocal, with lesions extending along a single bone or along an entire limb. Solitary lesions tend to be quite large at the time of presentation, depicted radiographically as an expansile "bubbly" lytic lesion or aggressive permeative lytic lesion with cortical breakthrough affecting adjacent bones. Multifocal lesions are present in nearly 40% of cases and lesions may be found in both medullary and intracortical locations. Cortical lesions have a spectrum of appearances from fusiform-shaped lytic lesions that produce endosteal scalloped erosions to frank cortical destruction with soft tissue masses. Computed tomography and magnetic resonance imaging are both valuable since these modalities are extremely sensitive for lesion detection and precise characterization of the pattern of bone destruction and soft tissue extent. Bone scintigraphy is useful in staging the disease.

Notes

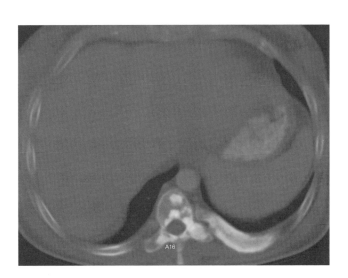
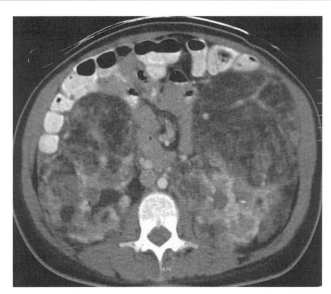

1. Describe the findings.

2. What is the diagnosis?

3. What is the leading cause of death in these patients? Second leading cause?

4. How do you acquire the disease?

Tuberous Sclerosis Complex

1. Sclerosis of a vertebra and adjacent left rib and bilateral renal angiomyolipomas.

2. Tuberous sclerosis.

3. Lesions of the nervous system (astrocytomas). Renal abnormalities.

4. Sixty-five percent are sporadic mutations and the remainder are linked to either gene TSC-1 (chromosome 9) or TSC-2 (chromosome 16).

References

Braffman BH, Bilaniuk LT, Naidich TP, et al: MR imaging of tuberous sclerosis: Pathogenesis of this phakomatosis, use of gadopentetate dimeglumine, and literature review. *Radiology* 183:227–238, 1992.

Narayanan V: Tuberous sclerosis complex: Genetics to pathogenesis. *Pediatr Neurol* 29:404–409, 2003.

Cross-Reference

Musculoskeletal Imaging: THE REQUISITES, 3rd ed, pp 644 and 646.

Comment

Tuberous sclerosis complex is an autosomal dominant neurocutaneous disorder characterized by development of hamartomatous lesions in multiple organs including the skin, kidney, heart, eyes, and other organs. The incidence is about 1 in 6000 live births and does not have a gender predilection. The cause is spontaneous mutation of genes TSC-1 (chromosome 9) or TSC-2 (chromosome 16). Lesions of the central nervous system are common, and patients may have seizures, mental retardation, and behavior problems. Lesions of the brain include cortical tubers, subependymal nodules, and giant cell astrocytomas. Renal abnormalities are common in this disease and often serious, resulting in hemorrhage or kidney failure. Renal manifestations are the second leading cause of death after lesions of the nervous system. Numerous fat attenuation angiomyolipomas result in an enlarged and deformed kidney. Renal cysts are common and vigilance for cancer is noteworthy. Cardiac rhabdomyomas, which are present at birth, may be large or multiple and can interfere with cardiac circulation and lead to death. Tuberous sclerosis causes patchy areas of sclerosis in the skeleton such as those seen in the vertebral body and adjacent rib in this patient. Cystlike changes in the bones of the hand and feet are also common. Early diagnosis is based on imaging of the brain and abdomen and close inspection of the eyes and skin.

Notes

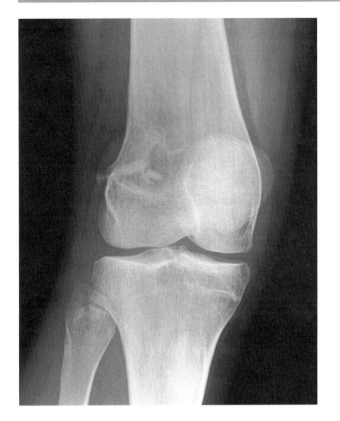

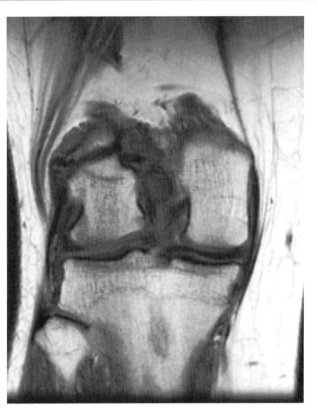

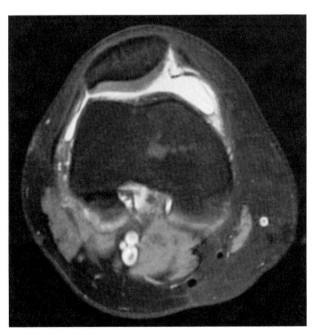

1. What surgical procedure did this patient have?

2. What happened in this patient?

3. What did you observe on the coronal magnetic resonance image?

4. What did you observe on the axial magnetic resonance image?

Fracture of ACL Reconstruction Transfemoral Pin

1. Anterior cruciate ligament (ACL) reconstruction with hamstring graft.

2. Graft failure due to fracture of the transfemoral pin.

3. Migration of the pin fragments.

4. Absence of the graft looping over the transfemoral pin ("empty" notch sign).

Reference

Cossey AJ, Kalairajah Y, Morcom R, Spriggins AJ: Magnetic resonance imaging evaluation of biodegradable transfemoral fixation used in anterior cruciate ligament reconstruction. *Arthroscopy* 22:199–204, 2006.

Cross-Reference

Musculoskeletal Imaging: THE REQUISITES, 3rd ed, p 237.

Comment

Reconstructive surgery using a hamstring tendon graft is a popular method of restoring biomechanical function in an ACL-deficient knee. It is a preferred method owing to both a lower complication rate and lower severity than seen in knees reconstructed with patellar tendon grafts. The hamstring is fixated proximally with a transfemoral pin that transversely bridges the femoral condyles, with the graft looping over the pin in the intercondylar notch. Most pins used today are biodegradable. The transfemoral pin may be evident radiographically as a linear continuous band of increased density on frontal radiographs of the knee but is depicted unequivocally on magnetic resonance imaging as a low signal intensity structure on all pulse sequences. One of the complications that can occur with a new injury to the knee or when there is too much tension on the hamstring graft is a fracture of the cross-pin, resulting in its deformation and, ultimately, failure of the graft when early in the postoperative course. Other important complications include stress fractures of the supracondylar area of the femur, graft impingement, bone plug or interference screw migration, and localized arthrofibrosis.

Notes

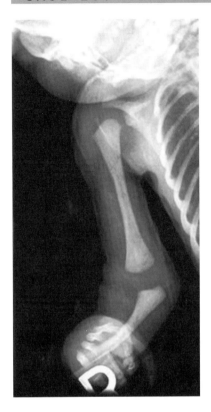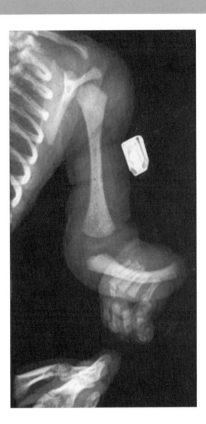

1. What is the name of the deformity seen in both arms of this neonate?

2. Are findings in the thumb helpful in naming the disorder?

3. Is there an association with other conditions? List some.

4. What abnormalities comprise the VACTERL syndrome?

Radial Clubhand

1. Radial clubhand.

2. Occasionally. Radial clubhand is associated with absence or hypoplasia of the thumb, Fanconi's anemia is associated with a hypoplastic thumb, and Holt-Oram syndrome has a triphalangeal thumb.

3. Atrial septal defect in Holt-Oram syndrome, thrombocytopenia in thrombocytopenia-absent radius syndrome, pancytopenia in Fanconi's anemia.

4. Vertebral, anal, cardiac, tracheoesophageal, renal, and limb anomalies.

Reference

Goldfarb CA, Wall L, Manske PR: Radial longitudinal deficiency: The incidence of associated medical and musculoskeletal conditions. *J Hand Surg* 31-A:1176–1182, 2006.

Cross-Reference

Musculoskeletal Imaging: THE REQUISITES, 3rd ed, pp 646–648.

Comment

A radial clubhand, also known as radial longitudinal deficiency, is a congenital deformity characterized by hypoplasia or aplasia of the radius. The deficiency usually involves the thumb. The wrist deviates markedly toward the radial side owing to the absence of the normal buttress afforded by the radius. The mode of inheritance is unknown and the disorder is bilateral in 70% of cases. Radiographically, the radial anomaly may vary from mild with absence of the distal radial epiphysis to severe with complete aplasia. The ulna bows toward the radial side and is usually thickened. The thumb may be hypoplastic or absent. As the child develops, carpal fusion or absence may become evident, and the humerus length may be shortened or deformed. Absence of the radius may be seen as part of several syndromes including thrombocytopenia-absent radius (TAR) syndrome; Holt-Oram syndrome; vertebral, anal, cardiac, tracheoesophageal, renal, and limb (VACTERL) syndrome; and Fanconi's anemia.

Notes